Understanding the Nursing Process: Concept Mapping and Care Planning for Students

Lynda Juall Carpenito-Moyet, RN, MSN, CRNP

Understanding the Nursing Process: Concept Mapping and Care Planning for Students

Lynda Juall Carpenito-Moyet, RN, MSN, CRNP

Family Nurse Practitioner
ChesPenn Health Services
Chester, Pennsylvania

Nursing Consultant
Mickleton, New Jersey

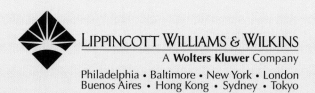

LIPPINCOTT WILLIAMS & WILKINS
A **Wolters Kluwer** Company

Philadelphia • Baltimore • New York • London
Buenos Aires • Hong Kong • Sydney • Tokyo

Senior Acquisitions Editor: Elizabeth Nieginski
Managing Editor: Michelle Clarke
Senior Production Editor: Marian A. Bellus
Director of Nursing Production: Helen Ewan
Senior Managing Editor / Production: Erika Kors
Art Director, Design: Joan Wendt
Art Director, Illustration: Brett MacNaughton
Manufacturing Manager: William Alberti
Indexer: Michael Ferreira
Compositor: Circle Graphics
Printer: R. R. Donnelley—Crawfordsville

9 8 7 6 5 4 3 2 1

Library of Congress Cataloging-in-Publication Data
Carpenito-Moyet, Lynda Juall.
   Understanding the nursing process : concept mapping and care planning for students / Lynda Juall Carpenito-Moyet.
       p. ; cm.
   Includes bibliographical references and index.
   ISBN 0-7817-5969-2 (alk. paper)
  1. Nursing assessment. 2. Nursing diagnosis. I. Title.
   [DNLM: 1. Nursing Assessment—standards. 2. Nursing Diagnosis—methods. WY 100.4 C294n 2006] I. Title.
RT48.C373 2006
616.07'5—dc22

                                                        2005029749

LWW.com

*It is fitting that my new book for beginning students of nursing
be dedicated to someone who is also beginning his life,
my grandson Olen Juall Carpenito Jr.*

*For all my readers who are grandparents,
I need not tell you what joy I experience with him.
For all of you, who have not experienced a grandchild,
you can look forward to the best that this life can give
as you grow in years.*

Acknowledgments

Thank you, Quincy McDonald for your provocative exchange with me the day the idea for this book was conceived. Thank you Michelle Clarke for your patience. Thank you to my daughter-in-law, Heather, who typed tirelessly even as her second pregnancy encumbered her. And to Marian Bellus and Helen Ewan for all their hard work on another "Carpenito" book.

Preface

In the winter of 2004, I met for the first time with Quincy McDonald, the new Senior Acquisition Editor in Philadelphia. I shared with him my frustration concerning the fact that, after 20 years, the teaching and learning of the nursing process and care planning was still very difficult and time consuming. There had to be a better method. On that day, this book was conceived. "Put the teacher in the book" I said.

This book is for beginning students of nursing. In Section One, the student will be guided through each step of the nursing process with interactive exercises and concept mapping. Concept mapping is used to analyze data, cluster data, and validate data and also for values clarification.

In the last chapter, the student will integrate the first 5 chapters in Putting It All Together in 11 Steps. This care planning system can reduce writing and increase critical thinking.

In Section Two, sixty nursing diagnoses approved by NANDA have been carefully selected to be appropriate for use by a beginning-nursing student. Each diagnosis has Definitions, Defining Characteristics or Risk Factors, Related Factors, Generic Considerations, Focus Assessment Criteria, Goals, and Interventions with Rationales.

In Section Three, seventeen collaborative problems appropriate for a beginning-nursing student are presented. Each collaborative problem has a Physiological Overview, Definitions, High-Risk Populations, Skill Checks, Nursing Goals with Indicators, and Nursing Interventions with Rationale.

Consistent throughout all these sections are Carp's Cues. Carp's Cues are suggestions, advice, and clarifications from this author to the student: "The teacher in the book."

The book concludes with three appendices: a Nursing Admission Database, a Generic Medical Care Plan, and a Generic Surgical Care Plan.

LYNDA JUALL CARPENITO-MOYET, RN, MSN, CRNP

Contents

Section Three: COLLABORATIVE PROBLEMS

Understanding the Nursing Process: Concept Mapping and Care Planning for Students

Lynda Juall Carpenito-Moyet, RN, MSN, CRNP

NURSING PROCESS AND CONCEPT MAPPING

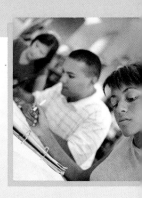

Section I takes the student through what is and how to use the nursing process and concept mapping. Each chapter is supplemented with Carp's Cues (tips from the author), Concept Maps (analysis tools), and Interactive Exercises (application opportunities).

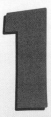

The Nursing Process and Concept Mapping

In many professions and jobs, the ability to problem solve is critical to success. You go to your nurse practitioner complaining of stomach pain. After answering a few questions and having your abdomen examined, your nurse practitioner tells you your pain is from a urinary tract infection. You take the medicine but have no improvement. When you return to the office, another nurse practitioner asks you many more questions. She also listens to your bowel sounds. She diagnoses that your pain is from constipation. She is right.

THE NURSING PROCESS

The Nursing Process is a term you will be hearing in almost every class in your nursing courses. Why does the nursing process have so much importance?

Here is another example. You take your car to a mechanic because it is making a strange noise. This noise disappears when your car is stopped. Your mechanic tells you that your car needs tires. You buy them. The noise is still there.

Identifying the right problem is dependent on knowing the possible causes of the problem. For example, when you complain of abdominal pain, the clinician should have identified possible causes of abdominal pain, such as

- ➤ Appendicitis
- ➤ Ovarian cyst
- ➤ Pelvic infection
- ➤ Urinary tract infection
- ➤ Constipation
- ➤ Gastritis

With these possible causes in mind, the clinician then asks questions to prove or disapprove each cause. If the clinician did not consider constipation, then he/she would not ask the question "When was your last bowel movement?"

The mechanic did not consider other possibilities for your car problem, like transmission or alternator, but went directly to replacing the tires.

The failure to know what causes could possibly be responsible for the problem led the first clinician and the mechanic to the wrong diagnoses.

Carp's Cue ▶ *In order for you to correctly diagnose a problem, you must first understand all the situations or factors that can cause the problem the person is complaining of. The more you understand what can cause a problem, the more likely you will identify the problem correctly.*

The nursing process is a problem-solving technique. It is organized to help the nurse logically approach situations that may lead to problems. It will help you to consider more possibilities. It will help you not to jump too quickly to one conclusion.

The nursing process has five steps:

1. Assessment
2. Diagnosis
3. Planning
4. Implementation
5. Evaluation

For convenience, these five steps are described separately and in step-like order. Assessment is the first step with evaluation as the last step.

For example, if you want to know whether your client has a sleep problem, you will ask the questions (assessment) to determine whether he has a sleeping problem (diagnosis). If the person does have a sleeping problem, then you would plan with the client what might help him to sleep better (planning). You instruct him on some things to do before bedtime (implementation). The next day you ask him how he slept (evaluation).

So the steps look like this:

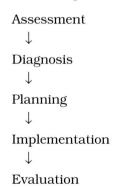

Assessment
↓
Diagnosis
↓
Planning
↓
Implementation
↓
Evaluation

Each step depends on the accuracy of the proceeding step.

Assessment

The first step of the nursing process is assessment. Assessment is a technique where you collect information (data) about a person, family, or group. You are looking for evidence of problems or risks for problems. You are also looking for strengths in the person or group.

Diagnosis

The second step is the judgment you make about the assessment data. The judgment can be a problem, risk for a problem, or strength.

Planning

Planning has several activities:

➤ Deciding which problems are priorities
➤ Determining the goals of care
➤ Selecting interventions
➤ Creating a plan of care

Implementation

The fourth step involves giving the care with interventions that are appropriate for the client. It also includes documentation of the care.

Evaluation

The last step of the nursing process involves deciding whether the interventions have helped the client. Do you need to change the plan?

The next five chapters will carefully explain each of these steps.

Even though evaluation is the fifth step of the nursing process, it is important to know that evaluation is also a part of each of the four other steps. Figure 1-1 shows the relationship.

For example, when you are assessing a person for a sleep problem, you will mentally note each piece of information as significant or not significant. This process is evaluation or analysis. In the chapter on evaluation, you will find more examples of evaluation.

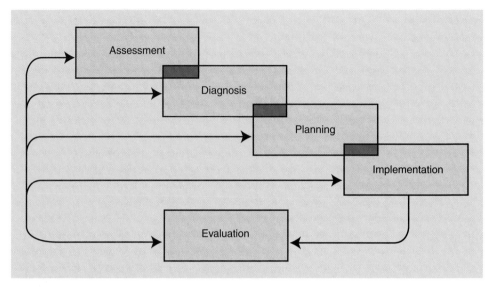

Figure 1-1. The nursing process (Carpenito-Moyet, 2002).

RELATIONSHIPS AMONG THE STEPS

As you learn more about each step of the nursing process in later chapters, you will learn that these steps are not separate from each other. They overlap. For example, while you are giving a woman a bath (implementation), you are also observing her skin (assessment). In another situation, you are writing a care plan (planning) and you determine if the person will agree with the plan and goals (evaluation). Another example is as you make a nursing diagnosis of constipation (diagnosis), you mentally check whether you have the signs or symptoms to support the data (evaluation).

As you provide care to an individual, you will be continually processing data and response to care. Through this continuous process, you will increase the likelihood that your data and judgments are correct.

CONCEPT MAPPING

Concept mapping is an educational technique that uses diagrams to demonstrate the relationship of one concept or situation to other concepts and situations. By linking a central concept to other concepts, you can be helped to understand the central concept better.

For example, examine the following diagram. The central concept is insomnia (difficulty sleeping). Surrounding the central concepts are factors (other concepts) that can cause or contribute to insomnia.

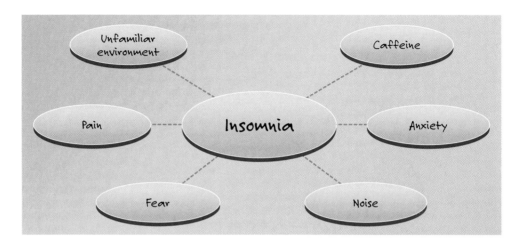

This diagram shows how a variety of factors can interfere with sleep. Remember the last time you could not sleep. What was causing your insomnia? This technique will increase your knowledge about relationships of data, causes, and effects. It will prompt you to look closer and to explore possibilities.

Consider another example. You failed a nursing quiz. What are some possible reasons for your failing grade? Examine this concept map with some reasons.

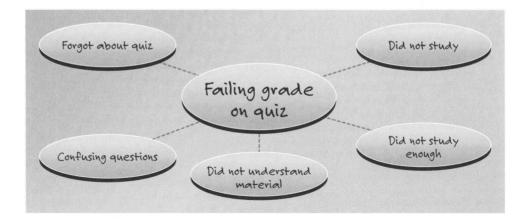

As you look at these reasons, they are different and require a different response from you. For example, if the quiz questions were confusing, sit down with your instructor and discuss them. If you did not study enough, design a plan to study regularly and not just before a test.

Decision Making

Concept mapping can also help you with decision making. For example, you are trying to decide whether you should live in the dormitory next semester or rent an apartment with two other students. Using a concept map, outline all the disadvantages of living in the dorm and all the disadvantages of living in an apartment.

Disadvantages of living in a dormitory:

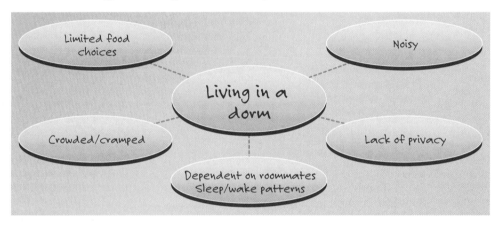

Disadvantages of living in an apartment:

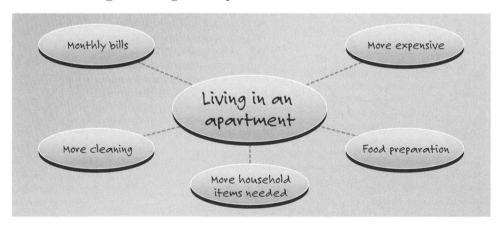

Now as you look at these maps, you have better information to base your decision.

Assessment

Concept mapping can assist you in exploring relationships of data. Consider this situation:

You know an elderly woman who lives alone. She has no car and no regular visitors. You wonder about her nutrition.

Let us look more closely using a concept map.

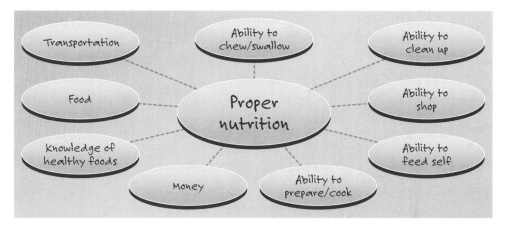

Now take one of these factors that influence proper nutrition and map it. For example, use ability to clean up. What factors will influence the elderly woman's ability to clean up?

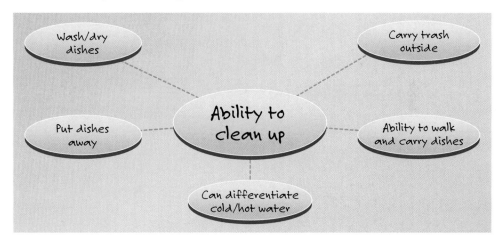

Proper nutrition requires many abilities. If the elderly lady were your client, you would probably request a home assessment by a nurse.

INTERACTIVE EXERCISE 1-1

Create a concept map with ability to shop in the middle. What factors can affect one's ability to shop? Refer to end of chapter for answers.

Diagnosis

Concept mapping can be used to help validate a diagnosis or to determine what factors have contributed to the diagnosis developing. For example, you are admitted to the hospital. You are anxious. What factors can cause anxiety when one is admitted to the hospital?

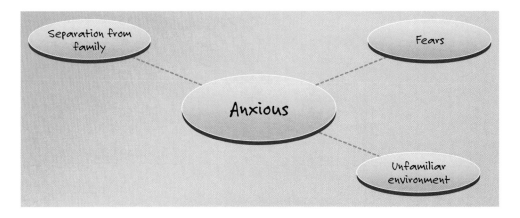

Let us look more closely at fears by mapping it.

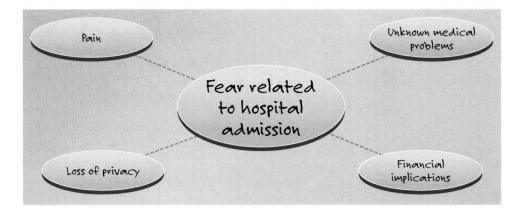

By mapping fears related to hospital admission, you will be more knowledgeable about these sources of fear. This knowledge will help you to intervene with clients on admission. You will offer explanations and strive to keep the client well–informed. You will always tell the truth, which sometimes means, "I do not know but I will try to find out for you."

Values Clarification

Concept mapping is a very effective tool for value clarification. All of us have values and prejudices. When you can identify a prejudice, sometimes you open yourself to think a different way. It is most important that you examine your values and prejudices as a student nurse.

Sometimes even if you try, you may not change how you feel, but you can always change how you behave. There is no such thing as bad thoughts, only bad actions.

As a nurse, you will be asked to care for people of all races and religions. You will be asked to care for a woman who tried to kill herself or for an adolescent drunk driver. You will care for a man with lung disease who continues to smoke or for a woman with hepatitis C who continues to drink alcohol. In one room is the president of a large bank. In another is a homeless man covered with sores. Can you be equally caring and professional in both rooms?

You will of course always have clients that you favor. There is nothing wrong with doing "extras" for a favorite client. What would be wrong is to deprive someone who is not your favorite of good nursing care.

So from this day forward, you will have to monitor your responses to clients. When you find you have negative feelings, ask yourself: "Did this person do or say something to disturb me?" Or "Did I bring my negative feelings with me?" Or "Did I allow the negative feelings of another staff member (or student) to influence me"?

Sometimes if you identify your prejudices as barriers, you can work around them and provide good nursing care.

INTERACTIVE EXERCISE 1-2

Review the following characteristics of clients. Which clients would you prefer not to care for? Why?

- A 400-pound woman
- A gay man with AIDS
- A woman with severe burns on her face and arms
- A wealthy young man who tried to commit suicide
- A homeless man who tried to commit suicide
- A man after cardiac surgery who has a wife and a girlfriend visit him
- A prostitute who was burned by a client
- An unmarried 20-year-old with four children on public assistance
- An experienced nurse with breast cancer

There are no right or wrong answers. Some of these people will evoke negative feelings in you. How will you manage these feelings? How can you prevent these feelings from interfering with your nursing care? You can try and learn more about this person beyond what you find offensive. Your interest in him or her can create a positive and caring environment. Remember that you probably are not the first person to have negative feelings toward him or her but you can be the first person to genuinely try to know him or her. When a nurse is a client or a family member, they too often intimidate nurses. Instead of giving a fellow nurse some extras, we respond to their requests and questions coldly and critically. Take charge of your practice and always hold yourself responsible for your actions or failure to act. When you are in a room and the door is closed, only you are responsible for the quality of care you provide. Make yourself proud.

SUMMARY ▽

The nursing process is a key competency in the practice of nursing. It is a systematic decision-making model.

Concept mapping was presented as a diagramming technique to demonstrate the relations of one central concept to other concepts. This technique helps clarify the central concept. The remaining five chapters address each step separately.

INTERACTIVE EXERCISE ANSWERS

Interactive Exercise 1-1

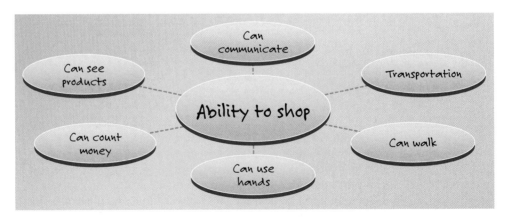

2 Nursing Process: Focus on Assessment

A cousin of yours brings a date to a family party. How would you "get to know him"? How would you form an opinion of him?

INTERACTIVE EXERCISE 2-1

On a sheet of paper create a concept map with "Getting to Know Him" in the center. Around the center, write the ways (or methods) you will use to form an opinion of your cousin's date. After you complete the activity, review the suggested answers at the end of this chapter.

The process of getting to know your cousin's date is a type of assessment. You will use four methods to collect information (observation, conversation, listening, direct questioning) to determine your opinion of him. The more information you have to help you make your opinion, the more likely your opinion is fair.

For example, if you used only one type of data collection (observation), your opinion would only be based on appearance.

Carp's Cue ▶ *Forming an opinion on appearance only is very problematic. Strategies to avoid these mistakes will be outlined throughout this chapter.*

NURSING ASSESSMENT

Assessment in nursing is the deliberate and systematic collection of information (data) about an individual, family, or group (community). As a beginning student, you will probably focus on the individual and family only.

The purpose of your assessment is to determine the person's

➤ Present health status
➤ Ability to function
➤ Strengths
➤ Limitations
➤ Ability to cope with stresses

With the information from your assessment, you will be able to form judgments about health problems and risks to health problems.

 These judgments are called diagnoses. These diagnoses will be discussed in Chapter 3.

ASSESSMENT PROCESS

To collect accurate data, you must be able to

➤ Communicate effectively
➤ Listen carefully
➤ Observe systematically
➤ Perform physical examinations
➤ Interpret data
➤ Validate data

Communicate Effectively

Through your nursing courses, you will learn communication techniques to encourage others to share information and feelings with you. These techniques are verbal and nonverbal. Verbal techniques are

➤ Open-ended questions
  These questions are used to encourage the sharing of opinions and feelings. The questions usually begin with how or what. Examples are: "How do you feel about that?" or "What do you want to be able to do when you go home?"
➤ Closed-ended questions
  This type of question is useful to acquire facts. Usually, these questions can be answered in one or two words. For example: "Do you have pain?" or "Where is your pain?"

 Open-ended questions are very useful because they require the person to describe a situation or to share their feelings. It would not be effective to ask only open-ended

questions because they are time-consuming. Close-ended questions are very useful because they are an efficient data collection method. If you want to assess feelings, ask how is the pain affecting your life? (open-ended). If you want a description of the pain intensity, ask to rate the pain on a 0–10 scale (0 = no pain, 10 = worst pain you ever had).

➤ Multiple-Choice Questions
These types of questions provide the person with a choice of answers to choose from. For example: "Do your headaches occur every day, every week, or every month? When you have chest pain, do you feel sweaty, sick to the stomach, or short of breath?"
➤ Rephrasing: Rephrasing what the person has said to you is a useful technique to encourage the person to share more information. It also helps to clarify what was said. For example, a man tells you "I am glad my mother is dead." You could rephrase this statement with "You are glad your mother is dead?" Doing so may elicit feelings of relief that his mother is no longer suffering.
➤ Inferring: Inferring is a technique used to help clarify information shared. For example, a young woman angrily reported vaginal symptoms of a bad odor and a yellowish discharge. You could respond, "You seem angry." She then starts to cry because she thinks her boyfriend has another girlfriend.
➤ Providing Information: When you are interviewing a person, you can take this opportunity to provide information related to the discussion. For example, after discussing how pain has affected her life, you respond with "continuous pain can be depressing."

INTERACTIVE EXERCISE 2-2

You want to assess the sleep patterns of a client. Write an example of each type of assessment question on a separate piece of paper:

➢ Open-ended question
➢ Closed-ended question
➢ Multiple-choice question
➢ Rephrasing

Listen Carefully

Learning to listen carefully is one of the most valuable skills to accomplish. Active listening is paying full attention to what is being said. Paying full attention to a person in need communicates a powerful message: "I am here to help you". Active listening involves

> ➤ Staying quiet within oneself
> ➤ Reducing or eliminating barriers to listening (noise, lack of privacy)
> ➤ Maintaining eye contact
> ➤ Positioning your body eye to eye and shoulder to shoulder to the other person
> ➤ Avoiding interruptions
> ➤ Allowing pauses to reflect on what was said
> ➤ Listening for feelings as well as words (Alfaro-LaFevre, 2002)

Active listening takes a lot of energy. Sometimes it is better to delay a discussion with a client when you are too distracted or stressed.

BARRIERS TO ACTIVE LISTENING

Besides environmental barriers to active listening, such as noise or lack of privacy, other things can prevent active listening, such as

> ➤ The client's views are different from the nurse's perceptions
> ➤ The client's appearance or accent is different or distracting
> ➤ The client is in pain or is anxious
> ➤ The client is telling the nurse something that he or she does not want to hear
> ➤ The nurse does not like the client
> ➤ The nurse is thinking of something else
> ➤ The nurse is planning the next statement
> ➤ The nurse is anxious or apprehensive
> ➤ The nurse is in a hurry

It is easy to listen to someone you like. It is very difficult to listen to someone who is very different from you such as someone with a foreign accent or someone with a bad facial scar. When you don't have the time to listen actively, tell the person you will come back when you can listen better.

How difficult would it be for you to actively listen to the following persons rating them as easy (1), somewhat difficult (2), or very hard (3). Place a 1, 2, or 3 next to each statement.

_____ A woman weighing over 400 pounds complaining of knee pain

_____ A man dressed as a woman

_____ A man with very strong body odor

_____ A prostitute with a broken arm
_____ A drug addict complaining of pain

There are not any right or wrong answers. This exercise is an opportunity for you to identify barriers to listening. As a nurse, you will not like every one you care for, but you must not deny a person good nursing care because of your problem. Sometimes if you force yourself to look past the barrier, you may be surprised with what you find.

Observe Systematically

Your ability to observe systematically is dependent on how much you know. As you progress in the nursing program, you will increase your knowledge base and therefore you will increase your observational skills.

For example, if you are performing your first skin assessment on a dark-skinned person, you may believe some variations of skin color are abnormal. For example, dark skin when scarred often heals lighter.

As a beginning nursing student, you will use guidelines to improve your observations. In Section II in this book, you will find signs and symptoms (defining characteristics or risk factors) for each nursing diagnosis.

Your faculty will give you a preprinted assessment form to be used for your initial assessment. This form will direct you to ask the best questions and to focus your physical assessment as a beginning student.

Perform Physical Assessment

In a separate course, you will learn and practice some physical assessment skills. As a beginning student, it is important that you become expert in certain physical assessment skills:

Physical System	Criteria
Sensory-perceptual	Vision and appearance of eyes
	Hearing
	Sense of touch
	Taste and smell
Skin	Condition (color, turgor, character)
	Lesions
	Edema
Respiratory	Rate, character
	Breath sounds
	Cough
	Abnormal sounds (crackles, wheezes)

(continued)

Cardiovascular	Pulses (rate, quality, rhythm)
	Apical
	Radial
	Carotid
	Dorsalis pedis
	Brachial
	Femoral
	Posterior tibial
	Blood pressure
	Circulation (mucous membranes, capillary refill)
Neurological	Pupillary reactions
	Perception of senses
	Grasp strength
Gastrointestinal	Mouth, gums, teeth, and tongue (color, condition)
	Gag reflex
	Bowel sounds
	Presence of distention, impaction, hemorrhoids (external)
Genitourinary	Lesions
	Presence of retention
	Discharge (vaginal, urethral)
Musculoskeletal	Muscle tone, strength
	Gait, stability
	Range of motion

These physical assessment skills are very important to evaluate a client's condition. Before going to the clinical setting, take time to review any assessment skill that you are not confident with. Practice these skills with each client. Learn well what normal findings are. Therefore, when you find something not normal, even though you do not know what it means, you do know that you need to report it to your instructor or another nurse. As you progress in the program, you will learn more detailed assessments such as cranial nerves and percussion of the liver.

Interpret Data

Every time you care for clients, you are faced with numerous amounts of data. During your student clinical experiences and in all your future encounters with clients and families, you will have to make a judgment about data and decide which data or information is significant and which is not.

For example, you are buying a new suit. You try one on and review its qualities as you look in the mirror:

➤ Sale price $38.00 (reduced from $68.00)
➤ Pants too long

➤ Jacket fits well
➤ Medium gray color

Now review the above data about this suit. Would you buy this pantsuit? Your answer will depend on the significance of each of the four pieces of information. The significance of each one is directly related to the importance of each.

For example, this author would find the price and the jacket fit very appealing. The length of the pants is easily corrected. However, gray is an unattractive color to this author. If this suit were purchased because of the great price, it would sit in the closet.

You, however, may find everything positive except the length of the pants. Having the pants altered is too much trouble and will add to the price of the suit.

The four characteristics of this suit can be interpreted differently depending on your values. When one interprets data about a client or a family, it is important to reduce the effect of your values on your interpretation.

When you are shopping for a suit, your opinion can be biased and nonscientific. When you are interpreting client data, every attempt should be made to recognize when one is biased negatively.

CUES VERSUS INFERENCES

Cues are pieces of data that you gather by seeing, touching, tasting, hearing, or smelling. Examples of these are as follows:

➤ Seeing   Dark skin
➤ Touching   Cool hands
➤ Tasting   Bitter drink
➤ Hearing   "I am cold."
➤ Smelling   Fishy smelling vaginal discharge

Inferences are judgments or the interpretation of the cues or data. Interpretation is based on your knowledge, values, and experiences.

INTERACTIVE EXERCISE 2-3

Look at these cues:

➢ 89 years old
➢ Fishy smelling vaginal discharge
➢ Height 5'1", weight 210 pounds
➢ Consumes four to six beers a day

Write next to each your judgment about each. Look at the end of the chapter for suggested answers.

It is impossible not to have values and opinions that can interfere with your judgments. The goal for each of us is to recognize our negative opinions and to keep them from interfering with our nursing care.

INTERACTIVE EXERCISE 2-4

Complete the following values clarification exercise.

1. You are standing in a crowded bus. Put 1 next to the person you would most like to stand next to and continue until number 6 is given to the person you would least like to stand next to.

   _____ Blind

   _____ Body odor

   _____ Very obese

   _____ Spastic muscular dystrophy

   _____ Amputated arm

   _____ Severely burn-scarred face

2. Check which of the following are associated with careless and/or bad character.

   _____ Bad breath

   _____ Body odor

   _____ Amputation

   _____ Obesity (20% over ideal weight)

3. Finish each statement with your own spontaneous thoughts.

   a. When I see a blind person I _____

   _____

   _____

   b. To me, getting around in a wheelchair _____

   _____

   _____

   c. If I had cancer of the tongue _____

   _____

   _____

4. Rank the disability or physical difference you would feel most distressed to have as 1 and continue until 6 are ranked.

   _____ Obesity

   _____ Deaf

_____ Paralyzed legs

_____ Bad scar on face

_____ Colostomy

_____ Laryngectomy

5. Interview a person with a physical difference (blind, deaf, obese, paralyzed, scarred, etc.)
   a. Ask the person how people respond to his or her physical difference.
   b. Ask the person how he or she would like people to respond.

Now carefully examine your answers. Identify the physical differences or disabilities that are distressing to you.

This exercise, if done honestly, can help you begin to identify potential barriers to providing care to a client. You cannot change how you feel, but you can control how your feelings affect your care.

Sometimes if the nurse sees a client's illness or injury as preventable, less sympathy is present. This bias can prevent the nurse from making clear valid judgments. It can also create an emotional wall that deprives the person of the professional nursing care he/she deserves. For example:

➤ A man with multiple injuries from an auto accident in which he was driving under the influence
➤ A woman with invasive cancer that could have been prevented by regular Pap screenings
➤ A young man with a head injury resulting from a car crash while racing his car
➤ A woman who had no prenatal care who delivers a dead baby
➤ A young wife with multiple injuries from her husband

It is impossible not to have negative opinions about these situations. Each nurse has a responsibility to quiet these negative opinions so they do not interfere with nursing care. Sometimes we are successful, and sometimes we are not. If you are willing to identify your negative biases, you may be able to reduce their influence on your nursing practice.

THE PROCESS OF INTERPRETING DATA

Interpreting data involves two cognitive activities:

➤ Recognizing the cue or inference as significant
➤ Assigning meaning to the significance

To interpret data as significant, you must have learned why these data are significant. For example, on your first day in clinical, you meet your assigned client. She is 77 years old and answers all your questions incorrectly. You determine she is confused. As a new student, you may know very little about confusion, so your inference is confusion related to old age. After you learn about confusion, you would approach this client differently. For now you know to assess for the following:

➤ Is this new?
➤ Is she sleep deprived?
➤ Are her medications the cause?
➤ Does she have an infection?

Clearly, you cannot make valid judgments about data if you do not have certain knowledge that determines whether the data are abnormal or diagnostic. Before you learned about confusion, this woman was just a confused elderly woman. After you acquired learning about confusion, you will assess for various causes.

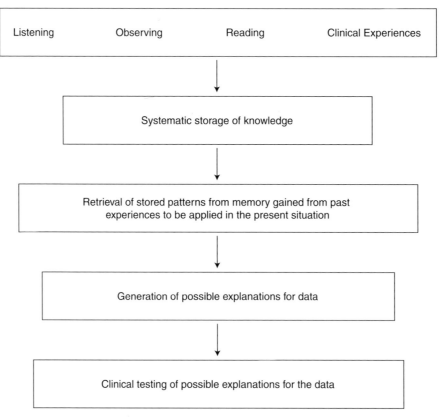

Figure 2-1. Acquisition of skilled clinical knowledge. From Weber & Kelley: Health Assessment in Nursing, 2e. Philadelphia: Lippincott Williams & Wilkins, 2003.

In other words you cannot make valid inferences if you do not know the significance of the data.

Let us examine three clinical situations:

Situation 1

You learn that four signs and symptoms can be present when someone has diabetes mellitus:

➤ Excess thirst
➤ Excess urination
➤ Blurred vision
➤ Weight loss

When a client complains of "being thirsty all the time," you think

➤ Possible diabetes mellitus
➤ Possible dehydration
➤ Possible excess salt intake

The next step is to ask more questions to narrow the possibilities to one or two:

Is your urine dark or clear colored? If the answer is no, you should request a urine sample to test for its concentration of water (specific gravity).
If the specific gravity is normal, she is probably not dehydrated. Now you have ruled out one of your possibilities.

As a beginning nursing student, you will be able to make inferences about data as normal or abnormal. You will not, however, be able to explain all data because you can only explain the significance of certain data if you have learned about it. This grouping or cluster of data signifies a particular health problem.

Situation 2

After you examine the feet of a client, you find a reddened area on each foot. You know this is not normal. You ask him about it and he tells you, "It must be from my new shoes." You report this to your instructor. For most people, this reddened lesion is not important, but if this man has diabetes mellitus or decreased circulation in his legs, then this is a very significant finding.

Even though you may have not known whether this foot lesion was significant or not, your decision to report the finding is key. As you acquire more knowledge of medical conditions and nursing diagnoses, clustering data will be easier.

Situation 3

You are assigned to a 35-year-old man who is scheduled for hernia surgery. When you review his laboratory findings, you note his hemoglobin (Hgb) is 11 and his hematocrit (HCT) is 38. Normal Hgb is 12–16 and normal HCT is 40–50%. Is this significant? Why? If this person were a female, would your judgment change? It is not unusual for women to be anemic due to the blood loss each month with menses (periods). Men, on the other hand, are not usually anemic. This finding will be investigated to evaluate if he is bleeding in his gastrointestinal tract or if he has a chronic disease not diagnosed (renal insufficiency, AIDS). Women are usually given iron supplements unless there are data to support more clinical studies. In both cases, a physician or nurse practitioner will be consulted.

It is not possible for you to understand the meaning of all abnormal data. As you learn more, you will make better inferences. It is critical, however, that you always report abnormal data even if you do not know what it means.

INTERACTIVE EXERCISE 2-5

1. Your friend meets you for dinner. She tells you that she has been having trouble sleeping. She says she has trouble falling asleep and wakes up several times a night. She looks tired. Underline all the above words that are cues. Circle all the words that are inferences (judgments).
2. Look at this picture.

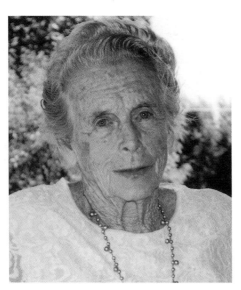

Circle the words that describe what you see:

Woman

Old

Gray hair

Pleasant

Tired

Well-groomed

The items you circled should be cues of what you see rather than judgments about what you see. There are two cues: woman and gray hair. Old is an inference (judgment) that you made based on what you saw: gray hair, wrinkled skin, shrinking face and neck muscles (cues). Pleasant, tired, and well-groomed are also inferences based on what you saw: combed hair and small smile (cues).

Create a concept map around the concept old. Write in boxes around the signs or cues that make you judge someone as old.

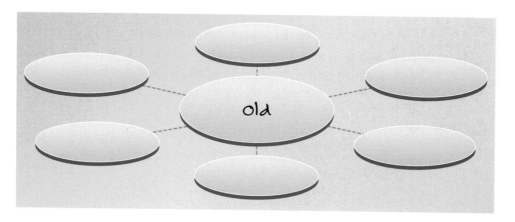

Look at your concept map. If you wrote gray hair, wrinkles, and loss of skeletal muscle, these are signs of aging. Old is a judgment based on your own age. If you are 20, then 50 may be old; if you are 50, then 80 may be old; and if you are 10, then 30 may be old.

Validating Data

To practice nursing well, you must learn to make valid rapid inferences. It is very important to have the data to support your inferences and decisions.

As you become more experienced, you will be able to collect, interpret, and validate data at the same time. For now you must proceed slowly, always asking yourself, "How do I know this? What data do I have to support my inference or judgment?"

As a beginning student, your goal should be to learn the nursing process as a problem-solving technique. Speed is not your goal. Practice validating your opinions in your private life. For example, when you make a judgment about someone in a store as helpful, rude, friendly, or ignorant, ask yourself on what cues did you base your opinion. Sometimes you can walk up to a counter and the person does not greet or acknowledge you. You may think that is rude. Try saying, "You seem to be having a bad day." Your answer may validate your judgment of rude behavior or it may change it.

Validating data with the client helps the nurse to avoid making incorrect inferences. Try to develop your own method of validation. Some examples are as follows:

➤ You seem sad.
➤ Why are you crying?
➤ You appear angry.
➤ Has something I said or did upset you?

Your goal is to help the person share their thoughts or feelings openly. Your goal is not to judge them for their responses but rather to use this information to better nurse them.

As a beginning nursing student, it is important that you share your inferences with an experienced nurse or your instructor. You are a learner; expect that you will make mistakes in inferences. Practice making judgments about cues. Make sure you have sufficient data to make an inference or judgment about it.

DATA COLLECTION

Data collection occurs during every encounter with a client or family. Data collection has two types: the nursing baseline (screening assessment) and focus assessment.

As a student, you will be given a form to guide your data collection during your baseline assessment. This form should help you focus on collecting predetermined data. Refer to Appendix A for an example of a Baseline Assessment Form.

During the data collection, you are also making inferences about the data as significant or insignificant. You can also ask other questions to help you better understand their responses. These other questions are focused questions. Focused assessments will be discussed later in this chapter.

The form that you will use should help you organize the data under one category like sleep, nutrition, or skin. After you finish one section, you can determine whether there are any problems in that section.

Remember your ability to recognize abnormal data will be directly related to how much you know about the problem.

Review the following two situations:

Situation 1
M.S. complains she is not sleeping well. She tosses and turns. She wakes up frequently. She looks tired.

Situation 2
S.M. complains that he is thirsty all the time and is urinating a lot. He also reports some weight loss.

As a beginning student, you probably will have no difficulty determining that M.S. has a sleep problem. For situation 2, you probably will not be able to interpret the data. You know that what he reports is not normal, but you do not know what it means. When you consult with your instructor, you will learn that these symptoms are common in diabetes mellitus. Specific laboratory tests will be needed to confirm the diagnosis.

Focus Assessment

Focus assessments are questions or observations that the nurse decides are necessary. Perhaps the client's condition has changed, which would require more assessment by the nurse. For example, after surgery the nurse would

- ➤ Check the incision
- ➤ Take temperature, pulses, and blood pressure
- ➤ Check urine output

This would be a focused assessment.

After walking into a room, your client says to you, "If my mother comes to see me, tell her I am sleeping." You respond "You do not want to see your mother today?" This is a focused assessment question.

During a baseline or screening assessment, sometimes you see or hear something that suggests a possible problem. You will ask additional questions. These additional questions are a focused assessment.

Admission Assessment
(baseline)

↓

Possible Problem

↓

Focus Assessment

↓

Rule out or confirm problem

Look at this diagram with data.

Admission Assessment

-Bowel movement 2 times a week
-Hard stools

↓

Possible Constipation

↓

Focus Assessment

-Is this usual for you?
-He responds, "No it started when I started taking pain
medicines 2-3 months ago

↓

Confirm Constipation

 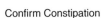

*In Section II, each nursing diagnosis will have some focus assessment criteria to help
you confirm or rule out the diagnosis.*

INTERACTIVE EXERCISE 2-6

Using a functional health pattern assessment, the following represents an admission assessment of Mrs. Patria, a 43-year-old woman who is 100 pounds overweight in the hospital with pneumonia (Display 2-1).

1. Review the data (Display 2.1, p. 30). Create a concept map of Mrs. Patria's strengths.

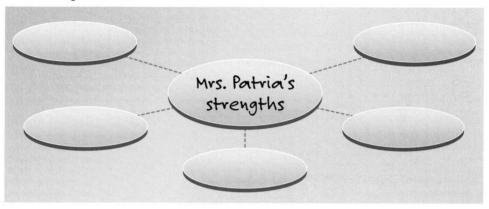

Strengths are a person's inner and external sources that promote positive coping. Strengths can be used to identify interventions to decrease the problem or to prevent a problem. As a college graduate, this client should be provided with a variety of resources to access (e.g., internet, community resources for weight loss, and tobacco cessation).

2. Review the data again and create a concept map of Mrs. Patria's limitations or risk factors.

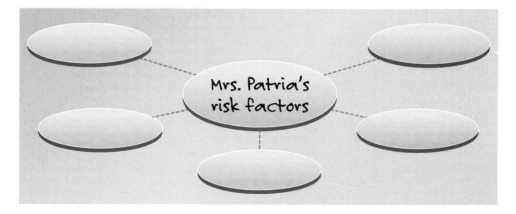

DISPLAY 2-1 FOR INTERACTIVE EXERCISE 2-6

NURSING ADMISSION DATA BASE

Name <u>Delia Patria</u>

Date <u>12-3-05</u> Arrival Time <u>6:30 p</u> Contact Person <u>husband Jorge</u> Phone <u>609 467 0022</u>

ADMITTED FROM: ___ Home alone ✓ Home with relative ___ Long-term care facility
___ Homeless ___ Home with ___
___ ER (Specify) ___ Other ___

MODE OF ARRIVAL: ✓ Wheelchair ___ Ambulance ___ Stretcher

REASON FOR HOSPITALIZATION: <u>c/o shortness of breath</u>
<u>Temperature > 101°F weakness, cough</u>

LAST HOSPITAL ADMISSION: Date <u>1990´</u> Reason <u>Birth of son</u>

PAST MEDICAL HISTORY: <u>negative</u>

MEDICATION (Prescription/Over-the-Counter)	DOSAGE	LAST DOSE	FREQUENCY
ASA	81 mg	yesterday	
Multivitamins	1	"	

HEALTH MAINTENANCE–PERCEPTION PATTERN

USE OF:
Tobacco: ___ None ___ Quit (date) ___ Pipe ___ Cigar ___ < 1 pk/day
✓ 1–2 pks/day ___ >2 pks/day Pks/year history ___
Alcohol: ___ Date of last drink ___ Amount/type
<u>4–6</u> No. of days in a month when alcohol is consumed
Other Drugs: ✓ No ___ Yes Type ___ Use ___
Allergies (drugs, food, tape, dyes): <u>Adhesive Tape</u> Reaction <u>local reaction</u>
Exercise: No regular program

ACTIVITY–EXERCISE PATTERN

SELF-CARE ABILITY:
0 = Independent 1 = Assistive device 2 = Assistance from others
3 = Assistance from person and equipment 4 = Dependent/Unable

	0	1	2	3	4
Eating/Drinking	✓				
Bathing	✓				
Dressing/Grooming	✓				
Toileting	✓				
Bed Mobility	✓				
Transferring	✓				
Ambulating	✓				
Stair Climbing	✓				
Shopping	✓				
Cooking	✓				
Home Maintenance	✓				

ASSISTIVE DEVICES: ✓ None ___ Crutches ___ Bedside commode ___ Walker
___ Cane ___ Splint/Brace ___ Wheelchair ___ Other

CODE: (1) Not applicable (2) Unable to acquire
(3) Not a priority at this time (4) Other (specify in notes)

NUTRITION–METABOLIC PATTERN

Special Diet/Supplements _none_

Previous Dietary Instruction: ___ Yes _✓_ No

Appetite: ___ Normal ___ Increased _✓_ Decreased _✓_ Decreased taste sensation
___ Nausea ___ Vomiting

Weight Fluctuations Last 6 Months: ___ None _5_ lbs. (Gained)/Lost

Swallowing difficulty: _✓_ None ___ Solids ___ Liquids

Dentures: _x_ None ___ Upper (___ Partial ___ Full) ___ Lower (___ Partial ___ Full)
With Person ___ Yes ___ No

History of Skin/Healing Problems: ___ None ___ Abnormal Healing ___ Rash
___ Dryness ___ Excess Perspiration

ELIMINATION PATTERN

Bowel Habits: ___ # BMs/day _2 days ago_ Date of last BM ___ Within normal limits
_✓_ Constipation ___ Diarrhea ___ Incontinence
___ Ostomy: Type: ___ Appliance ___ Self-care ___ Yes ___ No

Bladder Habits: _✓_ WNL ___ Frequency ___ Dysuria ___ Nocturia ___ Urgency
___ Hematuria ___ Retention

Incontinency: _✓_ No ___ Yes ___ Total ___ Daytime ___ Nighttime
___ Occasional ___ Difficulty delaying voiding
___ Difficulty reaching toilet

Assistive Devices: ___ Intermittent catheterization
___ Indwelling catheter ___ External catheter
___ Incontinent briefs ___ Penile implant type _____

SLEEP–REST PATTERN

Habits: _7_ hrs/night ___ AM nap ___ PM nap

Feel rested after sleep _✓_ Yes ___ No

Problems: _✓_ None ___ Early waking ___ Insomnia ___ Nightmares

COGNITIVE–PERCEPTUAL PATTERN

Mental Status: _✓_ Alert ___ Receptive aphasia ___ Poor historian
_✓_ Oriented ___ Confused ___ Combative ___ Unresponsive

Speech: _✓_ Normal ___ Slurred ___ Garbled ___ Expressive aphasia
Spoken language _____ Interpreter _____

Language Spoken: _✓_ English ___ Spanish ___ Other _____

Ability to Read English: _✓_ Yes ___ No _____

Ability to Communicate: _✓_ Yes ___ No _____

Ability to Comprehend: _✓_ Yes ___ No _____

Level of Anxiety: ___ Mild _✓_ Moderate ___ Severe ___ Panic

Interactive Skills: _✓_ Appropriate ___ Other _____

Hearing: _✓_ WNL ___ Impaired (___ Right ___ Left) ___ Deaf (___ Right ___ Left)
___ Hearing Aid

Vision: _✓_ WNL ___ Eyeglasses ___ Contact lens
___ Impaired ___ Right ___ Left
___ Blind ___ Right ___ Left
___ Prosthesis ___ Right ___ Left

Vertigo: ___ Yes ___ No memory intact ___ Yes ___ No

Discomfort/Pain: ___ None ___ Acute ___ Chronic ___ Description _____
Shortness of Breath, Cough

Pain Management: _____

COPING-STRESS TOLERANCE/SELF-PERCEPTION/SELF-CONCEPT PATTERN

Major concerns regarding hospitalization or illness (financial, self-care): _afraid I will get worse_
_____

Major loss/change in past year: _✓_ No ___ Yes _____

Fear of Violence ___ Yes _✓_ No Who _____

Outlook on Future _7_ (rate 1–poor–to 10–very optimistic)

_____

CODE: (1) Not applicable (2) Unable to acquire
(3) Not a priority at this time (4) Other (specify in notes)

DISPLAY 2-1 FOR INTERACTIVE EXERCISE 2-6 (continued)

SEXUALITY–REPRODUCTIVE PATTERN
LMP: <u>11-30-05</u>   Gravida ____<u>2</u>____   Para ____<u>2</u>____
Menstrual/Hormonal Problems: ___ Yes ✓ No _____
Last Pap Smear: <u>1 year ago</u>_____   Hx of Abnormal PAP <u>No</u>_____
Monthly Self-Breast/Testicular Exam: ___ Yes ✓ No Last Mammogram: <u>June 2005</u>_____
Sexual Concerns: <u>deferred</u>_____

ROLE–RELATIONSHIP PATTERN
Marital status: <u>Married</u>
Occupation: <u>Librarian</u>_____
Employment Status: ✓ Employed ___ Short-term disability
                   ___ Long-term disability ___ Unemployed
Support System: ✓ Spouse ✓ Neighbors/Friends ___ None
                ___ Family in same residence ✓ Family in separate residence
                ___ Other _____
Family concerns regarding hospitalization: <u>none specific</u>_____

VALUE–BELIEF PATTERN
Religion: <u>Roman Catholic</u>_____
Religious Restrictions: ✓ No ___ Yes (Specify) _____
Request Chaplain Visitation at This Time: ✓ Yes ___ No
<u>active in her church, teaches sunday school</u>

PHYSICAL ASSESSMENT (Objective)
1. CLINICAL DATA
Age __<u>43</u>__ Height <u>57½</u> Weight <u>245</u> (Actual/Approximate)
Temperature <u>101.2</u>
Pulse: ✓ Strong ___ Weak ___ Regular ___ Irregular rate <u>86</u>
Blood Pressure: <u>120/78</u>

2. RESPIRATORY/CIRCULATORY
Rate <u>22</u>
Quality: ✓ WNL ___ Shallow ___ Rapid ___ Labored ___ Other _____
Cough: ___ No ✓ Yes/Describe _____
Auscultation:
   Upper rt lobes ✓ WNL ___ Decreased ___ Absent ___ Abnormal sounds ___
   Upper lt lobes ✓ WNL ___ Decreased ___ Absent ___ Abnormal sounds ___
   Lower rt lobes ___ WNL ✓ Decreased ___ Absent ___ Abnormal sounds ___
   Lower lt lobes ___ WNL ✓ Decreased ___ Absent ___ Abnormal sounds ___
Right Pedal Pulse: ✓ Strong ___ Weak ___ Absent
Left Pedal Pulse: ✓ Strong ___ Weak ___ Absent

3. METABOLIC–INTEGUMENTARY
SKIN:
   Color: ___ WNL ✓ Pale ___ Cyanotic ___ Ashen ___ Jaundice ___ Other _____
   Temperature: ✓ WNL ✓ Warm ___ Cool
   Turgor: ✓ WNL ___ Poor
   Edema: ✓ No ___ Yes/Description/location _____
   Lesions: ✓ None ___ Yes/Description/location _____
   Bruises: ✓ None ___ Yes/Description/location _____
   Reddened: ✓ No ___ Yes/Description/location _____
   Pruritus: ✓ No ___ Yes/Description/location _____
   Tubes: Specify _____
   Changes _____ None, If Yes/Description/location _____
MOUTH:
   Gums: ✓ WNL ___ White plaque ___ Lesions ___ Other _____
   Teeth: ✓ WNL ___ Other _____

ABDOMEN:
    Bowel Sounds: _✓_ Present ___ Absent

4. NEURO/SENSORY
    Pupils: _✓_ Equal ___ Unequal
    Reactive to light:
      Left: _✓_ Yes ___ No/Specify _____
      Right: _✓_ Yes ___ No/Specify _____
    Eyes: _✓_ Clear ___ Draining ___ Reddened ___ Other _____

5. MUSCULAR–SKELETAL
    Range of Motion: _✓_ Full ___ Other _____
    Balance and Gait: _✓_ Steady ___ Unsteady
    Hand Grasps: _✓_ Equal _✓_ Strong ___ Weakness/Paralysis (___ Right ___ Left)
    Leg Muscles: _✓_ Equal _✓_ Strong ___ Weakness/Paralysis (___ Right ___ Left)

DISCHARGE PLANNING
Lives: Alone ___ With <u>husband</u> No known residence _____
Intended Destination Post Discharge: _✓_ Home ___ Undetermined ___ Other _____
Previous Utilization of Community Resources:
    ___ Home care/Hospice ___ Adult day care ___ Church groups ___ Other _____
    ___ Meals on Wheels ___ Homemaker/Home health aide ___ Community support group
Post-discharge Transportation:
    _✓_ Car ___ Ambulance ___ Bus/Taxi
    ___ Unable to determine at this time
Anticipated Financial Assistance Post-discharge?: _✓_ No ___ Yes _____
Anticipated Problems with Self-care Post-discharge?: _✓_ No ___ Yes _____
Assistive Devices Needed Post-discharge?: _✓_ No ___ Yes _____
Referrals: (record date)
    Discharge Coordinator _____ Home Health _____
    Social Service _____ V.N.A. _____
Other Comments: _____
          _____

SIGNATURE/TITLE <u>J. T. Juall RN</u>   Date <u>12-3-05</u>

3. Mrs. Patria has pneumonia. Look up pneumonia in your pathophysiology book. Complete the following concept map of s/s of pneumonia.

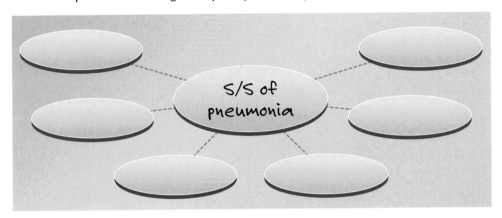

Re-examine the admission data on Mrs. Patria. Look for data to support the signs and symptoms of pneumonia.

4. Next, add another box for each sign and symptom and write in the specific data from Mrs. Patria that support a sign or symptom:

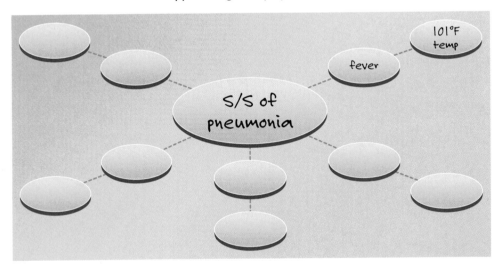

Because you do not know Mrs. Patria or her laboratory and x-ray results, you cannot support all signs and symptoms. In your actual clinical experiences, you can review her chart and correlate her diagnostic studies and laboratory results to the reference data. This activity helps you learn about medical diagnosis through practical analysis of your assigned client's clinical data.

SUMMARY ▼

> *Assessment is a critical component in the nursing process. Incomplete or incorrect assessment can lead to incorrect or missed diagnoses. Guidelines for assessment are important for a beginning student; they provide a system to ensure comprehensiveness and efficiency.*

INTERACTIVE EXERCISE ANSWERS

Interactive Exercise 2-1

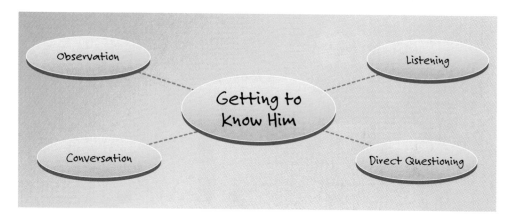

Interactive Exercise 2-2

Open-ended question: What do you do before you go to sleep every night? Any question that requires more than one- or two-word answers is correct.

Closed-ended question: Do you drink caffeine-type drinks (coffee or cola)? Any question that requires a one or two word answer is correct.

Multiple-choice question: Do you sleep with one, two, or three pillows or none? Any question that provides choices is correct.

Rephrasing: You reported you sleep poorly. What does that mean? Any question that uses information from a person's statement to elicit information is correct.

Interactive Exercise 2-3

Cue: Judgment
89 years old: elderly
Fishy smelling vaginal discharge: abnormal
Height 5'1", 210 pounds: obese
Consumes four to six beers per day: drinking problem

Interactive Exercise 2-5

Your friend meets you for dinner. She tells you <u>she is having trouble sleeping.</u> She says <u>she has trouble falling asleep</u> and <u>wakes up several times a night.</u> She (looks) (tired).

Interactive Exercise 2-6

1. Concept map of strengths

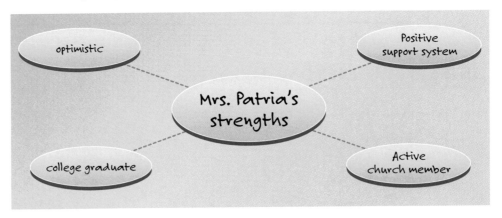

2. Concept map of risk factors

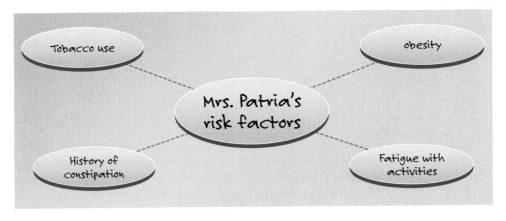

3. Concept map of s/s of pneumonia

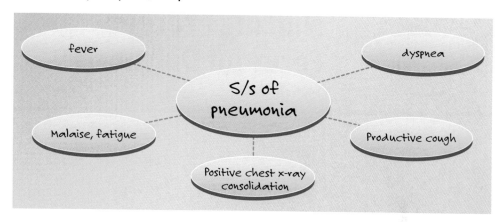

4. Concept map of s/s of pneumonia with supporting data from Mrs. Patria

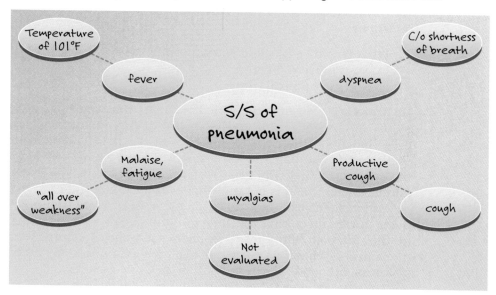

3

Nursing Process: Focus on Diagnosis

Y ou go to your nurse practitioner complaining of nausea, vomiting, and diarrhea. In his mind, your nurse practitioner reviews possible causes of your symptoms as food poisoning or viral gastroenteritis. He asks you more questions:

> What did you eat before you got sick?
> Do your muscles hurt?
> Do you have a headache?

He examines your abdomen. He concludes that you have a virus. No antibiotics are needed. He instructs you on dietary restrictions and gives you a prescription for treatment of the diarrhea. He made a diagnosis after careful assessment. Without this assessment, he may have ordered an antibiotic incorrectly if it was viral gastroenteritis or may have incorrectly ordered an antidiarrheal, which is not indicated with food poisoning.

Every diagnosis is only as good as the assessment that preceded it. Practicing nurses must have the ability to think of all explanations (or diagnoses) for the situation. With these possibilities in mind, the nurse will now proceed to confirm or eliminate these possibilities with questions and observations (assessment).

The word diagnosis has two meanings. Diagnosis is the second step of the nursing process. It involves analysis of data. Later in this chapter, the different types of diagnoses will be discussed.

Diagnosis is also a nursing diagnosis and is a label or statement about the health status of the client. Nursing diagnoses are specific labels used by nurses to describe a client or family's condition.

Nursing diagnoses were identified in 1973 at the first conference of the North American Nursing Diagnosis Association (NANDA). In 1990, NANDA approved the following definition:

> Nursing diagnosis is a clinical judgment about individual, family or community responses to actual or potential health problems or life processes. Nursing diagnosis provides the basis for selection

of nursing interventions to achieve outcomes for which the nurse is accountable (NANDA, 1990).

Every year, NANDA approves new diagnoses for clinical use. Presently, the classification has over 140 nursing diagnoses. Refer to www.nanda.org for more information regarding the purpose and work of the NANDA International Inc. (formerly NANDA).

DIAGNOSIS

You see an accident and stop. You find a woman in the front seat crying and with blood on her clothes. You ask a man who also stops to call 911. You believe she is anxious and bleeding, each requiring you to have two different approaches: one to calm her, and the other to find the source of the bleeding. You also assess the area (car, gasoline leak) to evaluate the danger of fire. In a short time you have

> ➤ Identified two problems
> ➤ Identified the risk for fire

At this accident site, you have identified (diagnosed) three problems: anxiety, bleeding, and risk for fire, from your assessment. You ordered an intervention when you requested a 911 call.

Not all diagnoses that a nurse makes are managed by the nurse. Some require a collaborative management by the nurse and physician (or a nurse practitioner or a physician's assistant). For convenience, physician-prescribed interventions will include all interventions that require a physician, advance practice nurse, or physician's assistant to order them.

Carp's Cue ➤ The accuracy of the care provided to a client depends on your ability to correctly identify the diagnosis or risk for a problem. The accuracy of your diagnosis is dependent on the completeness of your assessment.

The remainder of this chapter will discuss the types of diagnoses that nurses are responsible for.

In Chapter 2 you learned about assessment. After the data collection, you will now

> ➤ Review the data collected during the initial or focus assessment
> ➤ Look at each category on your assessment form like nutrition or sleep patterns
> ➤ Determine whether the client is functioning well or whether there is a problem
> ➤ Determine whether the client is vulnerable to developing a problem

BIFOCAL CLINICAL MODEL

In 1983, Carpenito (now Carpenito-Moyet) introduced a model for practice that describes the focus of professional nurses. This model identifies two types of client situations in which nurses intervene. In one situation, the nurse is the primary prescriber. In the other situation, the nurse must collaborate with a physician, nurse practitioner, or physician's assistant for cotreatment. Nurses are responsible for diagnosing and managing both nursing diagnoses and collaborative problems.

Examine the definitions of Nursing Diagnosis and Collaborative Problems:

Nursing Diagnosis is a clinical judgment about individual, family, or community responses to actual or potential health problems/life processes. Nursing diagnosis provides the basis for selection of nursing interventions to achieve outcomes for which the nurse is accountable (NANDA, 2005).

 This definition attempts to separate nursing diagnosis from medical diagnosis.

Look at this definition more closely. *Clinical judgment* is an opinion that the nurse makes based on the clinical data. *Individual, family, or community responses* are actually the nursing diagnoses. *Health problems/life processes* are situations such as surgery and diabetes mellitus, whereas life processes can be pregnancy, death of a relative, divorce, or aging.

 There are an endless number of examples of health problems, medical diagnoses, and life processes that can cause a problematic response for a person or family. As you learn more in each nursing course, you will expand your understanding of these situations.

Selection of nursing interventions to achieve outcomes is directly related to the nursing diagnosis selected. All nursing diagnoses have related interventions to treat them.

A nurse is accountable for nursing diagnoses. The nurse is responsible for correctly making nursing diagnoses. The nurse *is also* responsible for treatment.

 Naming a response a nursing diagnosis means that nursing has the primary responsibility to order the interventions for treatment.

Collaborative problems are certain physiologic complications that nurses monitor to detect onset or changes in status. Nurses manage collaborative problems using physician-prescribed and nursing-prescribed interventions to minimize the complications of the events (Carpenito, 1985).

A collaborative problem is a concept created by this author to explain problems that are important for the nurse to understand and manage. However, these problems are not nursing diagnoses. The difference between these diagnoses will be discussed for the remainder of this chapter.

Let us look more closely at the definition of collaborative problems. *Certain physiologic complications* signify that *all* collaborative problems are physiologic. *Certain* means that *all* physiologic problems are *not always* collaborative problems. Some physiologic problems are nursing diagnoses such as skin ulcers and difficulty swallowing. For example:

Nurses can prevent	**Nursing Diagnosis**
Pressure ulcers	Risk for Impaired Skin Integrity
Thrombophlebitis	Risk for Ineffective Peripheral
Complications of immobility	Tissue Perfusion
Aspiration	Disuse Syndrome
	Risk for Aspiration

Nurses can treat	**Nursing Diagnosis**
Stage I or II pressure ulcers	Impaired Skin Integrity
Swallowing problems	Impaired Swallowing
Ineffective cough	Ineffective Airway Clearing

Nurses cannot prevent	**Collaborative problems**
Seizures	Seizures
Bleeding	Bleeding

Nurses monitor to detect onset or change in status. This is a major responsibility of nurses. Nurses are constantly monitoring data, for example, vital signs, urine output, condition of wound to determine if there is a new problem or if a problem is worse.

Nurses manage collaborative problems using nurse-prescribed and physician-prescribed interventions. Collaborative problems require nursing *and* medical interventions. Neither nurses nor physicians can treat them without the other.

Minimizing complications of the events is a very important point. Nurses cannot prevent a collaborative problem from happening but can detect it *early* to reduce its seriousness. For example, a nurse can notice a small amount of bleeding on a dressing. This can be stopped before serious blood loss occurs.

WRITING COLLABORATIVE PROBLEMS

All collaborative problems begin with the label Potential Complication or PC. For example:

- ➤ PC: Bleeding
- ➤ PC: Pneumonia
- ➤ PC: High Blood Pressure

The label PC means that the person is at risk for the complication or has the complication and is at risk for it to worsen. For example:

Situation	Man is admitted after a myocardial infarction (heart attack) with a normal blood pressure ↓	Man is admitted after a myocardial infarction (heart attack) with high blood pressure ↓
Diagnosis	PC: Hypertension	PC: Hypertension
Nursing Focus	To monitor for a change in BP or onset of hypertension	To monitor the high BP for increases or decreases

Carp's Cue ▶ *This author describes two types of diagnoses that nurses manage—nursing diagnosis and collaborative problems. Both are very important. Some of the books you use may not use collaborative problems. Instead, they use only nursing diagnoses. This book will teach you both.*

INTERACTIVE EXERCISE 3-1

Read each statement. If the problem requires nurse-prescribed interventions, place an N before it. If the problem requires both nurse-prescribed and physician-prescribed interventions, put a C before it.

_____ 1. Person needs assistance eating

_____ 2. Child is afraid

_____ 3. Woman with high blood pressure

_____ 4. Man not drinking enough fluids

_____ 5. Woman with blood in urine

Answers are at the end of the chapter.

Let us look more closely at number 4, a man not drinking enough fluids. What assessment questions would help you find out more about this problem?

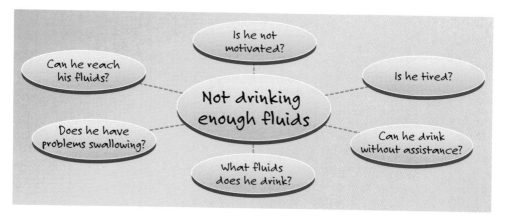

The answers to these questions will help you understand his problem better and will help you select the best interventions.

PREVENTION VERSUS MONITORING

Prevention differs from detection. Prevention interventions try to keep a problem from happening, such as washing your hands to prevent infection or turning a person regularly in bed to prevent skin problems. Monitoring interventions detect the presence of a problem to prevent it from becoming worse. For example, when you monitor a person's blood pressure and it is high, you did not prevent it from being too high. However, you will now consult with a physician for medications to reduce the blood pressure. Physicians cannot treat collaborative problems without nursing's knowledge, vigilance, and judgment.

TYPES AND COMPONENTS OF NURSING DIAGNOSES

There are five types of nursing diagnosis:

➤ Actual
➤ Risk
➤ Possible
➤ Wellness
➤ Syndrome

Actual Nursing Diagnosis

An actual nursing diagnosis is a problem that has been confirmed by the presence of major defining characteristics (signs and symptoms). An actual nursing diagnosis has a label, definition, defining characteristics, and related factors.

LABEL

These labels are concise clear terms that convey the meaning of the diagnosis. NANDA International is responsible for the labels. Refer to www.nanda.org for more information regarding the purpose and work of the NANDA International Inc. (formerly NANDA).

DEFINITION

The definition should add clarity to the diagnostic label. It should help to differentiate one diagnosis from another.

DEFINING CHARACTERISTICS

Defining characteristics are signs and symptoms that, when seen together, represent the nursing diagnosis. Defining nursing diagnoses are separated as major or minor:

➤ Major—at least one must be present to validate it
➤ Minor—they provide supporting evidence but may not be present

RELATED FACTORS

Related factors for actual nursing diagnoses are factors that have caused or contributed to the change in health status or problem. Related factors can be grouped into four categories:

1. Pathophysiologic (biologic or psychological disorders)
2. Treatment-related (medications, diagnostic studies, surgery, treatments, e.g., wound care)
3. Situational (environmental, home, community, institutions, personal, life experiences, roles)
4. Maturational (age-related issues)

These components diagram as follows:

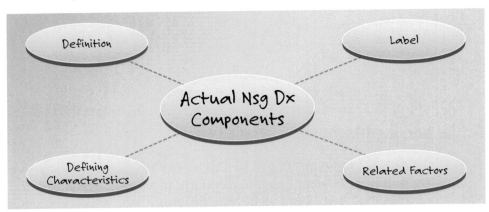

An actual nursing diagnosis may have only one related factor or it may have several. For example, a young man has a fractured (broken) left leg with a cast. He does not know how to use crutches. His nursing diagnosis is impaired physical mobility related to cast on left leg and lack of knowledge on use of crutches. A concept map for this diagnosis and its related factors is as follows:

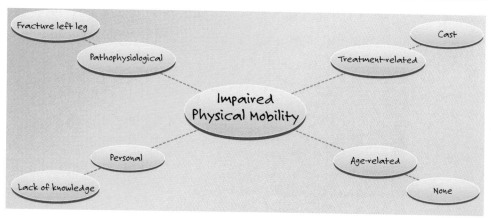

INTERACTIVE EXERCISE 3-2

Complete this concept map for insomnia. Write one example under each related factor category for a factor that can cause or contribute to insomnia.

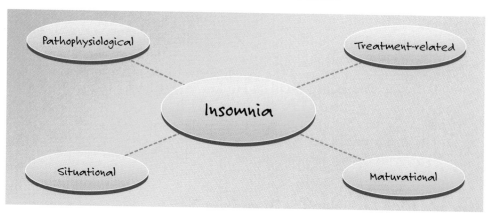

An example of an actual nursing diagnosis with a definition and defining characteristics is

Feeding Self-Care Deficit

Definition
Feeding Self-Care Deficit: a state in which a person experiences an impaired ability to perform or complete feeding activities for himself or herself.

Defining Characteristics

Unable to cut food or open food packages

Unable to bring food to mouth

These are many possible reasons for Feeding Self-Care Deficit. These are the related factors. Look at this concept map with a related factor under each category.

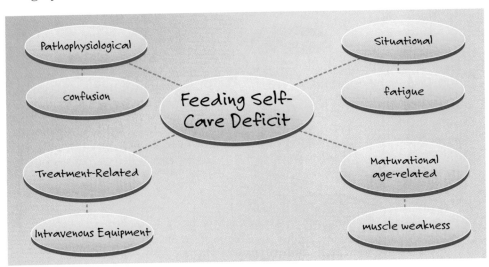

UNKNOWN ETIOLOGY

Sometimes you will have the defining characteristics to validate that a diagnosis is present but you do not know what the related factors are. You do not know what caused the problem. In these situations, you can write Feeding Self-Care Deficit related to unknown etiology.

Remember an actual nursing diagnosis needs defining characteristics for validation. Actual nursing diagnoses do not need related factors for validation.

Risk and High Risk Nursing Diagnoses

Risk Nursing Diagnosis is a clinical judgment that an individual, family, or community is more vulnerable to develop the problem than others in the same or similar situation (NANDA, 2005).

Risk nursing diagnoses are very clinically useful. They represent a person(s) who is(are) more susceptible to developing a problem. The focus of nursing care is to prevent the problem from occurring.

For example, all persons with a surgical incision are susceptible to infection. As a beginning nursing student, you will learn how to prevent infection and assess for early signs and symptoms. So Risk for Infection will be a frequently used nursing diagnosis.

HIGH RISK NURSING DIAGNOSIS

As mentioned before, all surgical clients will have the diagnosis of Risk for Infection. It is an expected diagnosis and considered standard.

Most hospitals have standardized care plans. These are care plans that apply to most persons with a certain medical condition (e.g., pneumonia) or surgical procedure (e.g., hysterectomy). The standardized care plans are preprinted or can be found in a computerized care plan system. When you have your clinical experiences, you will see these examples.

For experienced students and practicing nurses, risk nursing diagnoses are very common and well known. They are sometimes referred to as routine nursing care, which does not require them to be on an individual's care plan.

This author has created the option of using High Risk Nursing Diagnoses. For example, as mentioned earlier, all surgical clients have the nursing diagnosis Risk for Infection. This is standard. However, some surgical clients have other factors that make them more at risk for infection. Some factors are diabetes mellitus, malnutrition, cancer, and obesity. These persons would be High Risk for Infection because of surgical incision and malnutrition.

Ask your instructor about High Risk Nursing Diagnoses. You may be advised only to use Risk Diagnoses as a beginning student.

RISK NURSING DIAGNOSES COMPONENTS

Risk Nursing Diagnosis is a potential problem that is confirmed by the presence of risk factors. Risk diagnoses do not have defining characteristics (signs or symptoms). A Risk Nursing Diagnosis has a label, definition, and risk factors (or related factors) diagrammed as follows:

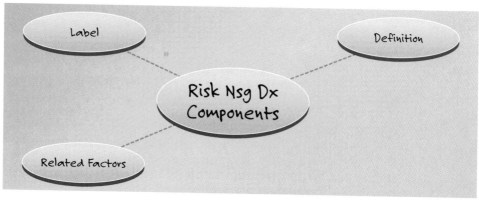

RISK FACTORS

Risk factors represent situations or factors that increase the vulnerability of the client or group. Related factors are the same as risk factors.

Remember that related factors for actual nursing diagnoses are what caused or contributed to the problem developing. The related factors for Risk Nursing Diagnoses are the situations and factors that make the person susceptible for a problem to occur.

	Actual	**Risk**
Related Factors	Cause or contribute to the problem	Increase vulnerability to acquire the problem
Focus on Nursing Care	To reduce or eliminate the problem	To prevent the problem
Proof or validation	Defining characteristics (signs and symptoms)	Risk factors

See Table 3-1.

Possible Nursing Diagnosis

Possible Nursing Diagnoses are statements that describe a suspected problem that requires more data collection. Possible nursing diagnoses are tentative nursing diagnoses. Possible nursing diagnoses are an option for a student

Table 3–1. TYPES OF DIAGNOSTIC STATEMENTS

One-Part Statement

Wellness nursing diagnoses (eg, *Readiness for Enhanced Parenting, Readiness for Enhanced Nutrition*)
Syndrome nursing diagnoses (eg, *Disuse Syndrome, Rape Trauma Syndrome*)

Two-Part Statement

Risk nursing diagnoses (eg, *Risk for Injury related to lack of awareness of hazards*)
Possible nursing diagnoses (eg, *Possible Disturbed Body Image related to isolating behaviors postsurgery*)

Three-Part Statement

Actual nursing diagnoses (eg, *Impaired Skin Integrity related to prolonged immobility secondary to fractured pelvis, as evidenced by a 2-cm lesion on back*)

and for clinical nurses. With possible nursing diagnoses, the nurse has some but not enough data to support a confirmed diagnosis. The related factors for possible nursing diagnoses are data that lead you to suspect the diagnosis *may* be present. Some diagnoses are so complex that they may require several interactions and assessments to confirm or rule out their presence. Some examples are powerlessness, disturbed self-concept, and spiritual distress. Using possible powerlessness allows you and other nurses to continue to collect data to confirm *or to rule out* the diagnosis.

As a beginning nursing student, you probably will not be able to make these more complex nursing diagnoses. You will learn about these in your nursing courses in your last year. You will then be more able to confirm and treat these diagnoses, as an experienced nurse will.

Using the word "possible" before a nursing diagnosis is also an option for you if you are creating a care plan for a client the night before you are going to care for him or her. You will have limited information about the person, perhaps only medical diagnoses and treatments. Technically, most of the nursing diagnoses you will make will be possible or tentative. Look again at the figure on page 22.

Ask your instructor about Possible Nursing Diagnoses. Can you use them as your preclinical diagnosis? You would collect more data while caring for the client. You would then be able to confirm or rule out the diagnosis. Be aware, however, that you may not have sufficient time with the client to assess for sufficient data to confirm or eliminate. Some nursing diagnoses take several interactions to confirm or eliminate, like Ineffective Coping and Spiritual Distress.

Wellness Nursing Diagnoses

A Wellness Nursing Diagnosis is a clinical judgment about an individual, group, or community in transition from a specific level of wellness to a higher level of wellness (NANDA, 2005). All Wellness Nursing Diagnoses have the same two criteria:

> ➤ A desire for increased wellness
> ➤ Is presently healthy

A person who is functioning well, if desired, can be assisted to function even better. For example, a couple reports they are effective parents. They ask the nurse for selected strategies to make them more effective. The diagnosis is Readiness for Enhanced Parenting.

WELLNESS NURSING DIAGNOSES COMPONENTS

Wellness Nursing Diagnoses do not need related factors because they would be the same for all Wellness Nursing Diagnoses as Readiness for Enhanced Parenting, that is, related to a desire to improve their present healthy or effective functioning.

So Wellness Diagnoses have a label and a definition only, diagrammed as follows:

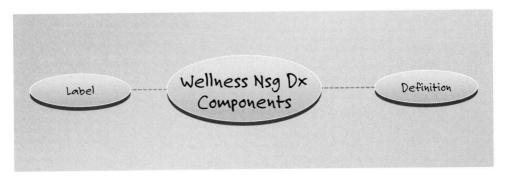

Syndrome Nursing Diagnosis

Syndrome Nursing Diagnoses are a group of predicted actual or risk nursing diagnoses related to a certain event or situation. Because these situations always produce this grouping, syndrome nursing diagnoses allow for very efficient documentation. Presently, NANDA has five syndrome nursing diagnoses: Rape Trauma Syndrome, Disuse Syndrome, Post-Trauma Syndrome, Relocation Stress Syndrome, and Impaired Environmental Interpretation Syndrome.

Syndrome Nursing Diagnoses have a label, definition, and group of predicted actual or risk nursing diagnoses.

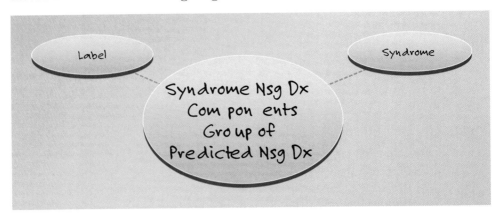

Syndrome Nursing Diagnoses should represent a cluster of actual or potential nursing diagnoses, not signs or symptoms. NANDA's syndrome diagnoses have clustered signs and symptoms. Syndrome Nursing Diagnoses in this author's work have been revised and will be discussed in more detail in Section II. As a beginning nursing student, one syndrome nursing diagnosis would be appropriate for your level: Disuse Syndrome. The others are too advanced for a beginning nursing student.

In review, the types of Nursing Diagnoses can be diagrammed as follows:

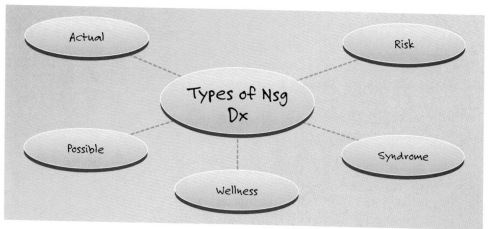

 ## INTERACTIVE EXERCISE 3-3

Match each type of nursing diagnosis in column A with the components in column B. Some will have more than one correct answer.

A	B
_____ **1.** Actual	a. Label and definition
_____ **2.** Risk	b. Contributing or causative factors
_____ **3.** Wellness	c. Risk factors
_____ **4.** Syndrome	d. Defining characteristics
	e. Predicted group of nursing diagnoses
	f. Desire to be healthy

DIAGNOSTIC STATEMENTS

Nursing Diagnostic Statements can be one, two, or three parts. One-part statements consist of a label only as in wellness or syndrome nursing diagnosis. Two-part statements contain the label and related factors as risk and possible nursing diagnosis. Three-part statements contain a label, contributing factors, and signs and symptoms of an actual nursing diagnosis. Examples of diagnostic statements are as follows:

> One Part
> Wellness—Readiness for Enhanced Nutrition
> Syndrome—Disuse Syndrome
> Two Part
> Risk—Risk for Infection related to a site for organism entry
> Possible—Possible Impaired Parenting related to inappropriate
>   interactions
> Three Part
> Actual—Anxiety related to scheduled surgery as evident by pacing and
>   rapid speech

Writing Diagnostic Statements

Three-part statements contain the following:

| Problem | | Etiology | Symptoms |
| Label | related to | Contributing factors | Signs/symptoms |

The "related to" reflects a relationship between the two parts. The contributing factors help the nurse select interventions for treatment. This will be discussed in Chapter 4.

Proof or validation of an actual nursing diagnosis is the last part of the three-part statement.

Impaired Skin Integrity related to immobility secondary to pain as evident by 2-cm lesion on left heel. The validation is the "evident by 2-cm lesion on left heel."

Risk for Impaired Skin Integrity related to immobility secondary to pain. The validation is "immobility secondary to pain."

In these examples, both diagnoses have the same related factors. The lesion on the heel has been caused by immobility. In the second diagnosis, immobility has not caused the diagnosis but instead made the person more vulnerable, that is, Risk.

Unknown Etiology

Sometimes for an actual nursing diagnosis, you may have defining characteristics (signs or symptoms) but do not know what caused the problem. In these situations, you can write, "Anxiety related to unknown etiology as evidenced by rapid speech and hyperalert state." Unknown etiology directs the nurse to assess for more data about the contributing factors.

Can unknown etiology be used for risk diagnosis such as "Risk for Impaired Skin Integrity related to unknown etiology?" No, because the proof of a risk diagnosis is the identification of risk factors.

INTERACTIVE EXERCISE 3-4

Review the following nursing diagnoses and underline which parts of the diagnosis validate or prove the diagnosis.

1. Risk for Infection related to compromised host defenses secondary to AIDS.
2. Disturbed Sleep Patterns related to unfamiliar noisy environment and emotional stress secondary to hospitalization as evident by fatigue during the day and reports of frequent awakening.
3. Risk for Constipation related to change in fluid and food intake and decreased activity secondary to hospitalization.
4. Possible Latex Allergy Response related to dry red hands.

Avoiding Errors in Diagnostic Statements

Writing diagnostic statements takes practice and knowledge. When a medical diagnosis is a related factor for an actual or risk diagnosis, avoid writing

➤ Anxiety related to cancer
➤ Impaired Sleep related to Multiple Sclerosis (MS)

Instead, ask yourself what has the medical diagnosis caused or contributed to the problem? Use this as the related factors. You can link the medical diagnosis with *secondary to*

➤ Anxiety related to perceived losses secondary to cancer.
➤ Impaired Sleep related to difficulty to achieve comfortable position secondary to spasms associated with MS.

For related factors, avoid using

Signs and Symptoms
➤ Disturbed Sleep Patterns related to difficulty falling asleep.
➤ Impaired Skin Integrity related to reddened lesion on leg.

Difficulty falling asleep and reddened lesion on leg are signs and symptoms and not related factors.

Needs
➤ Activity Intolerance related to need to walk every 4 hours
➤ Anxiety related to need to share feelings.

Goals

➤ Feeding Self-Care Deficit related to person should feed himself.

➤ Altered Parenting related to parents should hold child more.

Person should be able to feed himself and parents should hold their child are more goals and not related factors.

After you write your diagnosis, evaluate what you wrote for actual nursing diagnosis:

➤ Can you reduce or eliminate the factors after the *related to?*

➤ Do you have signs or symptoms after *as evidenced by?*

For risk diagnosis:

➤ Can you prevent the diagnosis from occurring by decreasing the related factors?

INTERACTIVE EXERCISE 3-5

Analyze the following diagnostic statements and write whether they are correctly or incorrectly written.

_____ 1. Anxiety related to AIDS.

_____ 2. Grieving related to crying and sleep problems.

_____ 3. Risk for Injury related to dizziness secondary to high blood pressure.

_____ 4. Risk for Constipation related to reports of hard dry stools.

_____ 5. Chronic confusion related to reports from daughter of disorientation and inability to focus.

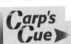

Carp's Cue ▶ *You may not be able to prevent all risk nursing diagnoses from occurring. It is your responsibility to try your best. Because you have a limited time with your clients, you may have limited data to support diagnoses. Remember, Possible Nursing Diagnoses are an option. When you use Possible Nursing Diagnoses, be prepared to support your decision with your instructor.*

INTERACTIVE EXERCISE 3-6

1. Review the Data Base Assessment of Delia Patria in Chapter 2. Under each Functional Health Pattern, write her strengths and risk factors.

➤ Health Perception-Health Management

➤ Activity-Exercise

➤ Nutritional–Metabolic
➤ Elimination
➤ Sleep-Rest
➤ Cognitive-Perceptual
➤ Self Perception
➤ Coping-Stress/Tolerance
➤ Sexuality-Reproductive
➤ Role-Relationship
➤ Value-Belief

2. Review the Physical Assessment data—list the abnormal data. Write one collaborative problem.

3. Review the nursing diagnoses under each pattern with problematic data. Select the actual diagnoses and complete the diagnostic statement with related to _____ and as evidenced by _____. Select risk diagnoses and complete the diagnostic statement as Risk for _____ related to _____.

SUMMARY ▽

Diagnosis is a professional responsibility. You can only diagnose those diagnoses that you understand. Gradually you will become more familiar with the diagnoses in Section II. Remember that even physicians must consult a reference when they encounter an unfamiliar finding. Use of references is a lifetime responsibility for all professionals. Nursing, like medicine, is very complex. The difference is that physicians focus on medical diagnoses, whereas nurses focus on nursing diagnoses and collaborative problems.

INTERACTIVE EXERCISE ANSWERS

Interactive Exercise 3-1

N 1. In this situation, the nurse will prescribe interventions to assist her to eat.

N 2. The nurse will prescribe interventions to reduce the child's fears

C 3. The nurse will continue to monitor the blood pressure and consult with the physician for medication prescriptions

N 4. The nurse will explore different strategies to help the man drink more, for example, preferred fluids

C 5. The nurse will continue to monitor the urine for blood and will consult a physician for physician-prescribed interventions.

Interactive Exercise 3-2

There are many possible examples. Share your responses with a fellow student or your instructor to check whether they are correct.

Interactive Exercise 3-3

A, B 1. Actual
A, C 2. Risk
A, F 3. Wellness
A, E 4. Syndrome

Interactive Exercise 3-4

1. Risk for Infection related to <u>compromised host defenses secondary to AIDS.</u>
2. Disturbed Sleep Patterns related to unfamiliar, noisy environment and emotional stress secondary to hospitalization <u>as evident by fatigue during the day and reports of frequent awakening.</u>
3. Risk for Constipation related to <u>change in fluid and food intake and decreased activity secondary to hospitalization.</u>
4. Possible Latex Allergy Response related to dry, red hands. Possible nursing diagnoses have no validation yet.

Interactive Exercise 3-5

1. Anxiety related to AIDS.

   INCORRECT
   This diagnosis is not specific enough. If this is a new diagnosis, the diagnosis can be written as Anxiety related to new diagnosis of AIDS. If it is not a new diagnosis, it is important for the nurse to explore specific factors with the client to determine their sources of anxiety.

2. Grieving related to crying and sleep problems.

   INCORRECT
   Crying and sleep problems are signs and symptoms of grieving not contributing factors. If you know what the loss is, write Grieving related to death of mother as evident by crying and sleep problems.

3. Risk for injury related to dizziness secondary to high blood pressure.

   CORRECT

4. Risk for Constipation related to reports of hard, dry stools.

   INCORRECT
   Hard, dry stools are signs and symptoms of constipation, not factors that contribute to constipation. Write Constipation related (factors) as evident by hard, dry stools. If you need more data, write Constipation related to unknown etiology as evident by dry, hard stools.

5. Chronic Confusion related to reports of daughter of disorientation and inability to focus.

INCORRECT

The reports by the daughter are signs and symptoms not related to factors. Until the related factors are unknown, write Chronic confusion related to unknown etiology as evident by reports of daughter of disorientation and inability to focus.

Interactive Exercise 3-6

1. Functional Health Problems
   Health Perception-Health Management Pattern
      Tobacco use
      Obesity
   Nutritional-Metabolic Pattern
      Fever
   Elimination Pattern
      History of constipation
   Activity-Exercise Pattern
      Fatigue with activities
      Shortness of breath
      Malaise
   Sleep-Rest Pattern
      Effective pattern
   Self-Perception Pattern
   Role-Relationship Pattern
      Positive support system
   Sexuality-Reproductive Pattern
      Positive pattern
   Coping-Stress Tolerance Pattern
      Optimistic
   Value-Belief Pattern
      Active church member
   Cognitive-Perceptual
      College graduate
2. Abnormal Physical Data
   ➢ Weight 245 lbs
   ➢ Temperature 101.2°F
3. Selecting Nursing Diagnoses and collaborative problems
   ➢ Ineffective Health Maintenance related to an unhealthy lifestyle as evident by obesity (weight 240 lb) and tobacco use
   ➢ Altered Comfort related to fatigue and fever as evidenced by temperature of 101°F
   ➢ Risk for constipation related to history of constipation and immobility.
   ➢ Activity Intolerance related to compromised oxygen transport system secondary to pneumonia and inactivity secondary to obesity as evidenced by c/o shortness of breath and malaise
   ➢ Potential complication: Respiratory Hypoxemia

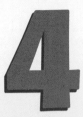

Nursing Process:
Focus on Planning Care

You receive a failing grade (62) on a biology test. If you shrug your shoulders and say, "Oh well," it is likely that you will not be successful on the next test. You could instead have a goal to pass your next test.

Using the nursing diagnosis statements described in Chapter 3, you could write the following:

> Failed Biology Test related to ? as evidenced by grade of 62.

You now need to determine what contributed to your failed test grade. Examine the concept map below:

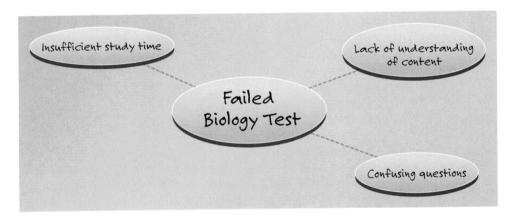

To increase your success to pass the next test, you must identify what caused your failing grade. Each factor in the concept map is different and so are the strategies to eliminate or decrease their influence on your next test. Let's say the diagnosis is

> Failed Biology Test related to lack of understanding of content as evident by grade of 62.

Now let us focus on the next test. Your goal is to pass the next test, maybe even achieve a grade of an A or B. You are at risk to fail another biology test. The diagnosis is now a Risk Diagnosis:

> Risk for a Failed Biology Test related to previous failed test and lack of understanding of the content.

Now you need to plan your strategies to improve your grade and prevent failing. These strategies will focus on activities needed to improve your understanding of the content. One strategy could be to request a fellow student who knows the material well to study with. Another strategy is to ask your instructor to review your test answers with you to increase your understanding of your wrong answers.

Look again at this example and you have an actual diagnosis and a risk diagnosis, a goal, and a plan. These are components of a care plan and will be discussed in this chapter.

CARE PLANS

Care plans are a method to provide directions for the nursing staff to care for a particular person. In health care settings, care plans can be handwritten, computerized, or preprinted. Experienced nurses do not need to create or read a care plan describing routine or predicted care. They know what it is. Instead, they will only need to read care directions that are not routine for the medical diagnosis or surgical procedure. If a care plan is changed or revised, the nurse will need to read it.

Students write care plans to learn what care is needed for a particular client. This care can be routine care and added care indicated by the assessment data. These care plans are also created for the faculty to evaluate as criteria to indicate your ability to use the nursing process.

It is important that you appreciate the efforts you put into the nursing process on paper. It is a vital activity to increase your cognitive ability to scientifically problem solve. Often students view this activity as a waste of time. As a practicing nurse, your problem-solving abilities (nursing process) are critical to your and your client's successes. As a student, you will train yourself to have data to support your decisions. Care planning provides you with a tool to ensure validation.

PLANNING

The planning phase of the nursing process has three components:

➤ Establishing priorities
➤ Formulating goals
➤ Prescribing nursing interventions

Establishing Priorities

Determining priorities can be grouped into three categories:

1. Urgent problems
    These problems cannot wait. They need immediate attention or the person's condition will worsen. For example, you assess there was no urine output for 1 hour through the catheter. You need to notify a nurse immediately.
2. Problems that must be on the plan of care
    These problems or risk problems must be managed in order for the person to progress. Some of these are standard for the client's condition. Other nursing diagnoses and collaborative problems have been added because of data about your client. For example, a client cannot turn himself. He must be assisted to turn in bed to prevent pressure ulcers.
3. Problems that are important but treatment can be delayed without compromising the person's health
    For example, a woman is recovering from surgery. She is obese. This problem does not need attention during the hospital stay, but the nurse can refer her to some community resources.

Carp's Cue ➤ *Priority identification is difficult for a beginning nursing student. Ask your instructor for help in selecting problems for the care plan. When in doubt, if a problem is urgent, always ask your instructor or a nurse.*

INTERACTIVE EXERCISE 4-1

Problems can be designated as urgent on the care plan and can be referred for assistance after discharge. Indicate "urgent," "care plan," or "refer" in front of each problem.

_____ 1. Bleeding from incision

_____ 2. Fear before surgery

_____ 3. Marital problems

_____ 4. Increasing pulse rate

_____ 5. Risk for falls

_____ 6. Transportation problems

CARE PLAN PROBLEMS

Nursing diagnoses and collaborative problems selected for a care plan are not all the problems a client has. Instead, they represent those that need nursing care now or else the person will get worse.

Most medical diagnoses or surgical conditions have a group of nursing diagnoses or collaborative problems that are present in all persons with that condition. In health care settings, these are considered standard.

For example, a group of nursing diagnoses and collaborative problems for someone after abdominal surgery would be as follows:

Nursing Diagnoses

➤ Risk for Ineffective Respiratory Function related to immobility secondary to postanesthesia state and pain.

➤ Risk for Infection related to a site for organism invasion secondary to surgery.

➤ Acute Pain related to surgical interruption of body structures, flatus, and immobility.

➤ Risk for Imbalanced Nutrition: Less Than Body Requirements related to increased protein and vitamin requirements for wound healing and decreased intake secondary to pain, nausea, vomiting, and diet restrictions.

➤ Risk for Constipation related to decreased peristalsis secondary to immobility and the effects of anesthesia and narcotics.

➤ Activity Intolerance related to pain and weakness secondary to anesthesia, tissue hypoxia, and insufficient fluid and nutrient intake.

➤ Risk for Ineffective Therapeutic Regimen Management related to insufficient knowledge of care of operative site, restrictions (diet, activity), medications, signs and symptoms of complications, and follow-up care.

Collaborative Problems

Potential complication (PC): Hemorrhage

PC: Hypovolemia/Shock

PC: Evisceration/Dehiscence

PC: Paralytic Ileus

PC: Infection (Peritonitis)

PC: Urinary Retention

PC: Thrombophlebitis

Nurses experienced with caring for surgical clients are very familiar with the needed care. They would not need to create a care plan with these problems. As a student, you will create care plans that are standard. You would then add or delete depending on your assessment of your assigned client. This will be discussed later in this chapter.

As a beginning nursing student, you will be able to access references to help you learn which nursing diagnoses and collaborative problems are associated with certain conditions.

Appendices B and C are examples of care plans for general medical and general surgical clients.

Due to your limited knowledge, you will find adding other nursing diagnoses and collaborative problems challenging. Focus on your data. If you have significant data, you probably have additional nursing diagnoses or collaborative problems.

For example, if you have a client having abdominal surgery, you will use the grouped diagnosis for abdominal surgery. If the person also has diabetes mellitus, you will add PC: Hypo/hyperglycemia because you will need to monitor blood glucose levels. If her blood glucose level drops below 70, you would know this is urgent and report it.

Urgent problems may be on the care plan, but they may not always be on the plan. These are often collaborative problems that have worsened and require immediate attention. Some urgent problems such as respiratory or cardiac problems may not be on the care plan but become urgent because the client's condition changes or worsens.

Formulating Goals

There are two types of goals:

1. Client goals or outcome criteria
2. Nursing goals

Goals are measures used to evaluate the client's process to improvement of the problem or that a problem has been prevented or managed.

CLIENT GOALS

Client goals are measurable behavior that signifies that a client, family, or group has changed to a favorable status or has continued to maintain a favorable status.

Client goals or outcomes are used

➤ To direct interventions
➤ To evaluate the effectiveness of the interventions

Client goals describe what you expect to see or hear to determine whether the client has improved or benefited from nursing care. Indications can be more specific to help you make a judgment about the client's condition. For example, for the nursing diagnosis grieving, the goals and indicators could be as follows:

Goal
The person will express his or her grief.

Indicators
➤ Describe the meaning of the death or loss to him or her
➤ Share his or her grief with significant others

In the literature, you will read other terms for goals and indicators as follows:

➤ *Goals: objectives, outcomes, long-terms goals*
➤ *Indicators: objectives, short-term goals*

Basically, they are all correct. Ask your instructor which terms are preferred.

NURSING GOALS

Nursing goals are statements describing measurable actions that describe the nurse's accountability for collaborative problems. The accountability for collaborative problems is shared with physicians and advanced nurses. Collaborative problems have nursing goals that reflect nursing's accountability to perform the following:

➤ Monitor for physiologic instability
➤ Initiate physician orders for the situation
➤ Notify the physician or advanced nurse for additional orders for interventions
➤ Perform specific actions to manage and reduce the severity of the event
➤ Evaluate the client's response and to respond appropriately if unsatisfactory

Nursing goals also have indicators, but they are different from indicators for nursing diagnoses. If a nursing goal represents accountability, it would not be correct to make nurses accountable to achieve the indicators. For example:

The client will maintain a blood pressure (BP) over 90/60 and under 140/90. If a person's BP is 170/100, what could the nurse order to change this? Nothing. Instead, a physician or nurse practitioner needs to be consulted. The nurse's accountability is to monitor the BP and report changes. Indicators for nursing goals represent physiological indicators of stability.

All nursing goals for collaborative problems are written as follows:

The nurse will detect early signs and symptoms of _____ and will intervene collaboratively to stabilize the client followed by indicators.

For example:

PC: Hypo/hyperglycemia
Nursing Goal: The nurse will monitor for early signs and symptoms of hypo/hyperglycemia and collaboratively intervene to stabilize the client.
Indicators: Fasting blood sugar 70–115 mg/dl; no ketones in urine

 INTERACTIVE EXERCISE 4-2

Read the following goals:

The client will
➤ Have a BP over 90/60 and under 140/90
➤ Have a regular cardiac rhythm and a rate between 60 and 100 beats per minute
➤ Have dry warm skin

While you are caring for your client, his cardiac rate increases to 130 while in bed and his BP drops to from 120/80 to 90/58. What would you do?

1. Change the nursing care plan
2. Revise the goals
3. Call the doctor or nurse-practitioner

Goals for Nursing Diagnoses

As earlier mentioned, nursing diagnoses have goals and outcomes that focus on a client's behavior. The essential characteristics of goals are as follows:

➤ Measurable behavior
➤ Specific in content and time
➤ Attainable during the care time period

MEASURABLE BEHAVIOR

To write goals with measurable behavior, the goal must either contain a verb that you can see or hear or have indicators that you can hear or see. For example, you cannot see or hear "the client will experience less fear" but can hear "the client will report less fear."

INTERACTIVE EXERCISE 4-3

Read the following goals. Write "Yes" if the goal is measurable or "No" if the goal is not measurable.

_____ 1. Understand the symptoms of low blood sugar

_____ 2. Share her feelings about the death of her mother

_____ 3. Administer an insulin injection correctly

_____ 4. Accepts the diagnosis of cancer

_____ 5. Identify two techniques to reduce fatigue

_____ 6. List food high in salt

SPECIFIC IN CONTENT AND TIME

The goal should indicate what the client needs to do, say, or learn. Modifiers can be added to indicate how, where, what, or how much. For example:

The client will drink more fluids.

What does *more* mean? One glass, six glasses? It would be more measurable if the goal were written:

The client will drink 1500 ml every 24 hours.

The goal should also have a time for achievement. Some examples are as follows:

➤ By discharge: The client will inject himself correctly by discharge.
➤ Continued: The client will demonstrate continued intact skin.
➤ By date: The client will walk unassisted by Friday evening.

Carp's Cue▸ *Determining a time for achievement of a goal is difficult for a student with a limited time on the clinical unit. Ask your instructor if you can write goals that can be achieved in the 1 or 2 days with your assigned client.*

ATTAINABLE

Make sure that the goal is realistic and attainable. Consider the following:

➤ Is there enough time?
➤ Does the client agree with the goal?
➤ Is the client capable of achieving the goal?

In summary, a concept map for criteria for goals or outcomes is shown below:

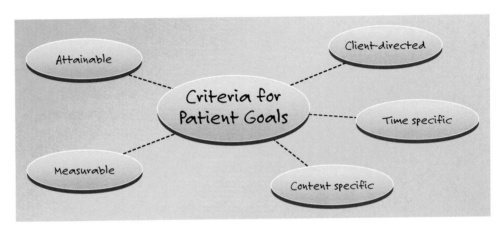

 ## INTERACTIVE EXERCISE 4-4

Using the following concept map, write examples under each criterion for goals that are present in the following goal. If there is none, write none.

The client demonstrates optimal hydration with a urine specific gravity between 1.005–1.030.

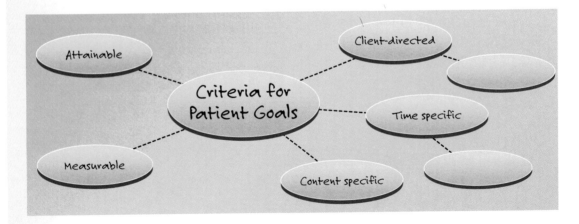

To write measurable correct goals:

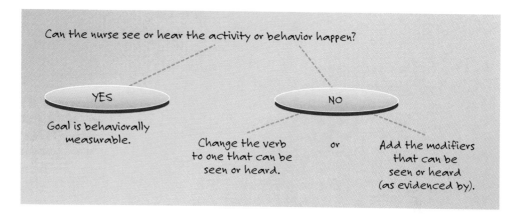

Can the nurse see or hear the activity or behavior happen?

YES

Goal is behaviorally
measurable.

NO

Change the verb
to one that can be
seen or heard.

or

Add the modifiers
that can be
seen or heard
(as evidenced by).

Write the activity or behavior that the client and nurse desire to occur after nursing care has been delivered.

Goals for Actual and Risk Nursing Diagnoses

Goals for actual nursing diagnoses represent the following:

1. Resolution of a problem: will drink less than two cups of caffeinated beverages a day
2. Evidence of progress toward resolution of a problem: will walk 25 feet with assistance
3. Progress toward improved health status: will walk ½ hour three times a day

Goals for Risk Nursing Diagnoses represent the following:

1. Continued maintenance of good health or functioning: will continue to bathe unassisted
2. Demonstrate no negative changes in health status or functioning: will demonstrate no evidence of pressure ulcers

Goals for Possible Nursing Diagnoses

You cannot write a client goal for possible nursing diagnoses because you do not know if there is a problem present or not. Possible nursing diagnoses actually direct the nurse to collect more data to confirm or to rule out the presence of the diagnosis. Nursing goals can be as follows:

The nurse will assess for more data to confirm or to rule out
the problem.

Prescribing Nursing Interventions

There are two types of nursing interventions: nurse-prescribed and physician-prescribed. Nurse-prescribed interventions are those that nurses formulate for themselves or other nurses to implement. Physician-prescribed or delegated interventions are interventions for the client formulated by physicians or advanced practice nurses for nurses to implement. Physician orders are not orders for nurses but rather are orders for the client that nurses implement if indicated.

Both types of interventions require independent nursing judgment because, legally, the nurse must determine whether it is appropriate to indicate the action, regardless if it is independent or delegated.

As a student and later as a practicing nurse, you will always be accountable for all your actions or failing to act. If you question a prescription from a physician or advanced practice nurse, you must ask for clarification and share your concerns. Never follow an order from any colleague or physician that you disagree with. If you give the wrong dose of a medication, both you and the person prescribing the medicine are responsible.

Focus of Nursing Interventions

The major focus on interventions differs from actual, risk, and possible nursing diagnoses and collaborative problems.

For *actual nursing diagnoses*, interventions seek to

➤ Reduce or eliminate contributing factors or the diagnosis
➤ Promote higher level wellness
➤ Monitor status

For risk nursing diagnoses, interventions seek to

➤ Reduce or eliminate risk factors
➤ Prevent the problem
➤ Monitor for onset

For possible nursing diagnoses, interventions seek to

➤ Collect additional data to rule out or confirm the diagnosis

For collaborative problems, interventions seek to

➤ Monitor for changes in status
➤ Manage changes in status with nurse-prescribed and physician-prescribed interventions
➤ Evaluate response

Nursing diagnoses can be treated or prevented using primarily nurse-prescribed interventions. Collaborative problems require both nurse-prescribed and physician-prescribed interventions.

INTERACTIVE EXERCISE 4-5

Read each intervention, and write an "N" if it is a nurse-prescribed intervention or a "P" if it is a physician-prescribed intervention.

_____ **1.** Monitor pulse and BP

_____ **2.** Assist with bath

_____ **3.** Increase intravenous intake

_____ **4.** Apply antibiotic cream to wound

_____ **5.** Monitor intake and output

_____ **6.** Administer an injection of a pain medicine

_____ **7.** Turn the person every 1½ hours

_____ **8.** Apply antiembolism stockings

_____ **9.** Avoid flexing neck when turning

_____ **10.** Avoid putting the bed flat

Interventions for nursing diagnoses can treat the diagnostic label and/or the contributing factors. For example:

Anxiety related to recent diagnosis of cancer.

Nursing interventions will

➤ Reduce anxiety
➤ Promote sharing of feelings about cancer
➤ Explore experiences with cancer in family or with friends
➤ Reduce misconceptions

Diagrammed, it would look like this:

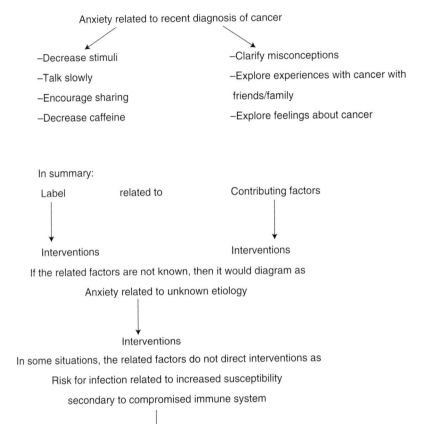

Anxiety related to recent diagnosis of cancer

–Decrease stimuli

–Talk slowly

–Encourage sharing

–Decrease caffeine

–Clarify misconceptions

–Explore experiences with cancer with friends/family

–Explore feelings about cancer

In summary:

Label   related to   Contributing factors

Interventions   Interventions

If the related factors are not known, then it would diagram as

Anxiety related to unknown etiology

Interventions

In some situations, the related factors do not direct interventions as

Risk for infection related to increased susceptibility secondary to compromised immune system

Interventions to reduce exposure to infectious agents

 INTERACTIVE EXERCISE 4-6

1. Refer to answers for Interactive Exercise 3-6.
2. For the four nursing diagnoses, write goals and interventions. Refer to Section II.
3. For the one collaborative problem, write nursing goals and interventions. Refer to Section III.

 Carp's Cue ▶ *This is a practice exercise. Limit your interventions to those that are major as:*

➤ *Teach risks of smoking and obesity.*
➤ *No rationale is needed for this exercise.*

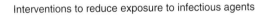

SUMMARY ▼

To plan care, you must learn how to determine priorities, formulate goals, and prescribe interventions. Even though care planning requires a time commitment, as a student, this activity can help you sharpen your problem-solving skills and require you to validate your judgments.

INTERACTIVE EXERCISE ANSWERS

Interactive Exercise 4-1

Urgent	1	Bleeding from incision
Care plan	2	Fear before surgery
Refer	3	Marital problems (If marital problems have reached crisis level during the hospital stay, then the problem should be on the care plan.)
Urgent	4	Increasing pulse rate
Care plan	5	Risk for falls
Refer	6	Transportation problems

Interactive Exercise 4-2

The appropriate action is to call the physician or nurse practitioner for immediate interventions. If physician-prescribed interventions are needed when goals are not achieved, then the problem is a collaborative problem.

Interactive Exercise 4-3

No	1	You cannot hear or see *understand* but you can hear *relate* or see *writes*
Yes	2	You can hear her
Yes	3	You can see this activity
No	4	You cannot see or hear *accept* but you can hear *shares feelings about diagnosis of cancer*
Yes	5	You can hear *identifies*
Yes	6	You can see or hear *list*

Interactive Exercise 4-4

Optimal hydration is a continuous goal. No time is needed in the goal.

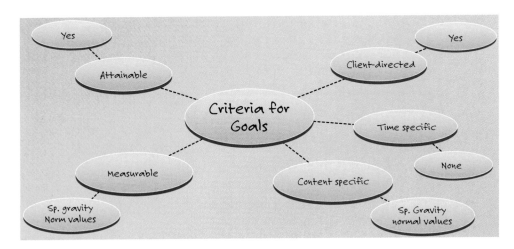

Interactive Exercise 4-5

1. N
2. N
3. P
4. P
5. N
6. P
7. N
8. P
9. N
10. N

Interactive Exercise 4-6

 ## Risk for Constipation related to history of constipation and immobility

GOALS

The person will report a bowel movement at least every 2–3 days.

Indicators

➤ Describe components for effective bowel movements

INTERVENTIONS

1. Explain the components for prevention of constipation, sufficient fluid intake, balanced diet high in fiber (fruits, vegetables, whole grains) and increased activity.
2. Establish a regular time for elimination.
3. Maintain hydration with water, at least 8–10 8 oz glasses a day.
4. Provide privacy.

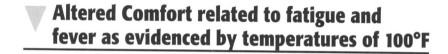

▼ Altered Comfort related to fatigue and fever as evidenced by temperatures of 100°F

GOALS

The person will report acceptable control of symptoms.

Indicators

➤ Describe factors that increase symptoms
➤ Describe measures to improve comfort

INTERVENTIONS

1. Keep room cool; avoid excess blankets.
2. Offer cool cloths to forehead.
3. Monitor temperature every 4 hours.
4. Stress importance of hydration.
5. Provide for periods of uninterrupted rest during each shift.

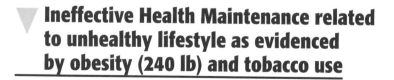

▼ Ineffective Health Maintenance related to unhealthy lifestyle as evidenced by obesity (240 lb) and tobacco use

GOALS

The person will verbalize intent to engage in a healthier lifestyle.

Indicators

➤ Identify risks of present lifestyle
➤ Commit to a weight loss program
➤ Commit to a smoking cessation program

INTERVENTIONS

1. Explain the risks of obesity on the cardiovascular system, the musculoskeletal system, and tissue healing.
2. Explain that excess weight contributes to hypertension, Type 2 diabetes, sleep apnea, osteoarthritis, gallstones, stress incontinence, and hypercholesteremia.
3. Refer to a program in the community, for example, Weight Watchers.
4. Review the effects of smoking on the heart, lung, vascular system, and oral cavity.
5. Provide with community literature and/or internet resources.

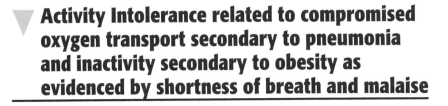

▼ Activity Intolerance related to compromised oxygen transport secondary to pneumonia and inactivity secondary to obesity as evidenced by shortness of breath and malaise

GOALS

The person will progress activity with less shortness of breath.

Indicators

➤ Identify methods to reduce activity intolerence.
➤ Identify factors that aggravate activity intolerance.
➤ Maintain blood pressure within normal limits 3 minutes after activity.

INTERVENTIONS

1. Monitor and evaluate response to activity (pulse, blood pressure, respirations) before, during, and after 3 minutes after.

2. Assess for complaints of chest pain, dizziness, or confusion.
3. Increase activity gradually if there are no abnormal responses.
4. Teach range of motion activities, leg exercises, and weight shifting when in bed.

▼ Potential Complication: Respiratory Hypoxemia

NURSING GOAL

The nurse will detect early signs and symptoms of respiratory insufficiency and will intervene collaboratively to stabilize the client.

Indicators

➤ Oriented, calm
➤ Heart rate 60–100 beats/min
➤ B/P >90/60, ≤140/90 mm Hg
➤ Minimal change in pulse pressure
➤ Respirations 16–20 breaths/min
➤ Urine output >30 ml/hr
➤ Capillary refill <3 seconds
➤ Skin warm; no pallor, cyanosis, or grayness
➤ Urine specific gravity 1.005–1.025
➤ Relaxed, regular, deep, rhythmic respirations
➤ No rales, crackles, wheezing
➤ Pulse oximetry >98%

INTERVENTIONS

1. Take pulse and respiratory rates.
2. Take pulse oximetry if available.
3. Take BP.
4. Assess respiratory pattern, and breath sounds.
5. Assess if short of breath, and presence of cough and sputum.
6. Teach effective coughing.

5

Nursing Process: Focus on Evaluation

After failing a science test, you create a plan to improve your next test grade. Your grade on the next test is a B. In your opinion, your plan worked. If, however, you just barely passed, you would re-evaluate your plan to determine whether you need to change it.

This is an example of evaluation. Evaluation in nursing is a judgment or opinion that is made about data. The data can be an inference (judgment) about a cue such as too high blood pressure (BP) or urine output too low.

To evaluate data or a situation, the nurse must know what the range of normal is for the data and what is the current data diagrammed as follows:

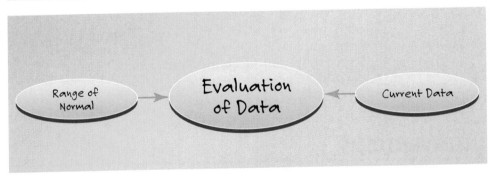

Carp's Cue▶ *As a student, you will be continually learning what the ranges of normal are for data. As a beginning student, you will learn normal ranges of vital signs, oral intake, urine output, and some physical assessment data like skin color and wound healing. Learning the normal range of data will take years. It is important to remember that if you do not know whether the data are normal or not, you always consult with your instructor or another nurse. Do not be afraid to say, "I don't know this yet."*

Knowing these two pieces of information, you form your opinion. After you measure urine output in the collection bag, you calculate 160 ml for 2 hours.

You know that an average urine output is 60 ml an hour with at least 30 ml an hour. This would diagram as follows:

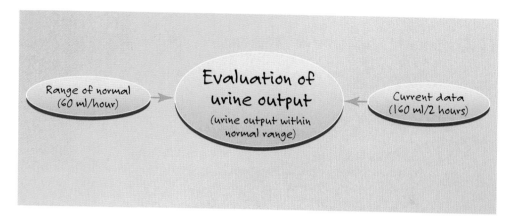

INTERACTIVE EXERCISE 5-1

After introducing yourself to your assigned client, BC age 47, you proceed to take his vital signs, which are temperature, 98.8°F; BP, 160/90; pulse, 84; and respirations, 18. Using these concept maps provided, write in the data for each of the two boxes to the right and left of the center box.

For example, for evaluation of temperature, the data are as follows:

Range of Normal [98.5–99°F]	→	Evaluation of Temperature [within normal limits]	←	Current Data [98.8°F]
1. Range of Normal [ ]	→	Evaluation of BP	←	Current Data [ ]
2. Range of Normal [ ]	→	Evaluation of Pulse	←	Current Data [ ]
3. Range of Normal [ ]	→	Evaluation of Respirations	←	Current Data [ ]

Carp's Cue ▶ *If you need help with these normal ranges, refer to Section III in this book under Cardiovascular and Respiratory Systems.*

TYPES OF EVALUATION

These are three types of evaluations that a nurse must complete as part of providing care:

➤ Evaluation of the Collaborative Problems
➤ Evaluation of Nursing Diagnosis and Progress to Goal Achievement
➤ Evaluation of the Care Plan's Status and Currency

Evaluation of Collaborative Problems

To evaluate collaborative problems, the nurse must

➤ Collect selected data
➤ Compare the data to the established norms
➤ Judge whether the data are within an acceptable range

This is what you did in Exercise 4-1. In Section III, collaborative problems have nursing goals with specific indicators. These indicators are the established norms. These data are what you use to determine the normal or abnormal. For example:

PC: Cardiovascular
Nursing Goal

The nurse will detect early signs and symptoms of cardiovascular problems and will intervene collaboratively to stabilize the client.

Indicators
Calm, alert, oriented
Pulse 60–100 beats/min, regular rhythm
BP >90/60 <140/90 mm Hg
Capillary refill < 3 seconds
Peripheral pulses full, equal
Skin warm and dry

These indicators are diagrammed as

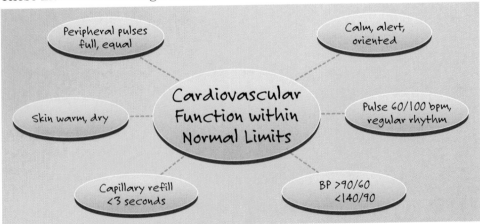

Indicators representing advanced cardiac assessment are not included as cardiac rhythm or dysrhythmias. You will learn this in later courses.

After you compare your assessed data to the established norm, you determine whether the client's condition is stable, within normal limits (WNL), improved, or worsened. Your evaluation will determine your next action. This decision tree can be diagrammed as follows:

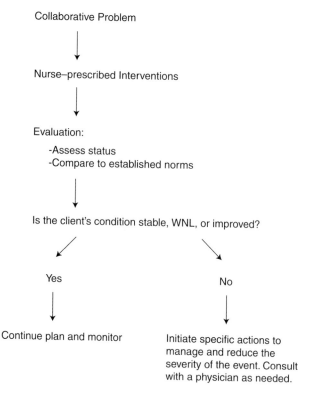

Collaborative Problem

Nurse–prescribed Interventions

Evaluation:
   -Assess status
   -Compare to established norms

Is the client's condition stable, WNL, or improved?

Yes / No

Continue plan and monitor

Initiate specific actions to manage and reduce the severity of the event. Consult with a physician as needed.

Let us look at a clinical example. You take Mr. P's BP, which is 100/62. What are his usual BP ranges? In the chart you find his BP to range from 130/84 to 160/90. Using the above decision tree to apply these data:

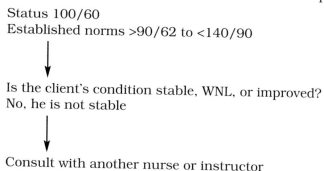

Status 100/60
Established norms >90/62 to <140/90

Is the client's condition stable, WNL, or improved?
No, he is not stable

Consult with another nurse or instructor

Even though the BP is within the normal range, it is a change that would be evaluated as unstable.

INTERACTIVE EXERCISE 5-2

The client you are caring for has an incision from abdominal surgery. Yesterday, you assessed the wound to

➤ Be healing with wound edges closed together
➤ Have no drainage
➤ Have minimal tenderness and redness

Today, the wound

➤ Has a 2-mm opening at wound edges
➤ Has no drainage
➤ Has increased redness and tenderness

What would you do next?

Evaluation of Nursing Diagnoses and Progress to Goal Achievement

Nurses need client goals (outcome criteria) to evaluate nursing diagnoses. After the nurse and client have established client goals, the nurse will provide the interventions. The nurse will then

➤ Assess the client's condition
➤ Compare the client's present condition to the goal
➤ Decide whether the client is progressing to outcome achievement

For example, your client has the following nursing diagnosis and goal:

Bathing Self-Care Deficit related to decreased motivation and endurance as evidenced by "I am too tired to wash myself."

Goal: The client will wash her face and arms today.

As you help the client with her morning hygiene, she brushes her hair, teeth, and washes her face, chest and arms. Based on these data, did she meet the goals for today? Yes.

Carp's Cue ▶ *It is important when forming outcome criteria for activities of daily living as hygiene, nutrition, and ambulation that the client agrees with the goals for them. Therefore, these goals are jointly made. Nursing diagnoses that are more psychologically oriented, such as anxiety and grieving, usually reflect sharing of feelings and therefore are not usually jointly made as: the client will communicate feelings regarding hospitalization.*

INTERACTIVE EXERCISE 5-3

On the care plan you created last night, you read the following:

1. Risk for Constipation related to change in fluid/food intake and activity level secondary to hospitalization.

   Goal: The client will maintain prehospital bowel pattern of bowel movement every other day.

2. Potential Complication: Respiratory Insufficiency

   Nursing Goal: The nurse will detect early signs and symptoms of respiratory insufficiency and will collaboratively stabilize the client.

   ### Indicators
   Calm, alert, oriented
   Respirations 16–20 breaths/min
   Breath sounds present all lobes
   No rales or wheezing

Focusing on these two diagnoses (one nursing diagnosis, one collaborative problem), you assess the client for data to help you evaluate his condition. He had a bowel movement yesterday that was soft and formed. He is cooperating in his care and asks questions. His respirations are regular, quiet, and at 17 per minute. You hear breath sounds in all lobes and hear no rales or wheezing.

1. What is your evaluation of Risk for Constipation?
2. What is your evaluation of Potential Complication: Respiratory Insufficiency?

Refer to answers at end of the chapter.

Evaluation of the Care Plan

Care plans require reviewing to update. Updating can be revising problems, goals, and interventions. Revising can be deletions or additions.

The student can do the evaluation of the care plan after providing care. In practice settings where the client will have longer relationships with a nurse such as rehabilitation, home care, and hospice, there will be an ongoing evaluation of the care plan with designated time frame for formal review. In the hospital, the short stay will make the evaluation a shift-to-shift requirement.

After you care for the client, you will evaluate each section of the care plan with the following questions:

Nursing Diagnosis
- ➤ Does the diagnosis still exist?
- ➤ Does a risk or high-risk diagnosis still exist?
- ➤ Has the possible diagnosis been confirmed or ruled out?
- ➤ Does a new diagnosis need to be added?

Goals
- ➤ Have they been achieved?
- ➤ Do they reflect the present focus of care?
- ➤ Can more specific modifiers be added?
- ➤ Are they acceptable to the client?

Interventions
- ➤ Are they acceptable to the client?
- ➤ Are they specific to the client?
- ➤ Do they provide clear instructions to the nursing staff?

Collaborative Problems
- ➤ Is continuing monitoring indicated?

In reviewing the problems and interventions, the nurse records one of the following decisions in the evaluation column or in the progress notes at the time prescribed for evaluation:

- ➤ **Continue.** The diagnosis is still present, and the goals and interventions are appropriate.
- ➤ **Revised.** The diagnosis is still present, but the goals or nursing orders require revision. The revisions are then recorded.
- ➤ **Ruled Out/Confirmed.** Additional data collection has confirmed or ruled out possible diagnosis. Goals and nursing orders are written.
- ➤ **Achieved.** The goals have been achieved, and that portion of the care plan is discontinued.
- ➤ **Reinstate.** A diagnosis that had been resolved returns.

SUMMARY ▽

Evaluation is part of the four other steps in the nursing process: assessment, diagnosis, planning, and implementation. Each step depends on the accuracy of the preceding step. For example, when you are assessing a client, you are evaluating whether the data are significant or not. You are evaluating the client's response. To validate a nursing diagnosis, you need to evaluate whether you have sufficient data to support it. Evaluation just may be the most difficult step in the nursing process.

INTERACTIVE EXERCISE ANSWERS

Interactive Exercise 5-1

1. Range of Normal ⟶ Evaluation of BP ⟵ Current Data
   [>90/60 <140/90]   [high]   [160/92]

   Even if the client's pressure had been higher, this reading is still too high. When clients are not in the hospital, the normal ranges for BPs are >90/60 and <130/85.

2. Range of Normal ⟶ Evaluation of Pulse ⟵ Current Data
   [60–100 beats/min]   [WNL]   [84]

   If the pulse rate is elevated and the client was just performing an activity, repeat the pulse again in 3 minutes.

3. Range of Normal ⟶ Evaluation of Respirations ⟵ Current Data
   [16–20]   [WNL]   [18]

Interactive Exercise 5-2

Asking the question, "Is the client's condition stable, within normal limits, or improved?

No, worsened

Consult with instructor or another nurse

Surgical wounds are expected to improve with time. These may be early signs of infection.

Interactive Exercise 5-3

1. Evaluation of Risk for Constipation.

   Because this is a risk diagnosis, is the client maintaining his bowel function with no signs or symptoms of constipation? Yes, continue plan.

2. Evaluation of Potential Complications: Respiratory Insufficiency

   Because this is a collaborative problem, is your assessment data about his respiratory function consistent with normal values? Yes, continue plan.

6 Putting It All Together in 11 Steps

N ow you have learned the five steps in the nursing process. You will have the tools to create a plan of care (or care plan) for your assigned client.

There are many types of formats of care plans. Each school has their own format. Health care facilities such as hospitals and home care agencies have their own format also. You will see care plans in the computer system in some of the hospitals that you will be practicing in.

STEP 1: ASSESSMENT

If you interview your assigned client before you write your care plan, complete your assessment using the form recommended by your faculty. If you need to write a care plan before you can interview the client, go to Step 2 now. After you complete your assignment, you will now need to identify

➤ Strengths
➤ Risk factors
➤ Problems in functioning

Strengths are qualities or factors that will help the person to recover, cope with stressors, and progress to his or her original health or as close as possible before hospitalization, illness, or surgery.

Examples of strengths are as follows:

➤ Positive spiritual framework
➤ Positive support system
➤ Ability to perform self-care
➤ No eating difficulties
➤ Effective sleep habits

➤ Alert, good memory
➤ Financial stability
➤ Relaxed most of the time
➤ Motivated

Create a concept map with the client strengths identified for your assigned client:

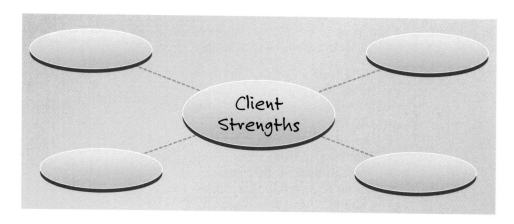

 For every client you are assigned, create a concept map of strengths. After you care for your client, you probably will discover some more strengths. Add them.

INTERACTIVE EXERCISE 6-1

Create a concept map of all your strengths as a person.

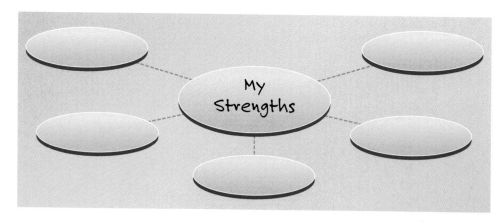

Risk factors are situations, personal characteristics, disabilities, or medical conditions that can hinder the person's ability to heal, cope with stressors, and progress to his or her original health before hospitalization, illness, or surgery. Examples of risk factors are as follows:

➤ No or ineffective support system
➤ No or little regular exercise
➤ Inadequate or poor nutritional habits
➤ Learning difficulties
➤ Denial
➤ Poor coping skills
➤ Communication problems
➤ Obesity
➤ Fatigue
➤ Limited ability to speak or understand English
➤ Memory problems
➤ Hearing problems
➤ Self-care problems before hospitalization
➤ Difficulty walking
➤ Financial problems
➤ Tobacco use
➤ Alcohol problem, substance abuse
➤ Moderate to high anxiety most of the time
➤ Frail, elderly
➤ Presence of chronic disease, such as

   Arthritis
   Diabetes mellitus
   Human immunodeficiency virus infection
   Multiple sclerosis
   Depression
   Cardiac disorder
   Pulmonary disease

Create a concept map of all your client's risk factors:

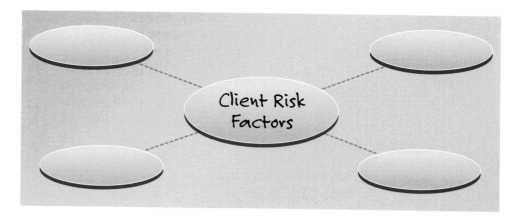

Carp's Cue For every client that you are assigned, create a concept map of his or her risk factors. You will be able to identify some of your client's risk factors before caring for him or her. You will probably discover more. Add them.

INTERACTIVE EXERCISE 6-2

Create a concept map of your risk factors to health:

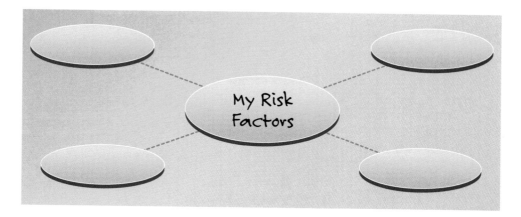

Carp's Cue Risk factors can negatively influence a person's health status. For example, diabetes mellitus will make a client more vulnerable to an infection after surgery.

STEP 2: SAME DAY ASSESSMENT

If you have not completed a screening assessment of your assigned client, determine the following as soon as you can by asking the client, family, or nurse assigned to your client.

Before hospitalization:

➤ Could the client perform self-care?
➤ Did the client need assistance?
➤ Could the client walk unassisted?
➤ Did the client have memory problems?
➤ Did the client have hearing problems?
➤ Did the client smoke cigarettes?

What conditions or diseases does the client have that make him or her more vulnerable to the following:

➤ Falling
➤ Infection
➤ Nutrition/fluid imbalance
➤ Pressure ulcers
➤ Severe or panic anxiety
➤ Physiological instability (e.g., electrolytes, blood glucose, blood pressure, respiratory function, healing problems)

When you meet the assigned client, determine whether any of the risk factors are present:

➤ Obesity
➤ Impaired ability to speak/understand English
➤ Cognitive difficulties
➤ High anxiety

Write significant data on an index card. Go to Step 3.

Carp's Cue➤ *In some nursing programs, students do not have the opportunity to see or to assess their assigned client before the clinical day. Therefore, they must assess the client on their first clinical day.*

STEP 3: CREATE YOUR INITIAL CARE PLAN

If your client is in the hospital for a medical problem, refer to the generic medical care plan in Appendix B. If your client is in the hospital for a surgical condition, refer to the generic surgical care plan in Appendix C.

Review each part of the care plan and delete anything that does not apply to your client. For example, if the person is not allowed to drink or eat anything, delete all that pertains to increasing eating and drinking. Add anything that will help the person meet goals, for example, adding their favorite beverages.

 Carp's Cue ▶ *These generic care plans reflect the usual predicted care a client needs. Ask your instructor how you can use them to prevent excessive writing. Refer to Appendices B and C for the generic care plans formatted to individualize.*

STEP 4: ADDITIONAL RISK, ACTUAL OR POSSIBLE PROBLEMS

After you have reviewed the generic medical or surgical problem, you may need to add additional problems that need attention now. Add them.

In Sections II and III, you will find a group of nursing diagnoses and collaborative problems that are pertinent for a beginning nursing student.

STEP 5: REVIEW THE COLLABORATIVE PROBLEMS ON THE GENERIC PLAN

Review the collaborative problems listed. These are the physiologic complications that you need to monitor. Do not delete any because they all relate to the condition or procedure that your client has had. You will need to add how often you should take vital signs, record intake and output, change dressings, and so forth. Ask the nurse you are assigned to for these times and review the Kardex, which also may have the time frames.

Review each intervention for collaborative problems. Are any interventions unsafe or contraindicated for your client? For example, if your client has edema and renal problems, the fluid requirements may be too high for him or her. Ask a nurse or instructor for help here.

Review the collaborative problems on the standard plan. Also review all additional collaborative problems you found that are related to any medical or treatment problems. For example, if your client has diabetes mellitus, you need to add

Potential Complication: Hypoglycemia/hyperglycemia

STEP 6: REVIEW THE NURSING DIAGNOSES ON THE STANDARD PLAN

Review each nursing diagnosis on the plan.

➤ Does it apply to your assigned client?
➤ Does your client have any risk factors (see your index card) that could make this diagnosis worse?

An example on the Generic Medical Care Plan is Risk for Injury related to unfamiliar environment and physical or mental limitations secondary to condition, medication, therapies, or diagnostic tests.

Now look at your list of risk factors for your assigned client. Can any factors listed contribute to the client sustaining an injury? For example, is he or she having problems walking or seeing? Is he or she experiencing dizziness?

If your client has an unstable gait related to peripheral vascular disease (PVD), you would add the following diagnosis: Risk for Injury related to unfamiliar environment and unstable gait secondary to peripheral vascular disease.

Review each intervention for each nursing diagnosis:

➤ Are they relevant for your client?
➤ Will you have time to provide them?
➤ Are any interventions not appropriate or contraindicated for your assigned client?
➤ Can you add any specific interventions?
➤ Do you need to modify any interventions because of risk factors (see index card)?

If you know your client has PVD but do not know how this can affect functioning, look up the diagnosis in another textbook and review what problems PVD causes. Examples include unstable gait, poor circulation to the legs, and risk for injury.

Review the goals listed for the nursing diagnosis:

➤ Are they pertinent to your client?
➤ Can the client demonstrate achievement of the goal on the day you provide care?
➤ Do you need more time?

Delete goals that are inappropriate for your client. If your client will need more time to meet the goal, add "by discharge." If the client can accomplish the goal this day, write "by (insert date)" after the goal.

Faculty and references may have different words to describe goals. Ask your faculty which terms they use.

Using the same diagnosis Risk for Injury related to unfamiliar environment and physical and mental limitations secondary to the condition, therapies, and diagnostic tests, consider this goal:

The client will not sustain an injury.

Indicators

➤ Identify factors that increase risk of injury.
➤ Describe appropriate safety measures.

If it is realistic for your client to achieve all the goals on the day of your care, you should add the date to all of them. If your client is confused, you can add the date to the main goal, but you would delete all the indicators because the person is confused. Or you could modify the goal by writing the following:

Family member will identify factors that increase the client's risk of injury.

Remember that you cannot individualize a care plan for a client until you spend time with him or her, but you can add or delete interventions based on your preclinical knowledge of this client (e.g., medical diagnosis, coexisting medical conditions).

STEP 7: PREPARE THE CARE PLAN (WRITTEN OR PRINTED)

You can prepare the care plan by

➤ Accessing the generic care plan from the website into your word processor and then deleting or adding specifics for your client (use another color or a different type font for additions/deletions)
➤ Photocopying a care plan from this book and then adding or deleting specifics for your client
➤ Writing the care plan

Ask your faculty person what options are acceptable. Using different colors or fonts allows your faculty person to clearly see your analysis. Be prepared to provide rationales for why you added or deleted items.

STEP 8: INITIAL CARE PLAN COMPLETED

Now that you have a care plan of the collaborative problems and nursing diagnoses, which ones are associated with the primary condition for which your client was admitted? If your assigned client is a healthy adult undergoing surgery or was admitted for an acute medical problem and you have not assessed any significant factors in Step 1, you have completed the initial care plan. Go to Step 10.

STEP 9: ADDITIONAL RISK FACTORS

If your client has risk factors (on the index card) that you identified in Steps 1 and 2, evaluate whether these risk factors make your assigned client more vulnerable to develop a problem. The following questions can help to determine whether the client or family has additional diagnoses that need nursing interventions:

- ➤ Are there additional collaborative problems associated with coexisting medical conditions that require monitoring (e.g., hypoglycemia)?
- ➤ Are there additional nursing diagnoses that if not managed or prevented now will deter recovery or affect the client's functional status (e.g., High Risk for Constipation)?
- ➤ What problems does the client perceive as priority?
- ➤ What nursing diagnoses are important but treatment for them can be delayed without compromising functional status?

You can address nursing diagnoses that are not on the priority list by referring the client for assistance after discharge (e.g. counseling, weight loss program).

Priority identification is a very important but difficult concept. Because of the shortened hospital stays and because many clients have several chronic diseases at once, nurses cannot address all nursing diagnoses for every client. Nurses must focus on those for which the client would be harmed or not make progress if they were not addressed.
  Ask your clinical faculty to review your list. Be prepared to provide rationales for your selections.

STEP 10: EVALUATE THE STATUS OF YOUR CLIENT (AFTER YOU PROVIDE CARE)

Collaborative Problems

Review the nursing goals for the collaborative problems:

- ➤ Assess the client's status.
- ➤ Compare the data to established norms (indicators).
- ➤ Judge whether the data fall within acceptable ranges.
- ➤ Conclude whether the client is stable, improved, unimproved, or worse.

Is your client stable or improved?

- ➤ If yes, continue to monitor the client and to provide interventions as indicated.
- ➤ If not, has there been a dramatic change (e.g., elevated blood pressure and decreased urinary output)? Have you notified the physician

or advanced practice nurse? Have you increased your monitoring of the client? Communicate your evaluations of the status of collaborative problems to your clinical faculty and to the nurse assigned to your client.

Nursing Diagnosis

Review the goals or outcome criteria for each nursing diagnosis. Did the client demonstrate or state the activity defined in the goal? If yes, then communicate (document) the achievement on your plan. If not and the client needs more time, change the target date. If time is not the issue, evaluate why the client did not achieve the goal. Was the goal

➤ Not realistic because of other priorities?
➤ Not acceptable to the client?

Ask your clinical faculty where to document evaluation of goal achievement.

STEP 11: DOCUMENT THE CARE ON THE AGENCY'S FORMS, FLOW RECORDS, AND PROGRESS NOTES

Ask your clinical faculty where you should document your evaluation of the client after you have provided care.
Care planning is a cognitive process that involves a great deal of data. Practice as much as you can. As a beginning student, do not be afraid to ask for help.

SUMMARY ▽

Chapter 6 is a condensed guideline that you can use with each of your clinical assignments. These 11 stages will help you organize your data and your analyses.

NURSING DIAGNOSES

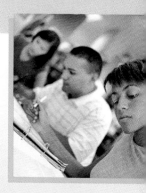

Section II contains 58 nursing diagnoses. Six are presented with an explanation describing their problematic clinical use. The remaining 52 contain the following:

- ➤ Definition
- ➤ Defining characteristics, signs and symptoms, or risk factors of the diagnosis
- ➤ Related factors, organized according to pathophysiologic, treatment-related, situational, and maturational, that may contribute to or cause the actual diagnosis

Additional components include the following:

- ➤ Carp's Cues, which clarify the concept and clinical use of the diagnosis by a beginning student
- ➤ Key Concepts, which list scientific explanations about the diagnosis and interventions, categorized as Generic, Geriatric, and Transcultural Considerations
- ➤ Focus Assessment Criteria, subjective and objective, which serve to guide specific data collection to help confirm or rule out the diagnosis

Each diagnosis has one group of interventions that focuses on the treatment associated with the diagnostic label, regardless of the etiologic and contributing factors, with outcome criteria. Interventions specifically direct a beginning nursing student to

- ➤ Clarify causative and contributing factors
- ➤ Reduce or eliminate the factors
- ➤ Promote selected activities
- ➤ Teach healthy choices and make referrals

For direction on creating a care plan for your assigned client, refer to Chapter 6.

▼ Activity Intolerance

Definition

Activity Intolerance: A state in which an individual experiences a reduction in one's physiologic capacity to endure activities to the degree desired or required (Magnan, 1987)

Defining Characteristics

MAJOR (SOME MUST BE PRESENT)

An altered physiologic response to activity
Assess for subjective (S) and objective (O) cues:

Respiratory

➤ Dyspnea (S)
➤ Shortness of breath (S)
➤ Excessively increased rate (O)
➤ Decreased rate (O)

Pulse

➤ Weak (O)
➤ Excessively increased (O)
➤ Rhythm change (O)
➤ Decreased (O)
➤ Failure to return to pre-activity level after 3 minutes (O)

Blood Pressure

➤ Failure to increase with activity (O)
➤ Increased diastolic pressure > 15 mm Hg (O)

MINOR (MAY BE PRESENT)

➤ Weakness (S)
➤ Pallor or cyanosis (O)
➤ Vertigo (S)
➤ Fatigue (S)
➤ Confusion (O)

Related Factors

Any factors that compromise oxygen transport, lead to physical deconditioning, or create excessive energy demands that compromise the person's physical and psychological abilities can cause activity intolerance. Some common factors are listed below.

PATHOPHYSIOLOGIC

Related to compromised oxygen transport system secondary to the following:

Cardiac examples

➤ Cardiomyopathies
➤ Dysrhythmias
➤ Myocardial infarction
➤ Congenital heart disease
➤ Congestive heart failure
➤ Angina
➤ Valvular disease

Respiratory examples

➤ COPD
➤ Atelectasis

Circulatory examples

➤ Anemia
➤ Hypovolemia
➤ Peripheral arterial disease

Related to increased metabolic demands secondary to the following:

Acute or chronic infections

➤ Viral infection
➤ Endocrine or metabolic disorders
➤ Mononucleosis
➤ Hepatitis

Chronic disease examples

➤ Renal failure
➤ Multiple sclerosis
➤ Cirrhosis
➤ Arthritis

Related to inadequate energy sources secondary to

➤ Malnourishment
➤ Inadequate diet

TREATMENT-RELATED

Related to increased metabolic demands secondary to

➤ Cancer
➤ Diagnostic studies
➤ Surgery
➤ Treatment schedule/frequency

Related to compromised oxygen transport secondary to

➤ Hypovolemia
➤ Prolonged bed rest

SITUATIONAL (PERSONAL, ENVIRONMENTAL)

Related to inactivity secondary to

➤ Depression
➤ Lack of motivation
➤ Sedentary lifestyle
➤ Obesity

Related to increased metabolic demands secondary to

➤ Assistive equipment
➤ Extreme stress
➤ Pain
➤ Environmental barriers (e.g., stairs)
➤ Climate extremes (especially hot, humid climates)
➤ Air pollution (e.g., smog)
➤ Atmospheric pressure (e.g., recent relocation to high-altitude living)

MATURATIONAL

Older adults may have decreased muscle strength and flexibility as well as secondary deficits. These factors can undermine body confidence and may contribute directly or indirectly to activity intolerance.

Activity Intolerance describes a person with compromised physical conditioning. This person can be helped to increase strength and endurance. In Activity Intolerance, the goal is to increase tolerance to activity; in Fatigue, the goal is to assist the person to adapt to the fatigue, not to increase the endurance.

Key Concepts

GENERIC CONSIDERATIONS

➤ Endurance is the ability to continue a specified task; fatigue is the inability to continue a specified task. Conceptually, endurance and fatigue are opposites. Nursing interventions, such as work simplification, aim to delay task-related fatigue by maximizing efficient use of the muscles that control movement, motion, and locomotion.

➤ The ability to maintain a given level of performance depends on personal factors, strength, coordination, reaction time, alertness, and motivation; and on activity-related factors, frequency, duration, and intensity.

➤ In normal people, the work of breathing is very limited. In those with COPD, however, it may increase 5 to 10 times above normal. Under such conditions, the oxygen required just for breathing may be a large fraction of total oxygen consumption.

➤ The effects of bed rest deconditioning develop rapidly and may take weeks or months to reverse. All people confined to bed are at risk for activity intolerance as a result of bed rest–induced deconditioning.

GERIATRIC CONSIDERATIONS

➤ Prolonged immobility and inactivity through self-imposed restrictions, mental status changes, or pathophysiologic changes can contribute to decreased activity tolerance (Cohen et al., 2000).

➤ Decreased muscle mass leads to decreased muscle strength, which, in turn, leads to decreased endurance. Muscle strength, which is maximal between 20 and 30 years of age, drops to 80% of that value by 65 years of age (Cohen, Gorenberg, & Schader, 2000).

➤ Increased chest wall rigidity with aging leads to decreased lung expansion, resulting in decreased tissue oxygenation. This immediately affects activity tolerance.

FOCUS ASSESSMENT CRITERIA

1. While the person sits or lies in bed, assess blood pressure, pulse, and respirations.
2. Evaluate rate, rhythm, and respiratory effort.
3. Evaluate pulse rate, rhythm, and quality.
4. Assist the person to the next level of activity that has been prescribed. For example, out of bed to chair, walking with assistance, and walking unassisted.
5. Take pulse, respirations, and blood pressure immediately after the activity.
6. Wait 3 minutes; take the vital signs again.
7. Assess for pale skin, cyanosis (grayish skin), confusion, or dizziness.
8. Evaluate response:

	Pulse	BP	Respirations
Resting			
Normal	60–90	<140/90	<20
Abnormal	>100	>140/90	>20
Immediately after activity			
Normal	↑ Strength, ↑ Rate	↑ Systolic	↑ Depth, ↑ Rate
Abnormal	Irregular rhythm	No change in systolic	Excessive ↓ rate
3 minutes after after			
Normal	Within 10 beats of resting pulse	Return to resting BP	Return to resting rate
Abnormal	>10 beats of resting pulse		

9. Assess for related factors. See Related Factors.

Carp's Cue ▶ *After you assess resting pulse, respirations, and blood pressure, evaluate whether they are within normal range. If they are not, consult with your instructor before beginning any activity.*

GOAL

The person will progress activity to (specify level of activity desired).

Indicators

➤ Identify factors that aggravate activity intolerance.
➤ Identify methods to reduce activity intolerance.
➤ Maintain blood pressure within normal limits 3 minutes after activity.

GENERAL INTERVENTIONS

1. Monitor the person's response to activity.

➤ Take resting pulse, blood pressure, and respirations.
➤ Consider rate, rhythm, and quality (if signs are abnormal, e.g., pulse above 100, consult with instructor about advisability of increasing activity).
➤ Have person perform the activity.
➤ Discontinue the activity and consult with instructor if the person responds with
   ➤ Complaints of chest pain, vertigo, or confusion
   ➤ Decreased pulse rate
   ➤ Failure of systolic blood pressure to increase
   ➤ Decreased systolic blood pressure
   ➤ Increased diastolic blood pressure by 15 mm Hg
   ➤ Decreased respiratory response
➤ Reduce the intensity or duration of the activity if
   ➤ The pulse takes longer than 3 to 4 minutes to return within six beats of resting pulse
   ➤ The respiratory rate increase is excessive after the activity

Rationale: Response to activity can be evaluated by comparing preactivity blood pressure, pulse, and respiration with postactivity results. These, in turn, are compared with recovery time.

2. Increase the activity gradually.

➤ Increase tolerance for activity by having the person perform the activity more slowly, for a shorter time with more rest pauses, or with more assistance.
➤ Allow for periods of rest before and after planned periods of exertion, such as treatments, ambulation, and meals.
➤ Encourage gradual increases in activity and ambulation to prevent a sudden increase in cardiac workload.
➤ Assess a person's perceived capability for increased activity.
➤ Assist person in setting short-term activity goals that are realistic and achievable.
➤ Reassure person that even small increases in activity will lift spirits and restore self-confidence.
➤ Minimize the deconditioning effects of prolonged bed rest and imposed immobility:
   ➤ Begin active range of motion (ROM) at least twice a day. For the person who is unable, the nurse should perform passive ROM.
   ➤ Encourage isometric exercise.
   ➤ Encourage the person to turn and lift self actively unless contraindicated.
   ➤ Promote optimal sitting balance and tolerance by increasing muscle strength.

> ➤ Gradually increase tolerance by starting with 15 minutes the first time out of bed.
>
> ➤ Have the person get out of bed three times a day, increasing the time out of bed by 15 minutes each day.

Rationale: Activity tolerance develops cyclically through adjusting frequency, duration, and intensity of activity until the desired level is achieved. Increasing activity frequency precedes increasing duration and intensity (work demand). Increased intensity is offset by reduced duration and frequency. As tolerance for more intensive activity of short duration develops, frequency is once again increased.

Rationale: People with impaired cardiac function often can increase both activity level and tolerance through adaptations in lifestyle, modifications in approach to activities, and careful monitoring of responses.

3. Determine adequacy of sleep.

> ➤ Plan rest periods according to the person's daily schedule. (They should occur throughout the day and between activities.)
>
> ➤ Encourage person to rest during the first hour after meals. (Rest can take many forms: napping, watching television, or sitting with legs elevated.)

Rationale: Rest relieves the symptoms of activity intolerance. The daily schedule is planned to allow for alternating periods of activity and rest and coordinated to reduce excess energy expenditure.

4. Promote a sincere "can-do" attitude.

> ➤ Identify factors that undermine person's confidence, such as fear of falling, perceived weakness, and visual impairment.
>
> ➤ Explore possible incentives with the person and family; consider what the person values:
>   > ➤ Playing with grandchildren
>   > ➤ Going fishing
>   > ➤ Performing a task, such as a craft
>   > ➤ Returning to work
>
> ➤ Allow person to set activity schedule and functional activity goals. If the goal is too low, negotiate (e.g., "Walking 25 feet seems low. Let's increase it to 50 feet. I'll walk with you.")
>
> ➤ Plan a purpose for the activity, such as sitting up in a chair to eat lunch, walking to a window to see the view, or walking to the kitchen to get some juice.
>
> ➤ Help the person to identify progress. Do not underestimate the value of praise and encouragement as effective motivational techniques. In selected cases, assisting the client to keep up a written record of activities may help to determine progress.

Rationale: Knowledge, values, beliefs, and perceived capability for action influence a person's decision to engage in a particular activity.

5. For a person with chronic lung disease:

➤ Teach controlled breathing (pursed-lip and diaphragmatic breathing) for use during increased activity or stress.
➤ Demonstrate the breathing technique, and then direct him or her to mimic your breathing pattern.
➤ For pursed-lip breathing, the person should breath in through the nose and then breathe out slowly through partially closed lips while counting to 7 and making a "pu" sound. (Often, people with progressive lung disease learn this naturally.)
➤ For diaphragmatic breathing:
   a. Place your hands on the person's abdomen below the base of the ribs and keep them there while he or she inhales.
   b. To inhale, the person relaxes the shoulders, breathes in through the nose, and pushes the stomach outward against your hands. The person holds the breath for 1 to 2 seconds to keep the alveoli open and then exhales.
   c. To exhale, the person breathes out slowly through the mouth while you apply slight pressure at the base of the ribs.
   d. Have the person practice this breathing technique several times with you; then, the person should place his or her own hands at the base of the ribs to practice alone.
   e. Once the person has learned the technique, have him or her practice it a few times each hour.

Rationale: Diaphragmatic breathing deters the shallow, rapid, inefficient breathing that usually accompanies COPD. Pursed-lip breathing slows expiration, keeps alveoli inflated longer, and provides some control over dyspnea.

   f. Explain activities and factors that increase oxygen demand:

➤ Smoking
➤ Extremes in temperature
➤ Excessive weight
➤ Stress

Rationale: Smoking, extremes in temperature, and stress cause vasoconstriction, which increases causes cardiac workload and oxygen requirements. Excess weight increases peripheral resistance, which also increases cardiac workload.

   g. Provide with ideas for conserving energy:

➤ Sit whenever possible when performing ADLs, for example, on a stool when showering.

➤ Pace activities throughout the day.
➤ Schedule adequate rest periods.
➤ Alternate easy and hard tasks throughout the day.

Rationale: Excessive energy expenditure can be prevented by pacing activities and allowing sufficient time to recuperate between activities.

h. Evaluate client's nutritional status. Refer to imbalanced nutrition for more interventions.

Rationale: The increased work of breathing causes decreased appetite and intake. Increased CHO intake increases CO_2 production. Decreased intake causes an energy deficit. Energy deficit causes malnutrition and muscle wasting, which decreases diaphragm and muscle strength.

i. Initiate health teaching and referrals.

➤ Initiate client and caregivers in ROM and therapeutic exercises.
➤ Consult physical therapist for an exercise program tailored to the client's needs.
➤ Consult dietitian for dietary evaluation and nutritional counseling.

Rationale: To increase endurance, the exercise program must be continued after discharge.

▼ Anxiety

Definition

Anxiety: A state in which the individual/group experiences feelings of uneasiness (apprehension) and activation of the autonomic nervous system in response to a vague nonspecific threat.

Defining Characteristics

MAJOR (SOME MUST BE PRESENT)

Assess for subjective (S) and objective (O) cues:

Physiologic

Increased heart and elevated blood pressure (O)
Increased respiratory rates (O)

Diaphoresis (O)
Voice tremors/pitch changes (O)
Palpitations (O)
Insomnia (S,O)
Body aches and pains (especially back, chest, neck) (S)
Dilated pupils (O)
Trembling, twitching (O)
Nausea, vomiting (O)
Diarrhea (O)
Fatigue and weakness (S)
Dry mouth (S)
Restlessness (O)
Faintness/dizziness (S)
Hot and cold flashes (S)
Poor appetite (S)

Remember anxiety is always present in all of us. It is a normal feeling. Anxiety becomes a problem only when it interferes with your ability to function or with your relationships with others.

Emotional

Person states feelings of

Apprehension (S)
Tension or being "keyed up" (S)
Nervousness (S)
Inability to relax (S)

Person exhibits

Irritability/impatience (O)
Crying (O)
Startle reaction (O)
Poor eye contact (O)
Angry outbursts (O)
Tendency to blame others (S)
Criticism of self and others (S)

Cognitive

–Inability to concentrate (S,O)
–Forgetfulness (S,O)
–Preoccupation (S,O)
–Diminished learning ability (S,O)

Related Factors

PATHOPHYSIOLOGIC

Any physiologic condition that interferes with the basic human needs for food, air, comfort, and security, for example, cancer, pain and difficulty breathing.

SITUATIONAL (PERSONAL, ENVIRONMENTAL)

Related to actual or perceived threat to self-concept secondary to

Change in status and prestige.
Failure (or success)
Loss of valued possession.
Ethical dilemma

Related to actual or perceived loss of significant others secondary to

Death/divorce
Temporary or permanent separation/moving

Related to actual or perceived threat to biologic integrity secondary to

Dying
Assault
Invasive procedures (e.g., surgery, chest tubes)

Related to actual or perceived change in environment secondary to

Hospitalization
Moving
Retirement
Safety Hazards

OLDER ADULT

Related to threat to self-concept secondary to

Sensory losses, motor losses
Financial problems, retirement changes
Pregnancy/parenting
Career changes
Loss of significant others

Key Concepts

> Fear and anxiety can look and feel the same, but what is causing these symptoms is different. Sometimes fear and anxiety are experienced at the same time by one person.
> Anxiety is an unclear feeling of uneasiness (mild) to terror (panic) in response to a threat to oneself. For example, hospitalization can be a source of threat, but the threats are what hospitalization can mean to you.
> Fear is a feeling of apprehension or dread to an identifiable source or danger as needles, snakes, and/or heights. Fear can be reduced or eliminated by removal from the situation.
> Normal anxiety is necessary for survival. It prompts constructive behaviors such as being on time or studying for a test.
> Acute or state anxiety is the response to an imminent loss or change that disrupts one's sense of security. Examples include apprehension before a speech or the death of a close relative or friend.
> The severely anxious person tends to overgeneralize, assume, and anticipate catastrophe with cognitive problems, including difficulty with attention and concentration and loss of objectivity and patience.

 For example, let's say you are upset when you see a snake or when you have to speak in front of the class. To deal with these feelings, you would try to avoid situations where snakes are. If you came upon a snake, you would quickly leave. These feelings are fear. Your uncomfortable feelings related to public speaking cannot be handled the same way as your fear of snakes. You must deal with your emotions. These emotions are anxiety. One technique you can use to reduce your anxiety is to use transparencies to help you focus and to decrease you from looking at your audience.

TRANSCULTURAL CONSIDERATIONS

> Clients and families from different cultures face many challenges when they seek health care in the dominant culture's health care delivery systems. In addition to usual sources of anxiety (e.g., unfamiliar people, unknown prognosis), they may be anxious about language difficulties, privacy, separation from support systems, and cost (Andrews & Boyle, 2003).
> Members of cultures that depend on kin for caring will expect more humanistic kinds of nursing care and less scientific-technologic care (Andrews & Boyle, 2003).

FOCUS ASSESSMENT CRITERIA

Assess for signs and symptoms of anxiety.

Mild

➤ Heightened perception and attention; alertness
➤ Ability to deal with problems
➤ Ability to integrate past, present, and future experiences
➤ Mild tension-relieving behaviors (nail biting, hair twisting)
➤ Sleeplessness

Moderate

➤ Slightly narrowed perception; selective inattention
➤ Slight difficulty concentrating; learning requires more effort
➤ Possible failure to notice what is happening around them; some difficulty adapting and analyzing
➤ Voice/pitch changes
➤ Increased respiratory and heart rates
➤ Tremors, shakiness

Severe

➤ Distorted perception; focus on scattered details
➤ Severely impaired learning; high distractibility and inability to concentrate
➤ View of present experiences in terms of past; almost cannot understand current situation
➤ Poor function; communication difficult to understand
➤ Hyperventilation, tachycardia, headache, dizziness, nausea
➤ Complete self-absorption

Panic

➤ Irrational reasoning; focuses on blown-up detail
➤ Inability to learn
➤ Inability to integrate experiences; focus only on present; inability to see or understand situation
➤ Inability to function; usually increased motor activity or unpredictable responses to minor stimuli; communication not understandable
➤ Feelings of impending doom (dyspnea, dizziness/faintness, palpitations, trembling, choking, hot/cold flashes, sweating)
➤ Thoughts related to loss of control, death, and illness

GOAL

The person will relate an increase in psychological and physiological comfort.

Indicators

Will verbalize feelings openly
Identify activities that increase comfort

GENERAL INTERVENTIONS

Nursing interventions for *Anxiety* can apply to anyone with anxiety regardless of causative and contributing factors.

1. Determine the level of anxiety.

Mild

➤ Increased ability to learn, problem solve
➤ Some restlessness, mild irritability
➤ Fidgeting, nail-biting
➤ Can identify things that are disturbing

Moderate

➤ Sees, hears, understands less information
➤ Can problem solve
➤ Can be directed by another
➤ Pounding heart, increased respirations
➤ Gastric discomfort, headache
➤ Shaking, voice tremors

Severe

➤ Can only focus on one thing at a time
➤ Cannot focus on environment
➤ Absorbed completely in one's self
➤ Cannot problem solve
➤ Confusion
➤ Purposeless activity
➤ Loud rapid speech
➤ Threats, demands

Panic

➤ Painful disturbed behavior
➤ Unable to process what is happening
➤ May see or hear things not there
➤ Extreme terror
➤ Cannot speak well
➤ Dilated pupils
➤ Sense of doom (dyspnea, choking, sweating)

Rationale: It is important to identify the level of anxiety because interventions are different for mild and moderate versus severe or panic. A person with severe or panic anxiety may not comprehend complex dialogue.

Remember that interventions that will help a moderately anxious person find alternative solutions to a problem will not help a person with severe or panic anxiety. Consult your instructor when you evaluate a person as having severe or panic anxiety.

2. Assist person to reduce present level of anxiety.

➤ Provide reassurance and comfort
  ➤ Stay with the person
  ➤ Do not make demands or ask the person to make decisions
➤ Support present coping mechanisms (e.g., allow client to talk, cry); do not confront or argue with defenses or rationalizations
➤ Speak slowly and calmly
➤ Convey empathic understanding (e.g., quiet presence, touch, allow crying, talking)
➤ Remind person that feelings are not harmful
➤ Respect personal space
➤ Enlist support from family, friends, and other sources. Limit the presence of those that increase the person's stress.

Rationale: Providing emotional support and encouraging sharing may help a client clarify and verbalize his or her fears, allowing the nurse to get realistic feedback and reassurance.

If anxiety is at severe or panic level:

➤ Provide quiet nonstimulating environment with soft lighting.
➤ Use short simple sentences; speak slowly.
➤ Give concise directions.
➤ Focus on the present.
➤ Remove excess stimulation (e.g., take the person to a quieter room); limit contact with others (e.g., other clients, family) who are also anxious.
➤ Provide physical measures that will aid in relaxation such as warm baths, back massage, aromatherapy, and music.
➤ Consult a physician/nurse practitioner for possible pharmacologic therapy if indicated.
➤ Provide opportunity to exercise (e.g., walk fast).

Rationale: An anxious client has a narrowed perceptual field with a diminished ability to learn. The client may experience symptoms caused by increased muscle tension and disrupted sleep. Anxiety tends to feed on itself, trapping the client in a spiral of increasing anxiety, tension, and emotional and physical pain (Arnold, 1997).

Do not try to solve a person's problems. Instead, learn to be comfortable with an anxious person. Speak slowly. Let them know their feelings are normal. You can help them look at options only when anxiety is mild or moderate.

3. When anxiety diminishes, assist person to recognize anxiety.

➤ Request validation of your assessment of anxiety (e.g., "Are you comfortable now?") If person says yes, continue with learning process. If the client cannot acknowledge anxiety, continue supportive measures until he or she can.

➤ When client can learn, determine usual coping mechanisms: "What do you usually do when you get upset?" (e.g., read, discuss problems, walk, use substances, and seek social support).

➤ Assess for unmet needs or expectations. Encourage recall and description of what the person experienced immediately before feeling anxious.

➤ Assist in reevaluation of perceived threat by discussing the following:
  ➤ Were expectations realistic?
  ➤ Was it possible to meet expectations?
  ➤ Where in the sequence of events was it possible to stop the anxiety from increasing?

➤ Encourage to recall and to analyze similar instances of anxiety.

➤ Explore alternatives the client might have used to replace maladaptive coping mechanisms.

➤ Teach anxiety interrupters to use when client cannot avoid stressful situations:
  ➤ Look up
  ➤ Control breathing
  ➤ Lower shoulders
  ➤ Slow thoughts
  ➤ Alter voice
  ➤ Give self-directions (out loud, if possible)
  ➤ Exercise
  ➤ "Scruff your face"—change facial expressions
  ➤ Change perspective: imagine watching situation from a distance (Grainger, 1990)

4. Refer for counseling for problematic coping mechanisms.

➤ Depression
➤ Violent behavior
➤ Denial
➤ Demanding behavior

Rationale: Professional counseling is needed after discharge.

5. Gently address the numerous physical complaints with no known organic base:

   ➤ Encourage expression of feelings.
   ➤ Give positive feedback when the person is symptom free.
   ➤ Acknowledge that symptoms must be burdensome.
   ➤ Encourage interest in external environment (e.g., volunteering, helping others).
   ➤ Listen to complaints.
   ➤ Evaluate secondary gains the person receives and attempt to interrupt cycle; see person regularly, not simply in response to somatic complaints.
   ➤ Discuss how others are reacting; attempt to have the client identify behavior when others react negatively (Withdrawal? Anger?)
   ➤ Avoid "doing something" to each complaint; set limits when appropriate.

Rationale: Excessive preoccupation with imagined diseases without any organic pathology can have roots in guilt and low self-esteem. The person believes he or she deserves an illness as a punishment.

Denial can serve as a protective function and is not always maladaptive. Anger is a response to frustration and anxiety. Not all anger is problematic. Uncontrolled anger is problematic.

6. Initiate health teaching and referrals as indicated.

   ➤ Instruct in nontechnical understandable terms regarding illness and associated treatments.
   ➤ Repeat explanations because anxiety may interfere with learning.
   ➤ Instruct in maintenance of physical well-being (i.e., nutrition, exercise, and elimination).
   ➤ Instruct in use of relaxation techniques (e.g., aromatherapy, hydrotherapy, music therapy and massage).
   ➤ Explain the benefits of foot massage and reflexology (Grealish et al., 2000; Stephenson et al., 2000).
   ➤ Instruct in constructive problem solving.

Rationale: Relaxation techniques enhance the client's sense of control over the body's response to stress (DeMarco-Sinatra, 2000). Complementary therapies such as massage, aromatherapy, and hydrotherapy are useful in managing stress and anxiety (Keegan, 2000; Wong, Lopez-Wahas & Molassiotis,

2001). Exercise can effectively reduce anxiety (Blanchard, Courneya & Laing, 2001). Music therapy is an effective nursing intervention in decreasing anxiety (Wong, Lopez-Nahas & Molassiotis, 2001). Exercise is an effective method for reducing state anxiety in breast cancer survivors (Blanchard, Courneya & Laing, 2001).

▼ Risk for Imbalanced Body Temperature

Definition

Risk for Imbalanced Body Temperature: The state in which the individual is at risk for failing to maintain body temperature within normal range (36°C to 37.5°C or 98°F to 99.5°F) (Smeltzer & Bare, 2004).

Risk Factors

Presence of risk factors (see Related Factors)

Related Factors

PATHOPHYSIOLOGIC

Related to impaired temperature control secondary to

Coma/increased intracranial pressure
Brain tumor/hypothalamic tumor/head trauma
Cerebrovascular accident
Infection/inflammation
Integument (skin) injury

Related to decreased circulation secondary to

Anemia
Neurovascular disease/peripheral vascular disease
Vasodilation/shock

Related to decreased ability to sweat secondary to (specify) the following:

TREATMENT RELATED

Related to cooling effects of

Parenteral fluid infusion/blood transfusion
Cooling blanket

Dialysis

Operating suite

SITUATIONAL (PERSONAL, ENVIRONMENTAL)

Related to

Exposure to cold, rain, snow, or wind; exposure to heat, sun, and
humidity extremes

Inappropriate clothing for climate

Inability to pay for shelter, heat, or air conditioning

Extremes of weight

Consumption of alcohol

Dehydration/malnutrition

MATURATIONAL

Related to ineffective temperature regulation secondary to extremes of age
(e.g., newborn, older adult)

*Changes in body temperature occur frequently in clients. Monitoring body
temperature is a regular nursing activity. Because a person's body temperature will
change sometimes in 1 day from normal to abnormal to normal again, using this
diagnosis is very useful. So when a person's temperature goes higher, you can still
keep the diagnosis as Risk. All hospitalized clients will have this diagnosis. As you
become a more experienced student, you will only use this with clients who are high
Risk for Imbalanced Body Temperature (e.g., head trauma).*

*Risk for Imbalanced Body Temperature includes those at Risk for Hypothermia,
Hyperthermia, Ineffective Thermoregulation, or all of these. If the person is only at
risk for one (e.g., Hypothermia but not Hyperthermia), then it is more useful to label
the problem with the specific diagnosis (Risk for Hypothermia). If the person is at risk
for more than one, then Risk for Imbalanced Body Temperature is more appropriate.
The focus of nursing care is preventing abnormal body temperatures by identifying
and treating those with normal temperature who demonstrate risk factors that nurse-
prescribed interventions (e.g., removing blankets, adjusting environmental temperature)
can control. If the imbalance is related to a pathophysiologic complication that requires
nursing and medical interventions, then the problem should be labeled as collaborative
problem (e.g., Potential Complication [PC]: Severe Hypothermia secondary to hypothalamus injury). The focus of concern then becomes monitoring to detect and report
significant temperature fluctuations and implementing collaborative interventions
(e.g., a warming or cooling blanket) as ordered.*

Key Concepts

GERIATRIC CONSIDERATIONS

➤ The body has two major compartments: the shell (skin and subcutaneous tissue) and the core (vital internal organs, intestinal tract, and large muscle groups). Heat transfer involves shell and core; it is possible for the shell to be warm while the core is cold, and vice versa.

➤ Regulation of body temperature is a dynamic process involving four mechanisms (Porth, 2002):

Conduction: Direct transfer of heat from the body to cooler objects without motion (e.g., from cells and capillaries to skin and onto clothing).

Convection: Transfer of heat by circulation (e.g., from warmer core areas to peripheral areas and from air movement next to the skin)

Radiation: Transfer of heat between the skin and the environment

Evaporation: Transfer of heat when skin or clothing is wet and heat is lost through moisture into the environment

➤ Heat production occurs in the core, caused by thermoreceptor regulation from the hypothalamus.

➤ Normothermia is defined as a core temperature of 36.6° to 37.5°C or 98° to 99.5°F (Smeltzer & Bare, 2004).

➤ Heat loss and gain vary in individuals and are influenced by body surface area, peripheral vasomotor tone, and quantity of subcutaneous tissue.

➤ Shivering, the body's physiologic attempt to create more heat, produces profound physiologic responses:

Increased oxygen consumption to two to five times the normal rate

Increased metabolic demand to as much as 400% to 500%

Increased myocardial work, carbon dioxide production, cutaneous vasoconstriction, and eventual lactic acid production

➤ The reliability of temperature depends on accurate temperature-taking technique, minimization of variables affecting the temperature measurement device, and the site chosen for measurement.

➤ Oral temperature readings may be unreliable (from such variables as poor contact between the thermometer and mucosa, air movement, and smoking and drinking before temperature-taking); oral temperatures measure 0.5° below core temperature (Giuliano et al., 2000).

➤ Rectal temperature readings, which have fewer affecting variables and are more reliable than oral readings, measure 0.5°C above core temperature at normothermia, and at temperatures less than 36.5°C measure peripheral temperature rather than core temperature. Rectal temperatures measure 1° higher than oral temperature readings.

➤ Axillary temperature readings are reliable only for skin temperature; they measure 1° lower than oral temperature readings.

➤ The body responds to hot environments by increasing heat dissipation through increased sweat production and dilation of peripheral blood vessels.

➤ Blood is the body's cooling fluid: low blood volume from dehydration predisposes to a fever.

➤ The body responds to cold environments with mechanisms aimed at preventing heat loss and increasing heat production:
Muscle contraction
Increased heart rate
Shivering and vasodilatation
Peripheral vasoconstriction
Dilation of blood vessels in muscles
Release of thyroxine and corticosteroids

GENERIC CONSIDERATIONS

➤ Older adults can become hypothermic in moderately cold or hot environments, compared with younger adults, who require exposure to severe cold or hot temperatures (Miller, 2004).

➤ Age-related changes that interfere with the body's ability to adapt to cold temperature include inefficient vasoconstriction, decreased cardiac output, decreased subcutaneous tissue, and delayed and diminished sweating (Miller, 2004).

➤ Older adults have a higher threshold for onset and decreased efficiency of sweating.

➤ Older adults have a dulled perception of cold and warmth and thus may lack the stimulus to initiate protective actions.

➤ The thirst mechanism becomes less efficient with aging, as does the kidney's ability to concentrate urine, increasing the risk of heat-related dehydration.

➤ Inactivity and immobility increase susceptibility to hypothermia by suppressing shivering and reducing heat-generating muscle activity.

➤ Seventy percent of all victims of heat stroke are older than 60 years (Robbins, 1989).

FOCUS ASSESSMENT CRITERIA

Assess for risk factors

Hyperthermia

➤ Dehydration
➤ Recent exposure to communicable disease without known immunity (e.g., measles without vaccine or previous illness)
➤ Recent overexposure to sun, heat, humidity

➤ Recent overactivity
➤ Radiation/chemotherapy/immunosuppression
➤ Alcohol use
➤ Impaired judgment
➤ Home environment
  ➤ Adequate ventilation?
  ➤ Air conditioning?
  ➤ Room temperature?

Hypothermia

➤ Recent exposure to cold/dampness
➤ Inactivity
➤ Impaired judgment
➤ Home environment
  ➤ Inadequate Heating, blankets
  ➤ Insufficient clothing (e.g., socks, hat, gloves)
  ➤ Homeless

Problems that may contribute to hyperthermia or hypothermia

➤ Smoking
➤ Diabetes
➤ Repeated infections
➤ Circulatory problems
➤ Mobility problems
➤ Neurologic disorders
➤ History of frostbite
➤ Cardiovascular disorders/peripheral vascular disease

INTERVENTIONS

1. Assess for risk factors.

➤ Refer to Focus Assessment Criteria

2. Monitor as often as directed for:

➤ Changes in vital signs
➤ Abnormal heart rate, rhythm
➤ Temperature < 35.5°C (96°F) or >37.8°C (100°F)
➤ Decreased or increased respirations
➤ Change in mental status
➤ Cool or flushed skin
➤ Increased or decreased urine specific gravity

Rationale: Normal body temperature varies among individuals with a range
of 0.5 to 1.0°F. Early detection of increasing or decreasing temperature can

prevent serious problems as dehydration, rapid heart rate, and decreased urine output.

3. Maintain intake as prescribed. Refer to Deficient Fluid Volume if oral intake is insufficient.

Rationale: Unless fluid intake is restricted, the average oral liquid intake for an adult for a 24-hour period should be at least 1,300 ml (Metheny, 2000).

4. Monitor urine output and urine specific gravity. Maintain a urine specific gravity between 1.005 and 1.030. Maintain urine output of at least 30 ml/hour.

Rationale: Normal specific gravity and urine output indicates that there is sufficient circulation to the kidneys.

5. If shivering occurs, provide more blankets. When shivering stops, remove extra blankets.

Rationale: Shivering raises body heat. When temperature is normal, too many blankets cause heat loss from sweating.

6. If temperature is subnormal:
   ➤ Avoid exposing large skin areas
   ➤ Remove wet clothing
   ➤ Warm blankets
   ➤ Provide warm fluids

Rationale: Interventions are provided to prevent heat loss, trap body heat next to skin, and conduct heat to internal organs (Timby, 2001).

▾ Decreased Cardiac Output

Definition

Decreased Cardiac Output: A state in which the individual experiences a reduction in the amount of blood pumped by the heart, resulting in compromised cardiac function.

Defining Characteristics

Low blood pressure (O)
Rapid pulse (O)
Restlessness (O)

Cyanosis
Dyspnea
Angina
Dysrhythmia
Oliguria
Fatigability
Vertigo
Edema (peripheral, sacral)

This author does not recommend the use of this diagnosis as a nursing diagnosis. This nursing diagnosis represents a situation in which nurses have multiple responsibilities. People experiencing decreased cardiac output may display various responses that disrupt functioning (e.g., activity intolerance, disturbed sleep–rest cycle, anxiety, and fear). Or they may be at risk for developing such physiologic complications as dysrhythmias, cardiogenic shock, and congestive heart failure.

When Decreased Cardiac Output is used clinically, associated goals are usually written as follows:

Systolic blood pressure is >100   Cardiac output is >5
Urine output is >30 ml/hour   Cardiac rate, rhythm are normal

These goals do not represent criteria for evaluating nursing care but for evaluating the person's status. Because they are monitoring criteria that the nurse uses to guide implementation of nurse-prescribed and physician-prescribed interventions, Decreased Cardiac Output is not appropriate as a nursing diagnosis. Refer to the Cardiac Collaborative Problems for this specific cardiac problem.

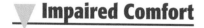 **Impaired Comfort**

Definition

Impaired Comfort: The state in which a person experiences an uncomfortable sensation in response to a noxious stimulus.

Defining Characteristics

MAJOR (MAY BE PRESENT)

The person reports or demonstrates discomfort (S,O); examples:

MINOR (MAY BE PRESENT)

Autonomic response in acute pain (O)
- ➤ Increased blood pressure
- ➤ Increased pulse
- ➤ Increased respirations
- ➤ Diaphoresis (sweating)
- ➤ Dilated pupils

Guarded position (O)
Facial mask of pain (O)
Crying, moaning (O)
Nausea (O)
Vomiting (O)
Fatigue (O)
Pruritus (S)

Related Factors

Any factor can contribute to impaired comfort. The most common are listed below.

BIOPATHOPHYSIOLOGIC

Related to tissue trauma and reflex muscle spasms secondary to the following:

Musculoskeletal disorders

- ➤ Fractures
- ➤ Contractures
- ➤ Spasms
- ➤ Arthritis
- ➤ Spinal cord disorders

Visceral disorders

- ➤ Cardiac
- ➤ Renal
- ➤ Hepatic
- ➤ Intestinal
- ➤ Pulmonary

Cancer
Vascular disorders

- ➤ Vasospasm
- ➤ Occlusion
- ➤ Phlebitis
- ➤ Cerebral vasodilatation

Related to inflammation of

Nerve
Tendon
Bursa
Joint
Muscle

Related to fatigue, malaise, or pruritus secondary to contagious diseases:

Rubella
Hepatitis
Pancreatitis
Chicken Pox
Mononucleosis

Related to effects of cancer on (specify)
Related to abdominal cramps, diarrhea, and vomiting secondary to

Gastroenteritis
Gastric ulcers
Influenza

TREATMENT-RELATED

Related to tissue trauma and reflex muscle spasms secondary to

Surgery
Burns
Accidents
Diagnostic tests (venipuncture, invasive scanning, biopsy)

SITUATIONAL (PERSONAL, ENVIRONMENTAL)

Related to fever
Related to immobility/improper positioning
Related to overactivity
Related to pressure points (tight cast, elastic bandages)
Related to allergic response
Related to chemical irritants
Related to unmet dependency needs
Related to severe repressed anxiety

A diagnosis not on the current NANDA list, Impaired Comfort can represent various uncomfortable sensations (e.g., pruritis, immobility, NPO status). For a person experiencing nausea and vomiting, the nurse should assess whether Nausea, Risk for Impaired Comfort or Risk for Imbalanced Nutrition: Less Than Body Requirements is

appropriate. Short-lived episodes of nausea, vomiting, or both (e.g., postoperatively) is best described with Nausea related to effects of anesthesia or analgesics. When nausea/vomiting may compromise nutritional intake, the appropriate diagnosis may be Risk for Imbalanced Nutrition: Less than Body Requirements related to nausea and vomiting secondary to (specify). Impaired Comfort also can be used to describe a cluster of discomforts related to a condition or treatment, such as radiation therapy.

Key Concepts

GENERIC CONSIDERATIONS

➤ Pruritis (itching) is the most common skin alteration. It can be a response to an allergen or a sign or symptom of a systemic disease, such as cancer, renal dysfunction, or diabetes.

➤ Pruritis, described as a tickling or tormenting sensation, originates exclusively in the skin and provokes the urge to scratch (Branov, Epstein & Grayson, 1989a).

➤ Although the same neurons are likely to transmit signals for itching as for pressure, pain, and touch, each sensation is perceived and mediated differently (Branov et al., 1989b).

➤ Pruritis arises from subepidermal nerve stimulation by proteolytic enzymes, which the epidermis releases as a result of either primary irritation or secondary allergic responses (Porth, 2002).

➤ The same unmyelinated nerves that act for burning pain also serve for pruritis. As a pruritic sensation increases in intensity, it may become burning (Porth, 2002).

➤ Areas that immediately surround body openings are most susceptible to itching. This apparently is related to a concentration of sensory nerve endings and vulnerability to external contamination (Porth, 2002).

GERIATRIC CONSIDERATIONS

Excessive dry skin is the most common cause of pruritis in older adults. Its incidence ranges from 40% to 80% as a result of varying criteria and climate differences. With scratching, small breaks in the epidermis can increase the risk of infection because of age-related changes in the immune system (Miller, 2004).

TRANSCULTURAL CONSIDERATIONS

➤ Pain is a universally recognized "private experience that is greatly influenced by cultural heritage" (Ludwig-Beymer, 1989, p. 283).

➤ US nurses are preponderantly white middle-class women socialized to believe "that in any situation self-control is better than open displays of strong feelings" (Ludwig-Beymer, 1989, p.294). Nurses should not stereotype members of a particular culture but instead should accept a wide range of pain expressions (Ludwig-Beymer, 1989).

➤ Families transmit to their children cultural norms related to pain (Ludwig-Beymer, 1989).

➤ Zborowski (1952), in his classic studies on the influence of culture on the pain experience, found that the pain event, its meaning, and responses are culturally learned and culturally specific. He reported the following cultural variations in interpretation and responses to pain:

Third-generation Americans: Unexpressive; concerned with implications; controlled emotional response

Jewish: Concerned about the implication of the pain; readily seek relief; frequently express pain to others

Irish: See pain as private; unexpressive; unemotional

Italian: Concerned with immediate pain relief; present-oriented

Japanese: Value self-control; will not express pain or ask for relief

Hispanic: Present-oriented; use folk medicine frequently; view suffering as a positive spiritual experience

Chinese: May ignore symptoms; use alternative health practices

Black Americans: May respond stoically because of dominant culture pressure or belief that pain is God's will

➤ Chinese women believe they will dishonor themselves and their family if they are loud during labor (Weber, 1996).

➤ Women from many South and Central American cultures believe the more intense the expression of pain during labor, the stronger the love toward the infant (Weber, 1996).

FOCUS ASSESSMENT CRITERIA

This nursing assessment of pain is designed to acquire data for assessing a person's adaptation to pain, not for determining the cause or existence of pain.

Subjective Data

Assess for the following:

Pain

➤ "Where is your discomfort located; does it radiate?" (Ask child to point to place)

➤ "When did it begin?"

➤ "Can you relate the cause of this discomfort?" or "What do you think has caused this discomfort?"
➤ "Describe the discomfort and its pattern."
  ➤ Time of day
  ➤ Duration
  ➤ Quality/Intensity
  ➤ Frequency (constant, intermittent, transient)
➤ Ask person to rate the pain: at its best, after pain-relief measures, and at its worst. Use consistent scale, language, or set of behaviors to assess pain.
➤ For adults, use an oral or visual analogue scale of 0 to 10 (0 = no pain, 10 = worst pain ever).
➤ "How do you usually react to pain (crying, anger, silence)?"
➤ "Are any other symptoms associated with your discomfort (nausea, vomiting, numbness)?"
➤ "What helps your pain? What makes it worse?"

Pruritis

➤ Onset
➤ Precipitated by what
➤ Site(s)
➤ Relieved by what
➤ History of allergy (individual, family)

Nausea/vomiting

➤ Onset/duration
➤ Vomitus (amount/appearance)
➤ Frequency/severity
➤ Relief measures

Assess for objective cues:

Behavioral manifestations

➤ *Mood*
  ➤ Calmness
  ➤ Moaning
  ➤ Crying
  ➤ Grimacing
  ➤ Pacing
  ➤ Restlessness
  ➤ Withdrawn

Musculoskeletal manifestations

➤ Mobility of painful part
➤ Full
➤ Limited/guarded
➤ No movement

➤ Muscle tone
➤ Tenderness
➤ Spasm
➤ Tenderness
➤ Tremors (in effort to hide pain)

Dermatologic manifestations

➤ Color (redness)
➤ Temperature
➤ Moisture/diaphoresis
➤ Edema

Cardiorespiratory manifestations

➤ *Cardiac*
　➤ Rate
　➤ Blood pressure
　➤ Palpitations present
➤ *Respiratory*
　➤ Rate
　➤ Rhythm
　➤ Depth

Sensory alterations

➤ Numbness
➤ Decreased sensation

For more information on Focus Assessment Criteria, visit http://connection.lww.com.

Chronic pain is a very complex experience. It affects all aspects of the person's life. As a beginning student, your focus should be on the present situation. You will focus on assessment and providing comfort measures; assessing how chronic pain affects a patient's life and assisting with adaptation are for a more experienced nurse.

GOAL

The client will report acceptable control of symptoms.

Indicators

Describe factors that increase symptoms.
Describe measures to improve comfort.

GENERAL INTERVENTIONS

    1. Assess for sources of discomfort.

➤ Pruritis
➤ Fever
➤ Nausea and vomiting
➤ Prolonged bed rest

    2. Reduce pruritis and promote comfort.

➤ Maintain hygiene without producing dry skin.
➤ Encourage frequent baths.
    ➤ Use cool water when acceptable.
    ➤ Use mild soap (Castile, lanolin) or a soap substitute.
    ➤ Blot skin dry; do not rub.
➤ Apply cornstarch lightly to skin folds by first sprinkling on hand (to avoid caking of powder); for fungal conditions, use antifungal or antiyeast powder preparations [Mycostatin (nystatin)], or miconazole cream.
    ➤ Massage pruritic scar tissue with cocoa butter daily (Field et al., 2000).
    ➤ Prevent excessive dryness.

Rationale: Massaging pruritic scars decreases itching, pain, and anxiety (Field et al., 2000).

➤ Lubricate skin with a moisturizer unless contraindicated; pat on with hand or gauze.
    ➤ Apply lubrication after bath, before skin is dry, to encourage moisture retention.
➤ Apply wet dressing continuously or intermittently to relieve itching and remove crusts and exudates.
➤ Provide 20- to 30-minute tub soaks of 32°F to 38°F; water can contain oatmeal powder, Aveeno, cornstarch, or baking soda (Branov et al., 1989b).

Rationale: Dryness increases skin sensitivity by stimulating nerve endings.

    ➤ Promote comfort and prevent further injury.
    ➤ Advise against itching; explain the scratch-itch-scratch cycle.
➤ Secure order for topical corticosteroid cream for local inflamed pruritic areas; apply sparingly and occlude area with plastic wrap at night to increase effectiveness of cream and prevent further scratching.
➤ Secure an antihistamine order if itching is unrelieved.
➤ Use mitts (or cotton socks), if necessary, on children and confused adults.
➤ Maintained trimmed nails to prevent injury; file after trimming.

➤ Remove particles from bed (food, crumbs, caked powder).

➤ Use old soft sheets and avoid wrinkles in bed; if bed protector pads are used, place draw sheet over them to eliminate direct contact with skin.

➤ Avoid using perfumes and scented lotions (Branov et al., 1989b).

➤ Avoid contact with chemical irritants/solutions.

➤ Wash clothes in mild detergent and put through a second rinse cycle to reduce residue; avoid use of fabric softeners (Branov et al., 1989b).

➤ Apply ointments with gloved or bare hand, depending on type, to lightly cover skin; rub creams into skin.

➤ Use frequent thin applications of ointment rather than one thick application.

Rationale: Excessive warmth or dryness, rough fabrics, fatigue, stress, and monotony (lack of distractions) aggravate pruritus (DeWitt, 1990; Thorns & Edmonds, 2000). Scratching stimulates histamine release, increasing pruritus.

3. Proceed with health teaching, when indicated.

➤ Explain causes of pruritus and possible prevention methods.

➤ Explain factors that increase symptoms (e.g., low humidity, heat).

➤ Explain interventions that relieve symptoms (e.g., fluid intake of 3,000 ml/day unless contraindicated).

➤ Advise about exposure to sun and heat and protective products.

➤ Teach person to avoid products that irritate skin (wool, coarse textures).

➤ Teach person to wear protective clothing (rubber gloves, apron) when using chemical irritants.

➤ Refer for allergy testing, if indicated.

➤ Provide opportunity to discuss frustrations.

Rationale: Excessive warmth or dryness, rough fabrics, fatigue, stress, and monotony (lack of distractions) aggravate pruritus (DeWitt, 1990; Thorns & Edmonds, 2000).

4. For excessive warmth, provide comfort measures as indicated.

➤ Keep the room cool; remove blankets as needed.

➤ Offer a cool washcloth for forehead; change frequently to maintain coolness.

➤ Provide tepid sponge baths or alcohol rubs; finish with powder to minimize moisture.

➤ Monitor bed linens (especially pillowcase) for dampness; change linens whenever moist.

➤ Encourage wearing absorbent cotton bedclothes rather that silk or nylon.

➤ Flip pillows and straighten linens frequently; assist with frequent repositioning.

➤ Provide for periods of uninterrupted rest.
➤ If requested, provide distractions (e.g., television, magazines, visitors).
➤ Consult with physician about the use of aspirin and acetaminophen on an alternating basis (aspirin q4h with acetaminophen q4h in between).

Rationale: Methods that interrupt pain also will interrupt pruritus. Examples include local anesthetics, cold, and peripheral nerve resection. Coolness reduces vasodilatation.

▼ Impaired Communication

Definition

Impaired Communication: The state in which a person experiences, or is at risk to experience, difficulty exchanging thoughts, ideas, wants, or needs with others.

Defining Characteristics

MAJOR (MUST BE PRESENT)

Inappropriate or absent speech or response (O)
Impaired ability to speak or hear (O)

MINOR (MAY BE PRESENT)

Incongruence between verbal and nonverbal messages (O)
Stuttering (O)
Slurring (O)
Word-finding problems (O)
Weak or absent voice (O)
Statements of being misunderstood or not understanding (S)
Dominant language not English (O)

Related Factors

PATHOPHYSIOLOGIC

Related to impaired motor function of muscles of speech

or

Related to ischemia of temporal frontal lobe secondary to the following:

Cerebrovascular accident
Oral or facial trauma
Brain damage (e.g., birth/head trauma)
CNS depression/increased intracranial pressure
Tumor (of the head, neck, or spinal cord)
Chronic hypoxia/decreased cerebral blood flow
Nervous system diseases (e.g., myasthenia gravis, multiple sclerosis, muscular dystrophy, Alzheimer's disease)
Vocal cord paralysis/quadriplegia

Related to impaired ability to produce speech secondary to

Respiratory impairment
Laryngeal deformities
Oral deformities

➤ Cleft lip or palate
➤ Malocclusion or fractured jaw
➤ Missing teeth
➤ Dysarthria

Related to auditory impairment

TREATMENT-RELATED

Related to impaired ability to produce speech secondary to

Endotracheal intubation
Surgery of the head, face, neck, or mouth
CNS depressants
Tracheostomy/tracheotomy/laryngectomy
Pain (especially of the mouth and throat)

SITUATIONAL (PERSONAL, ENVIRONMENTAL)

Related to decreased attention secondary to fatigue, anger, anxiety, or pain
Related to no access to or malfunction of hearing aid
Related to psychological barrier (e.g., fear, shyness)
Related to lack of privacy
Related to unavailable interpreter

MATURATIONAL

Older adult (auditory losses)
Related to hearing impairment
Related to cognitive impairments secondary to (specify)

> *Impaired communication may not be useful to describe communication problems that are a manifestation of psychiatric illness or coping problems. If nursing interventions focus on reducing hallucinations, fear, or anxiety, Disturbed Thought Processes, Fear, or Anxiety would be more appropriate.*

Key Concepts

GENERIC CONSIDERATIONS

➤ Effective communication is an interactive process involving the mutual exchange of information (thoughts, ideas, feelings, and perceptions) between two or more people. Problems with sending or receiving messages (or both) can hamper this process.

➤ Messages are sent more by body language and tone of voice than by words.

➤ After survival, perhaps the most basic human need is to communicate with others. Communication provides security by reinforcing that clients are not alone and others will listen. Poor communication can cause frustration, anger, hostility, depression, fear, confusion, and isolation.

➤ Speech represents the fundamental way for humans to express needs, desires, and feelings. If only one person expresses information without any feedback from a listener, effective communication cannot be said to have happened.

➤ Any of the following can cause problems with sending information:
  ➤ Inability or failure to send messages that the listener can clearly understand (e.g., language or word-meaning problems, failure to speak when listener is ready)
  ➤ Fear of being overheard, judged, or misunderstood (e.g., lack of privacy, confidentiality, trust, or nonjudgmental attitude)
  ➤ Concern over response (e.g., "I don't want to hurt or anger anyone.")
  ➤ Use of words that "talk down" to the receiver (e.g., talking to an elderly or handicapped person as if he or she were a child)
  ➤ Failure to allow sufficient time for listening or providing feedback
  ➤ Physical problems that interfere with the ability to see, talk, or move

➤ Any of the following can cause problems with receiving information:
  ➤ Language or vocabulary problems
  ➤ Fatigue, pain, fear, anxiety, distractions, attention span problems
  ➤ Not realizing the importance of the information
  ➤ Problems that interfere with the ability to see or hear

➤ Good communicators are also good listeners, who listen for both facts and feelings

➤ "Presencing" or just being present and available, even if one says or does little, can effectively communicate caring to another (Benner, 1984).

➤ Knowledge of a foreign language depends on four elements: how to speak, understand, read, and write the language.

➤ Dysarthria is a disturbance in the voluntary muscular control of speech. It is caused by conditions such as Parkinson's disease, multiple sclerosis, myasthenia gravis, cerebral palsy, and CNS damage. The same muscles are used in eating and swallowing. People with dysarthria usually do not have problems with comprehension.

➤ Expressive aphasia is a disturbance in the ability to speak, write, or gesture understandably.

➤ Receptive aphasia is a disturbance in the ability to comprehend written and spoken language. Those with receptive aphasia may have intact hearing but cannot process or are unaware of their own sounds.

➤ Emotional lability (swings between crying and laughing) is common in people with aphasia. This behavior is not intentional and declines with recovery.

➤ Ten percent of deaf people have the skill and language level to read lips. Only 40% of the English language is visible (Shelp, 1997).

➤ Successful interaction with deaf or hearing-impaired clients requires knowing background issues, including age of onset, choice of language, cultural background, education level, and type of hearing loss (Group for the Advancement of Psychiatry, 1997).

GERIATRIC CONSIDERATIONS

➤ Hearing loss is the third most prevalent condition affecting institutionalized older adults, exceeded only by arthritis and hypertension (Lindblade & McDonald, 1995). Only 18% of older adults with hearing loss own hearing aids. Many deny hearing loss because of fear of pressure to buy a hearing aid.

➤ About 40% of people older than 65 years have a significant hearing impairment that interferes with communication.

➤ Reduced auditory acuity correlates positively with social isolation. Understanding speech in group conversation has been identified as a prime area of difficulty for older adults. Some withdraw from social gatherings because they feel frustrated asking people to repeat things. Friends and family may refrain from entertaining hearing-impaired people because they misperceive their turning their heads away during conversation of failure to participate as disinterest. They may also misperceive hearing impairments as mental impairments because of inappropriate comments during conversation, irritability, and inattention.

➤ Older adults have a high prevalence of chronic conditions that can interfere with speech or understanding of speech.

TRANSCULTURAL CONSIDERATIONS

➤ The dominant US culture tends to conceal feelings and is considered low touch (Giger & Davidhizar, 2004). Difficulties can occur if the person or family does not communicate in a way that the nurse expects.

➤ In some cultures, a nod is a polite response meaning, "I heard you, but I do not necessarily understand or agree" (Giger & Davidhizar, 2004).

➤ Touch is a strong form of communication with many meanings and interpretations.

➤ Cultural uses of touch vary, with touch between same-sex people as taboo in some cultures but expected in others (Giger & Davidhizar, 2004).
  ➤ English and German cultures do not encourage touching.
  ➤ Some highly tactile cultures are Spanish, Italian, French, Jewish, and South American.
  ➤ All cultures have rules about who touches whom, when, and where.

➤ The dominant US culture views eye contact as an indication of a positive self-concept, openness, and honesty. It views lack of eye contact as low self-esteem, guilt, or lack of interest. Some cultures are not accustomed to eye contact, including Filipino, Native American, and Vietnamese (Giger & Davidhizar, 2004).

➤ The client and family should be encouraged to communicate their interpretations of health, illness, and health care (Giger & Davidhizar, 2004) within the context of their specific culture.

➤ African Americans speak English with varied geographic dialects. Some African Americans pronounce certain syllables or consonants differently (e.g., they may pronounce *th* as *d*, as in "des" for "these"). These different pronunciations should not be viewed as substandard or ungrammatical. In addition, some slang words may have different meanings, for example, "the birth of my daughter was a real bad experience." The person may mean it was unique and positive (Dillard, 1973).

➤ Mexican Americans speak Spanish, which has more than 50 dialects; thus, a nurse who speaks Spanish may have difficulty understanding a different dialect. Both men and women are very modest and restrict self-disclosure to those whom they know well. They consider direct confrontation and arguments rude; thus, agreeing may be a courtesy, not a commitment. A folk illness called *malojo* (evil eye) is thought to harm a child when the child is admired, but not touched, by a person thought to have special powers. When interacting with children, touch them lightly to avoid *malojo*. These clients may view kidding as rude and deprecating (Murillo, 1978).

➤ Chinese Americans value silence and avoid disagreeing or criticizing. Whereas many Americans of other cultural backgrounds naturally raise their voice to make a point, Chinese Americans associate raising the voice with anger and loss of control. They rarely use "no" and "yes" can mean "perhaps" or "no." Touching the head is a serious breach of etiquette. Hesitation, ambiguity, and subtlety dominate Chinese speech (Giger & Davidhizar, 2004).

FOCUS ASSESSMENT CRITERIA

Assess for subjective (S) and objective (O) data:

Note the usual pattern of communication as described by the person or family (O)

➤ Very verbal
➤ Sometimes verbal
➤ Uses sign language
➤ Writes only
➤ Responds inappropriately
➤ Does not speak/respond
➤ Speaks only when spoken to
➤ Gestures only

Does the person feel he or she is communicating normally today? (S)
If not, what does the client feel may help him or her to communicate better? (S)
Does the client have trouble hearing? (S)

➤ Hearing problem
➤ Both ears or one
➤ How long? Gradual? Sudden?
➤ Use of hearing aid
➤ Family history of hearing loss
➤ History of exposure to loud noises

Describe ability to form words (O)

➤ Not able
➤ Fair
➤ Good

Speech pattern (O)

➤ Slurred speech
➤ Lisping
➤ Stuttering
➤ Voice weakness (whisper)
➤ Language barrier

Ability to comprehend (O)

➤ Follows simple commands or ideas
➤ Can follow complex instructions or ideas
➤ Sometimes can follow instructions or ideas
➤ Follows commands and ideas only if hearing aid is working

Follows commands and ideas only if he or she can see speaker's mouth
  (reads lips)
Is eye contact maintained? (O)

➤ Yes
➤ No
➤ Occasionally
➤ Rarely
➤ Blind/Impaired vision

GOALS

The person will report improved satisfaction with ability to communicate.

Indicators

Demonstrate increased ability to understand.
Demonstrate improved ability to express self.
Use alternative methods of communication, as indicated.

GENERAL INTERVENTIONS

1. Use factors that promote hearing and understanding.

➤ Talk distinctly and clearly, facing the person.
➤ Minimize unnecessary sounds in the room.
  ➤ Have only one person talk.
➤ Be aware of background noises (e.g., close the door, turn off the television or radio)
➤ Repeat, and then rephrase, a thought if the person does not seem to understand the whole meaning.
➤ Use touch and gestures to enhance communication.
➤ If the person can understand only sign language, have an interpreter present as often as possible.
➤ If the person is in a group (e.g., diabetes class), place him or her in front of the room near the teacher.
➤ Approach the person from the side on which hearing is best (i.e., if hearing is better with the left ear, approach the person from the left).

> ➤ If the person can read lips, look directly at the person and talk slowly and clearly.
> ➤ Assess functioning of hearing aids (e.g., batteries).

Rationale: Many older adults with hearing impairments don't wear hearing aids. Those who wear them must be encouraged to use them consistently, clean and maintain them, and replace batteries. They should be assertive in letting significant others know about situations and environmental areas in which they experience difficulty because of background noise.

2. Provide alternative methods of communication.

> ➤ Use pad and pencil, alphabet letters, hand signals, eye blinks, head nods, and bell signals.
> ➤ Make flash cards with words or pictures depicting frequently used phrases (e.g., "Wet my lips," "Move my foot," glass of water, bedpan).
> ➤ Encourage the person to point and to use gestures and to pantomime.

Rationale: Using alternative forms of communication can help decrease anxiety, isolation, and alienation; promote a sense of control; and enhance safety.

3. Provide an atmosphere of acceptance and privacy.

> ➤ Do not rush.
> ➤ Speak slowly and in normal tone.
>> ➤ Decrease external noise and distractions.
>> ➤ Encourage client to share frustrations; validate client's nonverbal expressions.
> ➤ Provide client with opportunities to make decisions about his care when appropriate.
> ➤ Do not force client to communicate.
> ➤ If client laughs or cries uncontrollably, change subject or activity.

Rationale: Communication is the core of all human relations. Impaired ability to communicate spontaneously is frustrating and embarrassing. Nursing actions should focus on decreasing the tension and conveying an understanding of how difficult the situation must be for the client.

4. Make every effort to understand the client's communication efforts.

> ➤ Listen attentively.
> ➤ Repeat client's message back to him or her to ensure understanding.
> ➤ Ignore inappropriate word usage; do not correct mistakes.
> ➤ Do not pretend you understand; if you do not, ask client to repeat.
> ➤ Try to anticipate some needs (e.g., Do you need something to drink?).

Rationale: Nurse should make every attempt to understand the client. Each success, regardless of how minor, decreases frustration and increases motivation.

5. Teach the client techniques to improve speech.

➤ Instruct client to speak slowly and in short phrases.
➤ Initially ask questions that the client can answer with a "yes" or "no."
➤ With improvement, allow person to complete some phrases, e.g., "This is a _____."
➤ As the client is able, encourage her or him to share feelings and concerns.

Rationale: Deliberate actions can be taken to improve speech. As the client's speech improves, her or his confidence will increase and she or he will make more attempts at speaking.

6. Use strategies to improve the client's comprehension.

➤ Gain the client's attention before speaking; call client by name.
➤ Practice consistent speech patterns:
  ➤ Speak slowly.
  ➤ Use common words and use the same words consistently for a task.
  ➤ Repeat or rephrase when indicated.
➤ Use touch and behavior to communicate calmness.
➤ Add other nonverbal methods of communication.
  ➤ Point or use flash cards for basic needs.
  ➤ Use pantomime.
  ➤ Use paper/pen or spelling board.
  ➤ Display the most effective methods at the client's bedside.

▼ Impaired Verbal Communication

Definition

Impaired Verbal Communication: The state in which a person experiences, or is at high risk to experience, a decreased ability to speak but can understand others.

Defining Characteristics

MAJOR (ONE MUST BE PRESENT)

Inability to speak words but can understand others (O)
Articulation or motor planning deficits (O)

MINOR (MAY BE PRESENT)

Shortness of breath (O)

Related Factors

See *Impaired Communication.*

Key Concepts

See *Impaired Communication.*

FOCUS ASSESSMENT CRITERIA

See *Impaired Communication.*

GOAL

The person will demonstrate improved ability to express self.

Indicators

Relates decreased frustration with communication.
Uses alternative methods as indicated.

GENERAL INTERVENTIONS

1. Identify a method for communicating basic needs.

See *Impaired Communication.*

2. Identify factors that promote communication.

For clients with dysarthria:

➤ Reduce environmental noise (e.g., radio, television) to increase caregiver's ability to listen to words.
➤ Do not alter your speech or messages, because the client's comprehension is not affected; speak on an adult level.
➤ Encourage client to make a conscious effort to slow down speech and to speak louder (e.g., "Take a deep breath between sentences.").
➤ Ask client to repeat unclear words; observe for nonverbal cues to help understanding.
  ➤ If client is tired, ask questions that require only short answers.
➤ If speech is unintelligible, teach use of gestures, written messages, and communication cards.

3. Promote continuity of care to reduce frustration.

Observe for signs of frustration or withdrawal.

- ➤ Verbally address frustration over inability to communicate, and explain that both nurse and client must use patience.
- ➤ Maintain a calm positive attitude ("I can understand you if we work at it.").
- ➤ Use reassurance (e.g., "I know it's difficult, but I know you'll get it.").
- ➤ Maintain a sense of humor.
- ➤ Allow tears (e.g., "It's okay. I know it's frustrating. Crying can let it all out.").
- ➤ For the client with limited speaking ability (e.g., can make simple requests but not lengthy statements), encourage letter writing or keeping a diary to express feelings and share concerns.
- ➤ Anticipate needs and ask questions that need a simple yes or no.
- ➤ Maintain a specific care plan.
  - ➤ Write a method of communication that is used (e.g., "Uses word cards," "Points for bedpan").
  - ➤ Record directions for specific measures to reduce communication problems (e.g., allow him to keep urinal in bed).

Rationale: Language involves comprehension and transmission of ideas and feelings. Speech is the mechanics and articulations of verbal expression.

4. Initiate health teaching and referrals, as indicated.

- ➤ Teach communication techniques and repetitive approaches to significant others.
- ➤ Encourage family to share feelings concerning communication problems.
- ➤ Seek consultation with a speech pathologist early in treatment regimen.

Rationale: Assistance may be needed after discharge.

▼ Confusion

Definition

Confusion: The state in which a person experiences or is at risk of experiencing a disturbance in cognition, attention, memory, and orientation, of an undetermined origin or onset

Defining Characteristics

Assess for subjective (S) and objective (O) cues:

MAJOR (MUST BE PRESENT)

Disturbances of

Consciousness (O)
Attention (O)
Perception (S)
Sleep–wake cycle (O)
Memory (S)
Orientation (O)
Thinking (S)
Psychomotor behavior (reaction time, speed of movement, flow of speech, involuntary movements, handwriting) (O)

MINOR (MAY BE PRESENT)

Misperceptions (S)
Hypervigilance (S)
Agitation (O)

"The terms delirium and confusion are not interchangeable" (Anderson, 1999, p. 497). Confusion is a symptom of irreversible organic mental disorder; delirium is acute confusion of short duration and reversible when the underlying cause is treated (Anderson, 1999; Foreman et al., 1999). Refer to Key Concepts for descriptions of chronic confusion and acute confusion (delirium).

▼ Acute Confusion

Definition

Acute Confusion: The state in which there is an abrupt onset of a cluster of global, fluctuating disturbances in consciousness, attention, perception, memory, orientation, thinking, sleep-wake cycle, and psychomotor behavior (American Psychiatric Association, 2000).

Defining Characteristics

Assess for subjective (S) and objective (O) cues:

MAJOR (SOME MUST BE PRESENT)

Abrupt onset of

Reduced ability to focus (O)
Disorientation (O)

Incoherence (O)
Anxiety (O)
Hypervigilance (O)
Restlessness (O)
Fear (S)
Excitement (O)

Symptoms worse at nights or when fatigued

MINOR (MAY BE PRESENT)

Illusions (S)
Delusions (S)
Hallucinations (S)
Misperception of stimuli (S)

Risk Factors

Presence of risk factors (see Related Factors)

Related Factors

Related to abrupt onset of cerebral hypoxia or disturbance in cerebral metabolism secondary to the following (Miller, 2004):

Fluid and electrolyte disturbances

➤ Volume depletion
➤ Acidosis/alkalosis
➤ Hypocalcemia
➤ Hypokalemia
➤ Hyponatremia/hypernatremia
➤ Hypoglycemia/hyperglycemia

Nutritional deficiencies

➤ Folate or vitamin B12 deficiency
➤ Anemia
➤ Niacin deficiency
➤ Magnesium deficiency

Cardiovascular deficiencies

➤ Myocardial infarction
➤ Congestive heart failure

➤ Heart block
➤ Dysrhythmias
➤ Temporal arteritis

Respiratory disorders

➤ Chronic obstructive pulmonary disease (COPD)
➤ Pulmonary embolism
➤ Tuberculosis
➤ Pneumonia

Infections

➤ Sepsis
➤ Meningitis, encephalitis
➤ Urinary tract infection

Metabolic and endocrine disorders

➤ Hypothyroidism/hyperthyroidism
➤ Hypopituitarism/hyperpituitarism
➤ Parathyroid disorders
➤ Hypoadrenocorticism/hyperadrenocorticism
➤ Postural hypotension
➤ Hypothermia/hyperthermia
➤ Hepatic or renal failure

Central nervous system (CNS) disorders

➤ Multiple infarctions (strokes)
➤ Tumors
➤ Normal-pressure hydrocephalus
➤ Head trauma
➤ Seizures and postconvulsive states

TREATMENT-RELATED

Related to disturbance in cerebral metabolism secondary to the following:

Surgery
Therapeutic drug intoxication

➤ Narcotics
➤ Neuroleptics

General anesthesia
Side effects of medication (examples)

➤ Diuretics
➤ Digitalis
➤ Propranolol

- Atropine
- Oral hypoglycemics
- Antiinflammatories
- Antianxiety agents
- Phenothiazines
- Barbiturates
- Methyldopa
- Disulfiram
- Lithium
- Phenytoin
- Over-the-counter cough, cold, and sleeping preparations
- Sulfa drugs
- Ciprofloxin
- Metronidazole
- Acyclovir
- H2 receptor antagonists
- Anticholinergics

SITUATIONAL (PERSONAL, ENVIRONMENTAL)

Related to disturbance in cerebral metabolism secondary to the following:

Withdrawal from alcohol, sedatives, hypnotics
Heavy metal or carbon monoxide intoxication

Related to

Pain
Bowel impaction
Immobility
Depression

Related to chemical intoxications or substance abuse (specify):

Alcohol
Cocaine
Amphetamines
Opiates
Barbiturates
Hallucinogens

Carp's Cue ▶ *The addition of Acute Confusion and Chronic Confusion to the North American Nursing Diagnosis Association (NANDA) list provides the nurse with more diagnostic clarity than Disturbed Thought Process. Acute Confusion has an abrupt onset with fluctuating symptoms; Chronic Confusion describes long-standing or progressive degeneration. Disturbed Thought Processes is also a disruption of cognitive processes; however, the causes are coping problems or personality disorders.*

Key Concepts

GENERIC CONSIDERATIONS

➤ "Confusion" is a term nurses use frequently to describe an array of cognitive impairments. "Identifying a person as confused is just an initial step" (Roberts, 2001). Confusion is a biopsychological concept that indicates a disturbance in cerebral metabolism. Reduced cerebral metabolism decreases neurotransmitter levels in the brain, especially acetylcholine and epinephrine. Acetylcholine is necessary for attention, learning, memory, and information processing (Roberts, 2001).

➤ "The terms delirium and confusion are not interchangeable" (Anderson, 1999, p. 497). Confusion is a symptom of irreversible organic mental disorder; delirium is acute confusion of short duration and reversible when the underlying cause is treated (Anderson, 1999; Foreman et al., 1999).

➤ Acute confusion or delirium results from transient biochemical disruptions caused by medications, infections, dehydration, electrolyte imbalances, and metabolic disturbances (Foreman et al., 1999). It usually lasts less than 5 days when the underlying causes are treated. Early detection and treatment can prevent unnecessarily long hospital stays (Foreman et al., 1999).

➤ Clinical manifestations associated with depression, dementia, and delirium (Dellasega, 1998):

Depression

➤ Sudden or gradual onset
➤ Sleep difficulties
➤ Slowed motor behavior
➤ Sadness, loss of interest and pleasure
➤ Memory intact

Dementia

➤ Gradual insidious onset
➤ May sleep less; restlessness
➤ Wandering behavior
➤ Defensiveness
➤ Gradual loss of ability to remember

Delirium

➤ Sudden acute onset
➤ Behavior worsens at night
➤ Hypo/hyperarousal
➤ Hallucinations and illusions in attention
➤ Fluctuating performance

GERIATRIC CONSIDERATIONS

➤ Moderate to severe cognitive impairment in older adults can result from dementia, delirium, or depression. Nurses must approach their assessment carefully and cautiously; they should not base diagnosis on a single symptom or physical finding (Dellasega, 1998).

➤ Thinking and arithmetic abilities, memory, judgment, and problem solving are measured in older adults to give a general index of overall cognitive ability.

➤ With age, intelligence does not alter (perhaps until the very later years), but the person needs more time to process information. Reaction time is slowed. There may be some difficulty in learning new information because of increased distractibility, decreased concrete thinking, and difficulty solving new problems. Older adults usually compensate for these deficiencies by taking more time to process the information, screening out distractions, and using extreme care in making decisions (Miller, 2004).

➤ Most older adults exhibit no cognitive impairment. Severe cognitive impairment, a consequence of disease process, occurs only in 1% of people older than 65 years and 20% of people older than 85 years (Miller, 2004).

➤ Age-related changes can influence medication actions and produce negative consequences.

➤ Dementia describes impairments of intellectual, not behavioral, functioning. It refers to a group of symptoms, not a disease (Miller, 2004). Alzheimer's disease, the fourth leading cause of death in older adults, is one type of dementia.

➤ Blazer (1986) describes a multiple causation theory for late-life depression, which emphasizes the complex interactions of several etiologic factors. Examples identified include poor economic resources, decreased social support, and decreased physical health functioning.

➤ Suicide is always a possibility, especially in the early stage of dementia, for numerous reasons: depression, loss of self-worth, and impaired judgment.

FOCUS ASSESSMENT CRITERIA

Acquire data from client and significant others.

Subjective Data

History of the Individual
Lifestyle

➤ Interests
➤ Past and present coping
➤ Previous functioning
➤ Strengths and limitations
➤ Education
➤ Previous handling of stress
➤ Work history
➤ Use of alcohol/drugs

Support system (availability)

➤ History of medical problems and treatments (medications)
➤ Activities of daily living (ADLs; ability and desire to perform)

History of symptoms (onset and duration)

➤ Downward progression
➤ Time of day
➤ Continuous or intermittent
➤ Sudden or gradual

Assess for feelings of

➤ Extreme sadness
➤ Guilt for past actions
➤ Being rejected or isolated
➤ Worthlessness
➤ Others controlling client
➤ Excessive self-importance
➤ Mistrust or suspicion
➤ Apprehension
➤ Living in an unreal world

Assess for any hallucinations

➤ Visual
➤ Olfactory
➤ Auditory
➤ Tactile (includes objective component)
➤ Gustatory

Objective Data (Includes a Subjective Component)

General appearance

➤ Facial expression (alert, sad, hostile, expressionless)
➤ Dress (meticulous, disheveled, seductive, eccentric)

Behavior during interview

➤ Withdrawn
➤ Attentive

➤ Cooperative
➤ Anxious
➤ Apathetic
➤ Negativism
➤ Hostile
➤ Quiet
➤ Agitated

Communication pattern

➤ Appropriate
➤ Sexual preoccupations
➤ Denying problem
➤ Delusions
➤ Obsessions
➤ Suspicious
➤ Suicidal ideas
➤ Rambling
➤ Homicidal plans
➤ Worthlessness

Speech pattern

➤ Appropriate
➤ Topic jumping
➤ Loose connections
➤ Blocking (cannot finish idea)
➤ Cannot reach a conclusion

Rate of Speech

➤ Appropriate
➤ Slowed
➤ Rapid

Affect

➤ Appropriate of content
➤ Sad
➤ Flat
➤ Bright
➤ Inappropriate of content

Interaction skills
(With nurse)

➤ Inappropriate
➤ Hostile
➤ Demanding/pleading

➤ Withdrawn/preoccupied
➤ Relates well

(With significant others)

➤ Relates with all (some) family members
➤ Hostile toward one (all) member(s)
➤ Does not seek interaction
➤ Does not have visitors
➤ Does not recognize family

ADLs

➤ Capable of self-care (observed, reported)

Nutrition–hydration status

➤ Appetite
➤ Weight
➤ Eating patterns

Sleep–rest pattern

➤ Sleeps too much or too little
➤ Insomnia
➤ Early wakefulness
➤ Cycle reversed
➤ Fragmented sleep

Personal hygiene

➤ Cleanliness
➤ Clothes
➤ Grooming

Motor activity

➤ Within normal limits
➤ Increased
➤ Decreased/stuporous

GOAL

The person will have diminished episodes of delirium.

Indicators

Be less agitated
Participate in ADLs
Be less combative

GENERAL INTERVENTIONS

1. Assess for causative and contributing factors.

Ensure that a thorough diagnostic workup has been completed.

Laboratory

➤ Complete blood count (CBC) and electrolytes
➤ Vitamin B12 and folate, thiamine
➤ RPR
➤ Na and K
➤ AST, ALT, and bilirubin
➤ Urinalysis
➤ Thyroid-stimulating hormone, +4
➤ Serum thyroxine and serum-free thyroxine
➤ Calcium and phosphate
➤ Creatinine, blood urea nitrogen
➤ Serum glucose and fasting blood sugar
➤ Alcohol and drug levels
➤ Electroencephalogram

Diagnostic

➤ Computed tomography
➤ Electrocardiogram
➤ Chest x-ray
➤ Spinal tap

Psychiatric evaluation

➤ Evaluate for depression

Rationale: Differentiating between acute (reversible) and chronic (irreversible) confusion is important (Stolley & Buckwalter, 1992).

2. Promote client's sense of integrity.

➤ Examine attitudes about confusion (in self, caregivers, and significant others)
  ➤ Educate family, significant others, and caregivers about the situation and coping methods.
➤ Maintain standards of empathic respectful care.
  ➤ Be an advocate when other caregivers are insensitive to the client's needs
  ➤ Function as a role model with coworkers
  ➤ Provide other caregivers with up-to-date information on confusion
➤ Attempt to obtain information that provides useful and meaningful topics for conversation (likes, dislikes, interests, hobbies, work history). Interview early in the day.

➤ Encourage significant others and caregivers to speak slowly with a low voice pitch and at an average volume (unless hearing deficits are present), as one adult to another, with eye contact, and as if expecting person to understand.

➤ Provide and promote sharing.

➤ Reduce abrupt changes in schedule or relocation.

Rationale: Unconditional positive regard communicates acceptance and affection to a person who has difficulty interpreting the environment. Careful listening is critical to evaluate responses to prevent escalation of anxiety and to detect physiologic discomforts (Miller, 2004).

3. Provide sufficient and meaningful sensory input.

➤ Keep person oriented to time and place.

- ➤ Refer to time of day and place each morning
- ➤ Provide person with a clock and calendar large enough to see
- ➤ Use night lights or dim lights at night
- ➤ Use indirect lighting
- ➤ Single out holidays with cards or pins (e.g., wear a red heart for Valentine's Day)

➤ Use adaptive devices to diminish sensory impediments

➤ Encourage family to bring in familiar objects from home

➤ Discuss current events, seasonal events (snow, water activities); share your interests (travel, crafts)

➤ Assess if person can perform activity with his hands (e.g., latch rugs, wood crafts)

➤ In teaching a task or activity (e.g., eating), break it into small brief steps by giving only one instruction at a time

- ➤ Remove covers from plate and cups
- ➤ Cut foods
- ➤ Add sugar and milk to coffee
- ➤ Proceed with eating

➤ Explain all activities

Rationale: Sensory input is carefully planned to reduce excess stimuli, which increase confusion (Miller, 2004). People with dementia can be assisted to maximize their function level by reducing or eliminating certain factors. These factors include the following:

➤ Fatigue

➤ Change in routine, environment, caregiver

➤ Frustration from trying to function beyond capabilities or from being restrained

➤ Pain, discomfort, illness, or side effects from drugs

4. Increase person's self-esteem.

➤ Allow former habits (e.g., reading in the bathroom)
➤ Encourage the wearing of dentures
➤ Ask family to provide spending money
➤ Ask family members usual grooming routine and encourage it
➤ Provide for personal hygiene according to person's preferences (hair grooming, showers or baths, nail care, cosmetics, deodorants and fragrances)

Rationale: Unconditional positive regard communicates acceptance and affection to a person who has difficulty interpreting the environment.

5. Promote a well role.

➤ Discourage the use of nightclothes during the day. Have person wear shoes, not slippers.
➤ Promote mobility as much as possible.
➤ Have person eat meals out of bed
➤ Promote socialization during meals (set up lunch for four individuals in lounge)
➤ Schedule one or two rest periods daily.
➤ Plan an activity to look forward to

Rationale: Structured rest periods prevent fatigue and allow for lower stress periods.

6. Do not endorse confusion.

➤ Do not argue with person
➤ Never agree with confused statements
➤ Adhere to the schedule; if changes are necessary, advise person of them
➤ Provide simple explanations that cannot be misinterpreted
➤ Avoid opened-ended questions
➤ Replace five- or six-step tasks with two- or three-step tasks.

Rationale: Careful listening is critical to evaluate responses to prevent escalation of anxiety and to detect physiologic discomfort (Miller, 2004). Memory loss and intellectual functioning create a need for consistency.

7. Prevent injury to the individual.

➤ Discourage the use of restraints; explore other alternatives
➤ Refer to Risk for Injury for strategies for assessing and manipulating the environment for hazards.
➤ Register with an emergency medical system, including "wanderers list" with local police department.

Rationale: Restraints are a violation of a person's rights and increase anxiety. All attempts to protect the person should be used before selecting restraints. Restrained elderly have increased levels of confusion, especially at night (Rateau, 2000).

8. Assist family with effective coping (Young, 2001).

➤ Explain cause of confusion
➤ Explain person does not understand the situation
➤ Explain the need to remain patient
➤ Stress to respond to person as an adult
➤ Explain behavior is part of disorder and is not voluntary

▼ Chronic Confusion

Definition

Chronic Confusion: A state in which a person experiences an irreversible, long-standing, and/or progressive deterioration of intellect and personality.

Defining Characteristics

Assess for subjective (S) and objective (O) cues:

Cognitive or intellectual losses (S/O)

➤ Loss of memory
➤ Loss of time sense
➤ Inability to make choices, decisions

Inability to solve problems, reason (S)

➤ Poor judgment (S)

Affective or personality losses (O)

➤ Loss of affect
➤ Diminished inhibition
➤ Loss of tact, control of temper
➤ Loss of recognition (others, environment)
➤ Loss of general ability to plan
➤ Increasing self-preoccupation
➤ Antisocial behavior

Progressively lowered stress threshold

➤ Purposeful wandering
➤ Violent, agitated, or anxious behavior
➤ Purposeless behavior
➤ Compulsive repetitive behavior

Related Factors

PHYSIOLOGIC

Related to progressive degeneration of the cerebral cortex secondary to

➤ Alzheimer's disease
➤ Combination
➤ Multiinfarct disease

Related to disturbance in cerebral metabolism, structure, or integrity secondary to

➤ Pick's disease
➤ Toxic substance injection
➤ Brain tumors
➤ End-stage diseases
➤ Creutzfeldt-Jakob disease
➤ Degenerative neurologic disease
➤ Huntington's chorea
➤ Psychiatric disorders

Errors in Diagnostic Considerations
Refer to *Acute Confusion*

Key Concepts

➤ See *Acute Confusion*
➤ Progressive dementing illnesses have four clusters of symptoms (Hall, 1988, 1994):

Intellectual Losses

➤ Loss of memory
➤ Inability to make choices
➤ Loss of sense of time
➤ Inability to solve problems and reason
➤ Altered ability to identify visual or auditory stimuli
➤ Loss of receptive or expressive language

Affective Personality Losses

➤ Loss of affect
➤ Decreased attention span
➤ Decreased inhibitions
➤ Emotional lability
➤ Loss of tact
➤ Increased self-preoccupation

Cognitive or Planning Losses

➤ Loss of ability to plan
➤ Loss of instrumental functions
➤ Functional losses
➤ Loss of energy reserves
➤ Motor apraxia

Progressively Lowered Stress Threshold

➤ Confused or agitated night awakening
➤ Purposeful wandering
➤ Violent, agitated, anxious behavior
➤ Compulsive repetitive behavior

➤ Both depression and dementia cause cognitive impairments. Differentiating the underlying cause is critical, because depression is treatable (Miller, 2004).

FOCUS ASSESSMENT CRITERIA

Refer to *Acute Confusion.*

GOAL

The person will participate to maximum level of independence in a therapeutic milieu.

Indicators

Decreased frustration
Diminished episodes of combativeness
Decreased use of restraints
Increased hours of sleep at night
Stabilized or increased weight

GENERAL INTERVENTIONS

1. Refer to interventions under *Acute Confusion.* Assess who the person was before the onset of confusion.

➤ Educational level, career
➤ Coping styles
➤ Hobbies, lifestyle

2. Observe client to determine baseline behaviors (Hall, 1994).

- ➤ Best time of day
- ➤ Amount of distraction tolerated
- ➤ Insight into disability
- ➤ Routine
- ➤ Response time to a simple question
- ➤ Judgment
- ➤ Signs/symptoms of depression

Rationale: Assessing the client's personal history can provide insight into current behavior patterns and communicates the nurse's interest (Hall, 1994). Specific personal data can improve individualization of care (Hall, 1994). Baseline behavior can be used to develop a plan for activities and daily care routines (Hall, 1994).

3. Promote client's sense of integrity (Miller, 2004).

- ➤ Adapt communication to client's level
- ➤ Use positive statements
- ➤ Unless a safety issue is involved, do not argue
- ➤ Avoid questions you know the client cannot answer
- ➤ If possible, demonstrate to reinforce verbal communication
- ➤ Use touch to gain attention or show concern unless a negative response is elicited
- ➤ Maintain good eye contact and pleasant facial expressions

Rationale: Dysfunctional episodes are manifestations of fear; the goals of management are to prevent injury, provide a sense of serenity, and promote self-mastery (Hall, 1994). This demonstrates unconditional positive regard and communicates acceptance and affection to a person who has difficulty interpreting the environment.

4. Promote the client's safety.

- ➤ Ensure that client carries identification
- ➤ Adapt the environment so the client can pace or walk if desired
- ➤ Keep the environment uncluttered
- ➤ Keep medications, cleaning solutions, and other toxic chemicals in inaccessible places.
- ➤ Reduce abrupt locations

Rationale: Sensory input is carefully planned to reduce excess stimuli that increase confusion.

5. Discourage use of restraints; explore other alternatives (Quinn, 1994).

- ➤ If client's behavior disrupts treatment (e.g., nasogastric tube, urinary catheter, IV line), reevaluate whether treatment is appropriate.

Intravenous Therapy

➤ Camouflage tubing with loose gauze
➤ Consider an intermittent access device instead of a continuous IV therapy
➤ Use the less restrictive device

Urinary Catheters

➤ Evaluate causes of incontinence
➤ Institute specific treatment depending on type. Refer to *Impaired Elimination.*

Gastrointestinal (GI) Tubes

➤ Check frequently for pressure against nares
➤ Put person in a room with others who can help watch him or her
➤ Enlist aid of family or friends to watch person during confused periods
➤ Give person something to hold (e.g., stuffed animal)

Rationale: Research has validated that restraints increase fear, which increases confusion.

6. If combative, determine source of the fear and frustration.

➤ Fatigue
➤ Change in routine
➤ Physical stress
➤ Misleading or inappropriate stimuli
➤ Pressure to exceed functional capacity

Rationale: Physical stressors can precipitate a dysfunctional episode (e.g., urinary tract infections, caffeine, constipation).

7. Ensure physical comfort and maintenance of basic health needs.

➤ Refer to individual nursing diagnoses to assist with self-care.

8. Select modalities that provide favorable stimuli for the client.

Music Therapy

➤ Determine client's preferences. Play this music before usual level of agitation for at least 30 minutes; assess response.
➤ Provide soft familiar music during meals.
➤ Play music during other therapies.

Rationale: Music therapy at least 30 minutes before the person's usual peak level of agitation can reduce agitation (Gerdner, 1999).

Recreation Therapy

➤ Encourage arts and crafts
➤ Provide puzzles
➤ Suggest creative writing
➤ Organize group games

9. Implement techniques to lower the stress threshold (Hall & Buckwalter, 1987; Miller, 2004).

Reduce competing or excessive stimuli

➤ Keep environment simple and uncluttered
➤ Use simple wring cues to clarify directions for use of radio and television

Rationale: Overstimulation, understimulation, or misleading stimuli can cause dysfunctional episodes because of impaired sensory interpretation.

Plan and maintain a consistent routine

➤ Attempt to assign same caregivers
➤ Elicit from family members specific methods that help or hinder care
➤ Arrange personal care items in order of use (clothes, toothbrush, mouthwash, and so forth)
➤ Determine a daily routine with client and family
➤ Write down sequence for all caregivers
➤ Reduce the stress when change is anticipated

Rationale: Overstimulation, understimulation, or misleading stimuli can cause dysfunctional episodes because of impaired sensory interpretation.

Focus on client's ability level

➤ Do not request performance of function beyond ability
➤ Express unconditional positive regard for the person
➤ Do not ask questions that the person cannot answer
➤ Avoid open-ended questions
➤ Avoid using pronouns
➤ Use finger foods
➤ Offer simple choices

Rationale: Attempting to perform functions that exceed cognitive capacity will result in fear, anger, and frustration.

Minimize fatigue (Hall, 1994)

➤ Provide rest periods twice daily
➤ Determine with client a rest activity, such as reading or listening to music
➤ Allow person to cease an activity at any time
➤ Allow for wandering in safe environment

Rationale: Fatigue is the most frequent cause of dysfunctional episodes. Daytime rest periods help prevent night awakenings.

▼ Constipation

Definition

Constipation: The state in which a person experiences or is at high risk of experiencing stasis of the large intestine resulting in infrequent (two or less weekly) elimination and/or hard dry feces.

Defining Characteristics

Assess for subjective (S) and objective (O) cues:

MAJOR (MUST BE PRESENT)

Hard formed stool (S,O)
Prolonged and difficult evacuation (S)
Defecation fewer than two times a week (S)

MINOR (MAY BE PRESENT)

Decreased bowel sounds (O)
Reported feeling of rectal fullness (S)
Reported feeling of pressure in rectum (S)
Straining of defecation (S)
Palpable impaction (O)
Feeling of inadequate emptying (S)

Related Factors

PATHOPHYSIOLOGIC

Related to defective nerve stimulation, weak pelvic floor muscle, and immobility secondary to

Spinal cord lesions
Spinal cord injury
Spina bifida
Cerebrovascular accident (stroke)
Neurologic disease (multiple sclerosis, Parkinson's)
Dementia

Related to decreased metabolic rate secondary to

Obesity
Hypothyroidism
Hyperparathyroidism
Uremia
Hypopituitarism
Diabetic neuropathy

Related to decreased response to urge to defecate secondary to

Mental disorders

Related to pain (on defecation)

Hemorrhoids
Back injury

Related to decreased peristalsis secondary to hypoxia (cardiac, pulmonary)
Related to motility disturbances secondary to irritable bowel syndrome

TREATMENT-RELATED

Related to side effects of (specify):

Antidepressants
Antacids (calcium, aluminum)
Calcium channel blockers
Calcium
Iron
Barium
Aluminum
Aspirin
Phenothiazines
Anticholinergics
Anesthetics
Narcotics/opiates
Diuretics
Anti-Parkinson agents

Related to effects of anesthesia and surgical manipulation on peristalsis
Related to habitual laxative use
Related to mucositis secondary to radiation

SITUATIONAL (PERSONAL, ENVIRONMENTAL)

Related to decreased peristalsis secondary to

Immobility
Pregnancy
Stress
Lack of exercise

Related to irregular evacuation patterns
Related to cultural/health benefits
Related to lack of privacy
Related to inadequate diet (lack of roughage, fiber, thiamine)
Related to inadequate fluid intake
Related to fear of rectal or cardiac pain
Related to faulty appraisal
Related to inability to perceive bowel cues

 Constipation results from delayed passage of food residue in the bowel because of the factors that the nurse can treat (e.g., dehydration, insufficient dietary roughage, immobility). Perceived constipation refers to faulty perception of constipation with self-prescribed overuse of laxatives, enemas, and/or suppositories. Some individuals report they are constipated if they do not have a bowel movement everyday. The nurse will teach them that this is a normal pattern.

Key Concepts

GENERIC CONSIDERATIONS

> Bowel elimination is controlled primarily by muscular and neuralgic activity. Undigested food or feces passes through the large intestine propelled by involuntary muscles within the intestinal walls. At the same time, water that was needed for digestion is reabsorbed. The feces pass through the sigmoid colon, which empties into the rectum. At some point, the amount of stool in the rectum stimulates a defecation reflex, which causes the anal sphincter to relax and defecation to occur (Shua-Haim et al., 1999). Table II-1 illustrates the components needed for normal bowel elimination and the conditions that impede them.

> Bowel patterns are culturally or familially determined. Range of normal is wide, from three times a day to once every 3 days (Shua-Haim et al., 1999).

> Some medical conditions, such as brain disorders or spinal cord injuries, interfere with neurotransmission. Others, such as diabetes mellitus or rectal or anal trauma, cause rectal sphincter abnormalities. Inflammatory bowel disease, radiation proctitis, chronic constipation, and ileoanal surgery can decrease the fecal reservoir capacity and cause leaking (Shua-Haim et al., 1999).

> Three tablespoons of bran daily increases dietary fiber by 25% to 40% and eliminates constipation in 60% of individuals (Shua-Haim et al., 1999).

Table II–1. COMPONENTS FOR NORMAL BOWEL ELIMINATION AND CORRESPONDING BARRIERS

Components	Barriers
Daily diet of fiber (15–25 g)	Lack of access to fresh foods
	Financial constraints
	Insufficient knowledge*
8–10 glasses of water a day	Mobility problems
	Fear of incontinence
	Impaired thought process*
	Low motivation
Daily exercise	Minimal activity level
	Pain, fatigue
	Fear of falling
Cognitive appraisal	Impaired thought process
	Faulty appraisal
Toileting routine	Low motivation
	Change in routine
	Stress
Response to rectal cues	Mobility problems
	Decreased awareness
	Environmental constraints
	Self-care deficits

*These barriers can impede all the components.

➤ Diets high in unrefined fibrous food produce large soft stools that decrease the colon's susceptibility to disease. Diets low in fiber and high in concentrated refined foods produce small hard stools that increase the colon's susceptibility to disease.

➤ Undigested fiber absorbs water, which adds bulk and softness to the stool, speeding its passage through the intestines. Fiber without adequate fluid can aggravate, not facilitate, bowel function.

➤ Laxatives and enemas are not components of a bowel management program. They are for emergency use only (McLane & McShane, 1991).

➤ Chronic use of stool softeners can cause fecal incontinence and is not recommended for treatment of chronic constipation in nonambulatory individuals (Shua-Haim et al., 1999).

GERIATRIC CONSIDERATIONS

➤ Older adults experience reduced mucous secretion in the large intestines and decreases elasticity of the rectal wall (Miller, 2004).

➤ Sensory dysfunction in the anorectal area of older adults can reduce sensing rectal distention (Shua-Haim et al., 1999).

➤ Some older adults are prone to constipation due to such factors as decreased activity, insufficient dietary fiber and bulk, insufficient fluid intake, side effects of medications, laxative abuse, and inattention to defecation cues (Miller, 2004).

➤ Thirty percent of older adults complain of constipation compared with 2% of the general population (Shaefer & Cheskin, 1998).

FOCUS ASSESSMENT CRITERIA

Subjective Data

Assess for defining characteristics.

Elimination pattern

➤ Usual   Present

What frequency is considered normal?
Laxative/enema use

➤ Type   How often

Episodes of diarrhea

➤ How often?   Frequency?   Duration?

Precipitated by what?
Associated symptoms/complaints of

➤ Headache
➤ Pain
➤ Anorexia
➤ Thirst
➤ Lethargy
➤ Weight loss/gain
➤ Weakness
➤ Cramping
➤ Awareness of bowel cues

Assess for related factors

Lifestyle
Activity level
Occupation
Exercise (what? how often?)
Nutrition
24-hour recall of foods and liquid intakes

Carbohydrates
Fat
Current drug therapy

➤ Antibiotics
➤ Iron
➤ Steroids

Medical-surgical history

➤ Present conditions
➤ Surgical history (colostomy? ileostomy?)
➤ Protein
➤ Usual 24-hour intake
➤ Fiber
➤ Liquids
➤ Antacids
➤ Narcotics/opiates
➤ Past conditions
➤ Awareness of bowel cues

Objective Data

Assess for defining characteristics

Stool
Color, odor, consistency
Bowel sounds

➤ High-pitched, gurgling (5/min)
➤ Weak and infrequent
➤ High-pitched, frequent, loud pushing
➤ Absent

Perianal area/rectal examination

➤ Hemorrhoids
➤ Fissures
➤ Control of rectal sphincter (presence of anal wink, bulbocavernosus reflex)
➤ Irritation
➤ Impaction
➤ Stool in rectum

GOAL

The person will report on bowel movement at least every 2 to 3 days.

Indicators

Describe components for effective bowel movements.
Explain rationale for lifestyle change(s).

GENERAL INTERVENTIONS

Assess contributing factors

➤ Irregular schedule
➤ Side effects of medical regimen
➤ Stress
➤ Inadequate exercise
➤ Imbalanced diet
➤ A daily diet of fiber, six to eight glasses of water, and exercise maintain a normal bowel elimination pattern. In addition, the person must be able to appraise the need to evacuate and establish a toileting routine.

Promote Corrective Measures

➤ Regular time for elimination
   ➤ Review daily routine.
   ➤ Advise client to include time for defecation as part of daily routine.
   ➤ Discuss suitable time (based on responsibilities, availability of facilities, and so forth).
   ➤ Provide stimulus to defecation (e.g., coffee, prune juice).
   ➤ Advise client to attempt to defecate about 1 hour or so after meals and that remaining in the bathroom for a suitable length of time may be necessary.
   ➤ Use bathroom instead of bedpan if possible.
   ➤ Provide privacy (close door, draw curtains around bed, play television or radio to mask sounds, have room deodorizer available).
   ➤ Provide comfort (reading material and diversion) and safety (call button available).
   ➤ Allow suitable position (sitting, if not contraindicated).
   ➤ The gastrocolic and duodenocolic reflexes stimulate mass peristalsis two to three times a day, most often after meals.
➤ Adequate exercise
   ➤ Review current exercise pattern.
   ➤ Provide for frequent moderate physical exercises (if not contraindicated).
   ➤ Provide frequent ambulation of hospitalized client when tolerable.
   ➤ Perform ROM exercises for person who is bedridden.
   ➤ Teach exercises for increased abdominal muscle tone (unless contraindicated; Weeks et al., 2000).

➢ Contract abdominal muscle several times throughout the day.

➢ Do sit-ups, keeping heels on floor with knees slightly flexed.

➢ While supine, raise lower limbs, keeping knees straight.

➤ Turn and change positions in bed, lifting hips.

➤ Lift knees alternately to the chest, stretching arms out to side and up over head.

➤ Regular physical activity promotes muscle tonicity needed for rectal expulsion. It also increases circulation to the digestive system, which promotes peristalsis and easier feces evacuation.

➤ Balanced diet

➤ Review list of foods high in bulk:

➢ Fresh fruits and vegetables with skins

➢ Bran

➢ Nuts and seeds

➢ Beans (navy, kidney, lima)

➢ Whole-grain cereal

➢ Cooked fruits and vegetables

➢ Fruit juices

➤ Discuss dietary preferences.

➤ Consider any food intolerances or allergies.

➤ Include approximately 800 g of fruits and vegetables (about four pieces of fresh fruit and large salad) for normal daily bowel movement.

➤ Suggest moderate use of bran at first (may irritate GI tract, produce flatulence, cause diarrhea or blockage).

➤ Gradually increase bran as tolerated (may add to cereals, baked goods, and the like). Explain the need for fluids intake with bran.

➤ Suggest 30 to 60 ml daily of a recipe of 2 cups All Bran cereal, 2 cups applesauce, and 1 cup prune juice (Braun & Everett, 1990).

➤ Consider financial limitations (encourage the use fruits and vegetables in season).

➤ A daily diet of fiber, six to eight glasses of water, and exercise maintain a normal bowel elimination pattern. In addition, the person must be able to appraise the need to evacuate and establish a toileting routine.

➤ A well-balanced high-fiber diet stimulates peristalsis. Foods high in fiber should be avoided during episodes of diarrhea:

➢ Whole grains and nuts (bran, shredded wheat, brown rice, whole-wheat bread)

➢ Raw and coarse vegetables (broccoli, cauliflower, cucumbers, lettuce, cabbage, turnips, Brussels sprouts)

➢ Fresh fruits, with skins

➤ Adequate fluid intake

➤ Encourage intake of at least 2 liters (8 to 10 glasses) unless contraindicated.

➢ Discuss fluid preferences.

➢ Set up regular schedule for fluid intake.

➢ Recommend drinking a glass of hot water 30 minutes before breakfast, which may stimulate bowel evacuation.

➢ Advise avoiding grapefruit juice, coffee, tea, cola, and chocolate drinks as daily fluid intake.

➢ Sufficient fluid intake, at least 2 liters daily, is necessary to maintain bowel patterns and to promote proper stool consistency.

➢ Certain fluids act as diuretics: caffeine-containing drinks and grapefruit juice (Weeks et al., 2000).

➤ Optimal position

➢ Assist client to normal semisquatting position to allow optimum use of abdominal muscles and effect of force of gravity.

➢ Assist client onto bedpan if necessary; elevate head of bed to high Fowler's position or elevation permitted.

➢ Use fracture bedpan for comfort, if preferred.

➢ Stress the avoidance of straining.

➢ Encourage exhaling during straining.

➤ Chart results (color, consistency, amount).

➤ Elevate legs on footstool when on toilet.

➤ Voluntary contraction of the abdominal muscles aids in the expulsion of feces.

➤ Elevating the legs can increase the intraabdominal pressure (Shua-Haim et al., 1999).

Eliminate or reduce contributing factors.

➤ Administer mild laxative after oral administration of barium sulfate.*

➤ Assess elimination status while on antacid therapy (may be necessary to alternate magnesium-type antacid with other types).*

➤ Encourage increased intake of high-roughage foods and increased fluids intake as adjunct to iron therapy (e.g., fresh fruits and vegetables with skins; bran, nuts, and seeds; whole-wheat bread).

➤ Encourage early ambulation, with assistance if necessary, to counter effects of anesthetic agents.

➤ Assess elimination status while client receives certain narcotic analgesics (morphine, codeine) and alert physician if client experiences difficulty with defecation.

➤ Advise client about medications that cause constipation (e.g., antacids, bismuth, calcium channel blockers, clonidine, levodopa, iron, nonsteroidal antiinflammatories, opiates, sicralfate; Shua-Haim et al., 1999).

➤ Discuss laxative abuse (see *Perceived Constipation*).

*May require a primary care provider's order.

➤ Laxatives upset a bowel program, because they cause much of the bowel to empty and can cause unscheduled bowel movements. With constant use, the colon loses tone and stool retention becomes difficult. Chronic use of bowel aids can lead to problems in stool consistency, which interferes with the scheduled bowel program and bowel management. Stool softeners may not be necessary if diet and fluid intake are adequate. Enemas lead to overstretched bowel and loss of bowel tone, contributing to further constipation (Toth, 1998).

Conduct health teaching, as indicated.

➤ Explain the relationship of lifestyle changes to constipation.
➤ Explain interventions that relieve symptoms.
➤ Explain techniques to reduce the effects of stress and immobility.
➤ Frequency and consistency of stools are related to fluid and food intake. Fiber increases fecal bulk and enhances water absorption into stool. Adequate dietary fiber and fluid promote firm but soft well-formed stools and decrease hard, dry, constipated stools. Physical activity promotes peristalsis, aids digestion, and facilitates elimination (Shua-Haim et al., 1999).

▼ Compromised Family Coping

Definition

Compromised Family Coping: That state in which a usually supportive primary person (family member or close friend) is providing insufficient, ineffective, or compromised support, comfort, assistance, or encouragement that may be needed by the client to manage or master adaptive tasks related to his or her health challenge.

Defining Characteristics

SUBJECTIVE DATA

Client expresses or confirms a concern or complaint about significant other's response to his or her health problem.

Significant person describes preoccupation with personal reactions (e.g., fear, anticipatory grief, guilt, anxiety) to client's illness, disability, or to other situational or developmental crises.

Significant person describes or confirms an inadequate understanding or knowledge base, which interferes with supportive behaviors.

OBJECTIVE DATA

Significant person attempts assistive or supportive behaviors with less than satisfactory results.

Significant person withdraws or enters into limited personal communication with the client at time of need.

Significant person displays protective behavior disproportionate (too little or too much) to the client's abilities or need for autonomy.

 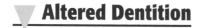 *This nursing diagnosis describes situations similar to the diagnosis Interrupted Family Processes. Until clinical research differentiates this diagnosis from the aforementioned diagnosis, use Interrupted Family Processes.*

▼ Altered Dentition

Definition

Altered Dentition: State in which a person experiences a disruption in tooth development/eruption patterns or structural integrity of individual teeth.

Defining Characteristics

Excessive plaque
Halitosis (foul breath)
Toothache
Excessive calculus
Malocclusion or tooth misalignment
Premature loss of primary teeth
Missing teeth or complete absence
Asymmetric facial expression
Crown or root caries
Tooth enamel discoloration
Loose teeth
Incomplete eruption for age (may be primary or permanent teeth)
Tooth fracture(s)
Erosion of enamel

▼ Diarrhea

Definition

Diarrhea: The state in which a person experiences or is at risk of experiencing frequent passage of liquid stool or unformed stool.

Defining Characteristics

Assess for subjective (S) and objective (O) cues:

MAJOR (MUST BE PRESENT)

Loose liquid stools and/or (S,O)
Increased frequency (more than three times a day) (S)

MINOR (MAY BE PRESENT)

Urgency (S)
Increased frequency of bowel sounds (O)
Cramping, abdominal pain (S)
Increased fluidity or volume of stools (O, S)

Related Factors

PATHOPHYSIOLOGIC

Related to malabsorption or inflammation secondary to

Colon cancer
Diverticulitis
Irritable bowel

Crohn's disease
Peptic ulcer
Gastritis
Spastic colon
Ulcerative colitis

Related to lactose deficiency
Related to increased peristalsis secondary to increased metabolic rate
(hyperthyroidism)
Related to infectious process secondary to

Parasites
Bacteria
Infectious hepatitis
Virus

Related to excessive secretion of fats in stool secondary to liver dysfunction
Related to inflammation and ulceration of gastrointestinal mucosa secondary
to high levels of nitrogenous wastes (renal failure)

TREATMENT-RELATED

Related to malabsorption or inflammation secondary to surgical intervention of
the bowel
Related to side effects of (specify)

Thyroid agents
Analgesics
Stool softeners
Chemotherapy
Laxatives
Iron sulfate
Antacids
Cimetidine
Antibiotics

Related to solute tube feedings

SITUATIONAL (PERSONAL, ENVIRONMENTAL)

Related to stress or anxiety
Related to irritating foods (fruits, bran cereals)
Related to changes in water and food secondary to travel
Related to change in bacteria in water
Related to hot weather
Related to increased caffeine consumption

FOCUS ASSESSMENT CRITERIA

Refer to *Constipation.*

GOAL

The person will report less diarrhea.

Indicators

Describe contributing factors when known
Explain rationale for interventions
Report less diarrhea

GENERAL INTERVENTIONS

1. Assess causative contributing factors.

➤ Tube feedings
➤ Dietetic foods
➤ Foreign travel
➤ Dietary indiscretions/contaminated foods
➤ Food allergies

2. Eliminate or reduce contributing factors.

➤ Side effects of tube feeding (Fuhrmann, 1999)
   ➢ Control infusion rate (depending on delivery set)
   ➢ Administer smaller more frequent feedings
   ➢ Change to continuous-drip tube feedings
   ➢ Administer more slowly if signs of GI intolerance occur
   ➢ Control temperature
   ➢ If refrigerated, warm in hot water to room temperature
   ➢ Dilute strength of feeding temporarily
   ➢ Follow standard procedure for administration of tube feeding
   ➢ Follow tube feeding with specified amount of water to ensure hydration
➤ Be careful of contamination/spoilage (unused but opened formula should not be used after 24 hours; keep unused portion refrigerated)
➤ Contaminated foods (possible sources)
   ➢ Raw seafood
   ➢ Raw milk
   ➢ Shellfish
   ➢ Restaurants

- ➤ Excess milk consumption
- ➤ Improperly cooked/stored food
- ➤ Dietetic foods: eliminate foods containing large amounts of the hexitol, sorbitol, and mannitol used as sugar substitutes in dietetic foods, candy, and chewing gum

Rationale: High solute feedings may cause diarrhea if not followed by sufficient water. Dietetic foods contain sugar substitutes that cause diarrhea from slow absorption and rapid small bowel mobility. Diminished intestinal absorption must be compensated for through gradual progressive introduction of enteral supplements. Administering cold formula can cause cramping and possibly lead to elimination problems. These precautions can minimize growth of microorganisms.

3. Reduce diarrhea.

- ➤ Discontinue solids
- ➤ Avoid milk (lactose) products, fat, whole grains, fried and spicy foods, and fresh fruits and vegetables.
- ➤ Gradually add semisolids and solids (crackers, yogurt, rice, bananas, and applesauce)
- ➤ Avoid opiate-containing antidiarrheal drugs with acute infectious diarrhea (e.g., Lomotil, Imodium)
- ➤ For mild or moderate diarrhea, advise to use bismuth subsalicylate (Pepto-Bismol), 30 ml or two tablets every 1/2 to 1 hour, up to eight doses in 24 hours. Avoid in individuals with salicylate contraindications.
- ➤ Instruct to seek medical care if blood in stool and fever greater than 101°F

Rationale: Foods with complex carbohydrates (e.g., rice, toast, cereal) facilitate fluid absorption into the intestinal mucosa (Bennett, 2000). Opiate-containing antidiarrheals do not alter the natural cause of the disease and are harmful if invasive pathogens are the cause (Bennett, 2000). Bismuth subsalicylate (Pepto-Bismol) has been found safe in a variety of diarrheal illnesses and to have antibacterial activity as well. It is also effective in controlling symptoms of traveler's diarrhea (Bennett, 2000).

4. Replace fluids and electrolytes.

- ➤ Increase oral intake to maintain a normal urine specific gravity or to approximate volume of diarrhea losses.
- ➤ Encourage liquids (tea, water, apple juice, flat ginger ale).
- ➤ When diarrhea is severe, use an oral rehydration solution, either over-the-counter packets or homemade (½ teaspoon salt, ½ teaspoon baking soda, 4 tablespoons sugar in 1 liter of water; discard in 24 hours)

➤ Teach to monitor the color of urine to determine hydration needs.

➤ Caution against very hot or very cold liquids

➤ Avoid soft drinks or sport drinks.

➤ Refer to Deficient Fluid Volume for more interventions.

Rationale: Soft drinks (nondietetic and dietetic) and sport drinks are unsatisfactory for fluid replacement for moderate or severe fluid loss because of their sugar and salt content (Bennett, 2000).

This diagnosis focuses on acute and chronic diarrhea. Chronic diarrhea is a condition that needs both medical and nursing treatment with the nursing focus on the collaborative problem, for example, PC: Fluid/Electrolyte Imbalances. The major focus is to provide optimal nutrition and prevent dehydration and electrolyte imbalances, for example, potassium and sodium. With individuals with chronic diarrhea, the nurse would also prevent rectal tissue damage using the diagnosis Risk for Impaired Skin Integrity.

Key Concepts

GENERIC CONSIDERATIONS

➤ Diarrhea can be acute or chronic. Causes of acute diarrhea include drug reactions, bacteria, heavy metal poisoning, fecal impaction, and dietary changes. Causes of chronic diarrhea include irritable bowel syndrome, lactose deficiency, colon cancer, inflammatory bowel disease, malabsorption disorders, alcohol, medication side effects, and laxatives.

➤ Drugs that can induce diarrhea are laxatives, antacids, certain antibiotics (e.g., tetracyclines), certain hypertensives (e.g., reserpine), cholinergics, certain antivirals, and select cardiac agents (e.g., digoxin).

➤ Rapid transit of feces through the large intestine results in decreased water absorption and unformed liquid stool. Ongoing diarrhea leads to dehydration and electrolyte imbalance

➤ Hyperperistalsis is the motor response to intestinal irritants.

➤ Diarrhea may be related to an inflammatory process in which the intestinal mucosal wall becomes irritated, resulting in increased moisture content in the fecal masses.

➤ Older people are more vulnerable to dehydration related to diarrhea.

5. Cleanse perineal area after each diarrheal episode, followed by the application of a moisture barrier ointment (e.g., Desitin, Vaseline, A & D Ointment, BAZA).

Rationale: A moisture barrier is a petroleum-based ointment that repels urine and fecal material and moisturizes the skin to assist in healing reddened irritated areas resulting from incontinence.

6. Conduct health teaching as indicated.

➤ Explain the interventions required to prevent future episodes.
➤ Explain the effects of diarrhea on hydration.
➤ Teach precautions to take when traveling to foreign lands.
   ➢ Avoid foods served cold, salads, milk, fresh cheese, cold cuts, and salsa.
   ➢ Drink carbonated or bottled beverages; avoid ice.
   ➢ Peel fresh fruits and vegetables
   ➢ Avoid foods not stored at proper temperature
➤ Consult with primary health care provider for prophylactic use of bismuth subsalicylate (e.g., Pepto-Bismol) 30 to 60 ml or two tablets qid during travel and 2 days after return; or antimicrobials, for prevention of traveler's diarrhea.
➤ Explain how to prevent food-borne diseases at home.
   ➢ Refrigerate all perishable foods.
   ➢ Cook all food at high temperature and boil for at least 15 minutes before serving
   ➢ Avoid allowing food to stand at warm temperatures for several hours
   ➢ Thoroughly clean kitchen equipment after contact with perishable foods (e.g., meats, dairy, fish)
➤ Caution about foods at picnics in hot summer
➤ Explain that a diet primarily made up of dietetic foods containing sugar substitutes (hexitol, sorbitol, and mannitol) may cause diarrhea

Rationale: Dietetic foods contain sugar substitutes that cause diarrhea from slow absorption and rapid small bowel mobility.

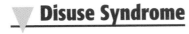

▼ Disuse Syndrome

Definition

Disuse Syndrome: The state in which a person is experiencing or is at risk for deterioration of body systems or altered functioning as the result of prescribed or unavoidable musculoskeletal inactivity

Defining Characteristics

Presence of a cluster of actual or risk nursing diagnoses related to inactivity:

> *Risk for Impaired Skin Integrity*
> *Risk for Constipation*
> *Risk for Altered Respiratory Function*
> *Risk for Ineffective Peripheral Tissue Perfusion*
> *Risk for Infection*
> *Risk for Activity Intolerance*
> *Risk for Impaired Physical Mobility*
> *Disturbed Sensory Perception*
> *Powerlessness*
> *Disturbed Body Image*

Related Factors

PATHOPHYSIOLOGIC

Related to (optional) immobility secondary to

> *Decreased sensorium*
> *Unconsciousness*
> *Neuromuscular impairment examples:*

- ➤ Multiple sclerosis
- ➤ Partial/total paralysis
- ➤ Muscular dystrophy
- ➤ Guillain-Barre syndrome
- ➤ Parkinsonism
- ➤ Spinal cord injury

> *Musculoskeletal impairment examples:*

- ➤ Fractures
- ➤ Rheumatic diseases

End-stage disease examples:

➤ Acquired immunodeficiency syndrome (AIDS)
➤ Cardiac
➤ Renal

Cancer
Psychiatric/mental health disorders examples:

➤ Major depression
➤ Catatonic state
➤ Severe phobias

TREATMENT-RELATED

Related to (optional)

Surgery (amputation, skeletal)
Traction/casts/splints
Prescribed immobility
Mechanical ventilation
Invasive vascular lines

SITUATIONAL (PERSONAL, ENVIRONMENTAL)

Related to (optional)

Depression
Fatigue
Debilitated state
Pain

MATURATIONAL

Related to (optional)

Newborn/infant/child/adolescent
Down syndrome
Juvenile arthritis
Cerebral palsy
Risser-Turnbuckle jacket
Osteogenesis imperfecta
Mental/physical disability
Legg-Calve-Perthes disease
Autism
Spina bifida
Older adult

➤ Decreased motor agility
➤ Muscle weakness
➤ Presenile dementia

Remember from Chapter 3 that syndrome nursing diagnoses represent a group of nursing diagnoses related to a certain event or situation. Disuse Syndrome describes a person experiencing or at risk for the problem effects of immobility. The clusters of risk or actual nursing diagnoses are the defining characteristics for a syndrome nursing diagnosis. For Disuse Syndrome, there are 11 risk or actual nursing diagnoses. If a person with Disuse Syndrome develops an actual skin problem related to immobility, add Impaired Skin Integrity to the care plan. Continue to use Disuse Syndrome also so other body systems do not deteriorate.

Key Concepts

GENERIC CONSIDERATIONS

➤ "Immobility is inconsistent with human life." Mobility provides control over the environment; without mobility, the person is at the mercy of the environment (Christian, 1982).

➤ Prolonged immobility decreases motivation to learn and ability to retain new material. Affective changes are anxiety, fear, hostility, rapid mood shifts, and disrupted sleep patterns (Porth, 2002).

➤ Immobility restricts the ability to seek out sensory stimulation. Conversely, immobile people may be unable to remove themselves from a stressful or noisy environment (Christian, 1982).

➤ Musculoskeletal inactivity or immobility adversely affects all body systems (Table II-2).

➤ A muscle loses about 3% of its original strength each day it is immobilized.

➤ Prolonged immobility adversely affects psychological health, learning, socialization, and ability to cope. Table II-3 illustrates these effects.

➤ Possible long-term complications in people with traumatic spinal cord injury are pneumonia, atelectasis, autonomic dysreflexia, deep vein thrombosis, pulmonary embolism, pressure ulcers, fractures, and renal calculi (McKinley et al., 1999).

GERIATRIC CONSIDERATIONS

➤ Aging affects muscle function because of progressive loss of muscle mass, strength, and endurance.

➤ Age-related changes in joint and connective tissues include impaired flexion and extension movements, decreased flexibility, and reduced cushioning protection for joints (Miller, 2004).

➤ After menopause, women experience an accelerated loss of trabecular and cortical bone of 9% to 10% per decade (Miller, 2004).

➤ Bed rest can cause an average vertical bone loss of 0.9% per week (Maher et al., 1998).

Table II–2. ADVERSE EFFECTS OF IMMOBILITY ON BODY SYSTEMS

System	Effect
Cardiac	Decreased myocardial performance
	Decreased aerobic capacity
	Decreased heart rate and stroke volume
	Decreased oxygen uptake
Circulatory	Venous stasis
	Orthostatic intolerance
	Dependent edema
	Decreased resting heart rate
	Reduced venous return
	Increased intravascular pressure
Respiratory	Stasis of secretions
	Impaired cilia
	Drying of sections of mucous membranes
	Decreased chest expansion
	Slower, more shallow respirations
Musculoskeletal	Muscle atrophy
	Shortening of muscle fiber (contracture)
	Decreased strength/tone (eg, back)
	Decreased bone density
	Joint degeneration
	Fibrosis of collagen fibers (joints)
Metabolic/Hemopoietic	Decreased nitrogen excretion
	Decreased tissue heat conduction
	Decreased glucose tolerance
	Insulin resistance
	Decreased red blood cells
	Decreased phagocytosis
	Hypercalcemia
	Change in circadian release of hormones (eg, insulin, epinephrine)
	Anorexia
	Decreased metabolic rate
	Obesity
	Elevated creatine levels
Gastrointestinal	Constipation
Genitourinary	Urinary stasis
	Urinary calculi
	Urinary retention
	Inadequate gravitational force
Integumentary	Decreased capillary flow
	Tissue acidosis to necrosis
Neurosensory	Reduced innervation of nerves
	Decreased near vision
	Increased auditory sensitivity

Porth, 2002; Tyler, 1984; Wong, 2004.

Table II–3. PSYCHOSOCIAL EFFECTS OF IMMOBILITY

Psychological	Increased tension
	Negative change in self-concept
	Fear, anger
	Rapid mood changes
	Depression
	Hostility
Learning	Decreased motivation
	Decreased ability to retain, transfer learning
	Decreased attention span
Socialization	Change in roles
	Social isolation
Growth and development	Dependency

Porth, 2002; Zubek & McNeil, 1967.

FOCUS ASSESSMENT CRITERIA

Assess for related factors

Neurologic
Musculoskeletal
Cardiovascular
Respiratory
History of recent trauma or surgery
Debilitating disease
History of symptoms

➤ (Complaints) of pain, muscle weakness, fatigue

Subjective and Objective Data

Assess for subjective (S) and objective (O) cues:

Motor Function (O)

Right arm:	strong	weak	absent	spastic
Left arm:	strong	weak	absent	spastic
Right leg:	strong	weak	absent	spastic
Left leg:	strong	weak	absent	spastic

Mobility (O)

Ability to turn self	yes	no	Assistance needed (specify)
Ability to sit	yes	no	Assistance needed (specify)
Ability to stand	yes	no	Assistance needed (specify)

Ability to transfer   yes   no   Assistance needed (specify)
Ability to ambulate   yes   no   Assistance needed (specify)

Weight bearing (assess both right and left sides) (O)
Full   partial   as tolerated   non–weight bearing

Gait (O)
Stable   unstable

ROM of shoulders, elbows, arms, hips, and legs (O)
Full   limited (specify)   none

Assess for related factors.

Assistive devices (O)

➤ Crutches
➤ Prosthesis
➤ Walker
➤ Wheelchair
➤ Braces
➤ Cane
➤ Other

Restrictive devices (O)

➤ Cast or splint
➤ Intravenous line
➤ Ventilator
➤ Foley
➤ Braces
➤ Dialysis
➤ Traction
➤ Monitor
➤ Drain

Motivation (as perceived by nurse, reported by person, or both) (S)
Excellent   satisfactory   poor

GOAL

The client will not experience complications of immobility.

Indicators

Demonstrate intact skin and tissue integrity
Demonstrate maximum pulmonary function

Demonstrate maximum peripheral blood flow
Demonstrate full ROM
Demonstrate adequate bowel, bladder, and renal functions
Explain rationale for treatments
Make decisions regarding care when possible
Share feelings regarding immobile state

INTERVENTIONS

1. Explain the effects of immobility on body systems and the reason for interventions as indicated.

Rationale: Understanding may help to elicit cooperation in reducing immobility.

2. Take steps to promote optimal respiratory function.
   a. Vary bed position, unless contraindicated, to change the horizontal and vertical positions of the thorax gradually.
   b. Assist with repositioning, turning from side to side every hour if possible.
   c. Encourage deep breathing and controlled coughing exercises five times an hour.

Rationale: Immobility contributes to stasis of secretions and possible pneumonia or atelectasis. These measures help increase lung expansion and the ability to expel secretions (Hickey, 2002).

3. Encourage increased oral fluid intake as indicated.

Rationale: Optimal hydration liquefies secretions for easier expectoration and prevents stasis of secretions that provide a medium for microorganism growth.

4. Explain the effects of daily activity on elimination. Assist with ambulation when possible.

Rationale: Activity influences bowel elimination by improving muscle tone and stimulating appetite and peristalsis.

5. Promote factors that contribute to optimal elimination.
   a. Balanced diet

➤ Review a list of foods high in bulk (e.g., fresh fruits with skins, bran, nuts and seeds, whole-grain breads, cooked fruits and vegetables, and fruit juices)
➤ Discuss dietary preferences

➤ Encourage intake of approximately 800 g of fruits and vegetables (about four pieces of fresh fruit and a large salad) for normal daily bowel movement

Rationale: A well-balanced diet high in fiber content stimulates peristalsis.

    b. Adequate fluid intake

➤ Encourage intake of at least 8 to 10 glasses (about 2,000 ml) daily unless contraindicated
➤ Discuss fluid preferences
➤ Set up a regular schedule for fluid intake

Rationale: Sufficient fluid intake is necessary to maintain bowel patterns and promote proper stool consistency

    c. Regular time for defecation

➤ Identify normal defecation pattern before onset of constipation
➤ Review daily routine
➤ Include time for defecation as part of the regular daily routine
➤ Discuss suitable time based on responsibilities, availability of facilities, and so forth.

Rationale: Taking advantage of circadian rhythms may aid in establishing a regular defecation schedule

➤ Suggest that client attempt defecation about an hour after meal and remain in the bathroom a suitable length of time
    d. Stimulation of the home environment

➤ Have client use the bathroom instead of a bedpan if possible; offer a bedpan or commode if client cannot use the bathroom
➤ Assist client into position on the toilet, commode, or bedpan if necessary
➤ Provide privacy (close the door, draw the curtains around the bed, play a television or music to mask sounds, and make room deodorizer available)
➤ Provide for comfort (e.g., provide reading materials as a diversion) and safety (make a call bell readily available)

Rationale: Privacy and a sense of normalcy can promote relaxation, which can enhance defecation.

    e. Proper positioning

➤ Assist client to a normal semisquatting position on toilet or commode if possible
➤ Assist onto a bedpan if necessary, elevating the head of the bed to high Fowler's position or to the elevation permitted
➤ Stress the need to avoid straining during defecation efforts

Rationale: Proper positioning uses the abdominal muscles and the force of gravity to aid defecation.

6. Institute measures to prevent pressure ulcers. (Refer to the Pressure Ulcers care plan for specific interventions).

Rationale: The immobile client is at risk for pressure ulcers, which are localized areas of cellular necrosis that tend to occur when soft tissue is compressed between a bony prominence and a firm surface for a prolonged period (Maklebust & Sieggreen, 2001).

7. Promote optimum circulation when the client is sitting.
   a. Limit sitting time for a client at high risk for ulcer development
   b. Instruct client to lift self every 10 minutes using chair arms if possible or assist client with this maneuver

Rationale: Capillary flow is increased if pressure is relieved and redistributed. Prolonged compromised capillary flow leads to tissue hypoxia and necrosis (Maklebust & Sieggreen, 2001).

8. With each position change, inspect areas at risk for developing ulcers:
   a. Ears
   b. Elbows
   c. Occiput
   d. Trochanter
   e. Heels
   f. Ischia
   g. Scapula
   h. Sacrum
   i. Scrotum

Rationale: Certain areas over bony prominences are more prone to cellular compression (Maklebust & Sieggreen, 2001).

9. Observe for erythema and blanching, palpate for warmth and tissue sponginess, and massage vulnerable areas lightly with each position change.

Rationale: Erythema and blanching are early signs of tissue hypoxia. Deep massage can injure capillaries, but light massage stimulates local circulation (Maklebust & Sieggreen, 2001).

10. Teach the client to do the following:
   a. Elevate legs above level of the heart (may be contraindicated if severe cardiac or respiratory disease is present)
   b. Avoid standing or sitting with legs dependent for long periods

    c. Consider using Ace bandages or below knee elastic stockings

    d. Avoid using pillows behind the knees or a gatch on the bed elevated at the knees

    e. Avoid leg crossing

    f. Change positions, move extremities, or wiggle fingers and toes every hour

    g. Avoid garters and tight elastic stockings above the knees

    h. Perform leg exercises every hour when advisable

Rationale: Immobility reduces venous return and increases intravascular pressure that contributes to venous stasis and thrombophlebitis. Elastic stockings reduce venous pooling by exerting even pressure over the leg; they increase flow to deeper veins by reducing the caliber of the superficial vein. External venous compression impedes venous flow. Leg exercises promote the muscle pumping effect on the deep veins.

11. Measure baseline circumference of calves and thighs daily if the client is at risk for deep venous thrombosis or if it is suspected.

Rationale: Thrombophlebitis causes edema, which increases leg measurements.

12. Institute measures to increase limb mobility.

    a. Perform ROM exercises as frequently as the client's condition warrants

    b. Support limbs with pillows to prevent or reduce swelling

    c. Encourage client to perform exercise regimens for specific joints as prescribed

Rationale: Joints without ROM exercise develop contractures in 3 to 7 days because flexor muscles are stronger than extensor muscles.

13. Take steps to maintain proper body alignment.

    a. Use a footboard

Rationale: This measure prevents foot drop.

    b. Avoid prolonged periods of sitting or lying in the same position

Rationale: This measure prevents hip flexion contractures.

    c. Change position of the shoulder joints every 2 to 4 hours

Rationale: This measure can help prevent shoulder contractures.

    d. Support the hand and wrist in natural alignment

Rationale: This measure can help prevent dependent edema and flexion contracture of wrist.

e. Use a small pillow or no pillow when client is in Fowler's position

Rationale: This measure prevents flexion contracture of the neck.

f. If client is supine or prone, place a rolled towel or small pillow under the lumbar curvature or under the end of the rib cage

Rationale: This measure prevents flexion or hyperflexion of lumbar curvature.

g. Place a trocanter roll or sandbags alongside hips and upper thighs

Rationale: This prevents external rotation of the femurs and hips.

h. If client is in the lateral position, place a pillow(s) to support the leg from groin to foot and a pillow to flex the shoulder and elbow slightly

Rationale: These measures prevent internal rotation and adduction of the femur and shoulder and prevent foot drop.

i. Use hand–wrist splints

Rationale: Splints prevent flexion or extension contractures of fingers and abduction of the thumbs.

14. Monitor for and take steps to reduce bone demineralization.
    a. Monitor for signs and symptoms of hypercalcemia
    b. Provide weight bearing whenever possible; use a tilt table if indicated

Rationale: Lack of motion and weight bearing results in bone destruction that releases calcium into the bloodstream and results in hypercalcemia (Bullock & Henze, 2000).

15. Take measures to prevent urinary stasis and calculi formation.

Rationale: Peristaltic contractions of the ureters are insufficient in a reclining position and result in urine stasis in the renal pelvis.

a. Provide daily intake of fluid of 2,000 ml or greater (unless contra-indicated)

Rationale: Stones form more readily in concentrated urine.

b. Maintain urine pH below 6.0 (acidic) with acid ash foods (e.g., cereals, meats, poultry, fish, cranberry juice, and apple juice)

Rationale: These measures reduce the formation of calcium calculi.

   c. Teach client to avoid these foods:

➤ Milk, milk products, and cheese
➤ Bran cereals
➤ Cranberries, plums, raspberries, gooseberries, olives
➤ Asparagus, rhubarb, spinach, kale, swiss chard, turnip greens, mustard greens, broccoli, beet greens
➤ Legumes, whole grain rice
➤ Sardines, shrimp, oysters
➤ Chocolate
➤ Peanut butter

Rationale: These foods are high in calcium and oxalate and can contribute to stone formation.

  16. Maintain vigorous hydration unless contraindicated (adult, 2,000 ml/ day; adolescent, 3,000 to 4,000 ml/day).

Rationale: Optimal hydration reduces the blood coagulability, liquefies secretions, inhibits stone formation, and promotes glomerular filtration of body wastes.

  17. Refer to Self-Care Deficits for specific interventions.
  18. Encourage client to wear desired personal adornments (baseball cap, colorful socks) and clothes rather than pajamas.

Rationale: Street clothes allow the client to express his or her individuality, which promotes self-esteem and reduces feelings of powerlessness.

  19. Plan strategies to reduce the monotony of immobility.
    a. Vary daily routine when possible.
    b. Have client participate in daily planning when possible.
    c. Try to make the routine as normal as possible (have dress in street clothes during the day).
    d. Encourage visitors.
    e. Alter physical environment when possible (update bulletin boards, change pictures on wall).
    f. Maintain a pleasant environment. Position client near a window if possible.
    g. Provide various reading materials, a television, and radio.
    h. Discourage excessive television watching.
    i. Plan some "special" activity daily to give client something to look forward to.
    j. Consider enlisting volunteer to read to the client or help with activities if necessary.
    k. Encourage client to devise his or her own strategies to combat boredom.

Rationale: These measures may help to reduce the monotony of immobility and compensate for psychological effects of immobility.

20. Provide opportunities for client to make decisions regarding surroundings, activities, and routines, and short-and long-term goals as appropriate.

Rationale: Mobility enables client to actualize decisions (when to eat, where to go, what to do). Loss of mobility can affect autonomy and control.

21. Encourage family members to request the client's opinions when making family decisions.

Rationale: The family can provide opportunities for client to maintain role responsibilities; this can help minimize feelings of powerlessness.

▼ Interrupted Family Processes

Definition

Interrupted Family Processes: State in which a usually supportive family experiences, or is at risk to experience, a stressor that challenges its previously effective functioning.

Defining Characteristics

Assess for subjective (S) and objective (O) cues:

MAJOR (MUST BE PRESENT)

Family system cannot or does not (S,O)

➤ Adapt constructively to crisis
➤ Communicate openly and effectively between family members

MINOR (MAY BE PRESENT)

Family system cannot or does not (S,O)

➤ Meet physical needs of all its members
➤ Meet emotional needs of all its members
➤ Meet spiritual needs of all its members
➤ Express or accept a wide range of feelings
➤ Seek or accept help appropriately

Related Factors

Any factor can contribute to Interrupted Family Processes. Common factors are listed below.

Interrupted Family Processes
Pathophysiologic
Related to effects of illness (specify)
Related to change in the family member's ability function

TREATMENT-RELATED

Related to the following:

Disruption of family routines because of time-consuming treatments
(e.g., home dialysis)
Physical changes because of treatments of ill family member
Emotional changes in all family members because of treatment of ill
family member
Financial burden of treatments for ill family member
Hospitalization of ill family member

SITUATIONAL (PERSONAL, ENVIRONMENTAL)

Related to loss of family member

➤ Death
➤ Incarceration
➤ Going away to school
➤ Desertion
➤ Separation
➤ Hospitalization
➤ Divorce

Related to addition of new family member

➤ Birth
➤ Marriage
➤ Adoption
➤ Elderly relative
➤ Interrupted family processes

Related to losses associated with

➤ Poverty
➤ Economic crisis
➤ Change in family roles
➤ Birth of child with defect
➤ Relocation (e.g., retirement)
➤ Disaster

Related to conflict (moral, goal, cultural)
Related to breach of trust between members
Related to social deviance by family member (e.g., crime)

Interrupted Family Processes describes a family that reports usual positive constructive functioning but is experiencing a change from a current stress-related challenge. The family is viewed as a system, with interdependence among members. Thus, life challenges for individual members also challenge the family system. Certain situations may negatively influence family functioning; examples include illness, an older relative moving in, relocation, separation, and divorce. Risk for Interrupted Family Processes can represent such a situation. Interrupted Family Processes differs from Caregiver Role Strain. Certain situations require one or more family members to assume a caregiver role for a relative.

Interrupted Family Processes can vary from ensuring an older parent has three balanced meals daily to providing for all hygiene and self-care activities for an adult or child. Caregiver Role Strain describes the mental and physical burden that the caregiver role places on individuals, which influences all their concurrent relationships and role responsibilities. It focuses specifically on the individual or individuals with multiple direct caregiver responsibilities. Caregiver Role Strain may be a too complex diagnosis for a beginning student.

Key Concepts

GENERIC CONSIDERATIONS

➤ Each family has a personality to which each member contributes.

➤ Families change with time. They must accomplish specific tasks that originate from the needs of their members. Table II-4 illustrates the tasks of the family.

➤ Each family responds to life challenges in ways that reflect past experiences and future goals.

➤ Within a family, members interact in various roles that result from individuals and group needs: parent, spouse, child, sibling, friend, teacher, and so forth. Illness of one member may precipitate great changes, putting the family at high risk for maladaptation (Clemen-Stone et al., 2002).

➤ Each family member influences the entire family unit. Thus, the health of an individual influences the health of the family. Family equilibrium depends on a balance of roles in the family and reciprocation (Clemen-Stone et al., 2002; Duval, 1977).

➤ Stress is defined as the body's response to any demand made on it. Stress has the potential to become a crisis when the person or family cannot cope constructively. A crisis is when a person's usual problem-solving methods are inadequate to resolve the situation.

Table II–4. STAGE-CRITICAL FAMILY DEVELOPMENTAL TASKS THROUGH THE FAMILY LIFE CYCLE

Stage of the Family Life Cycle	Positions in the Family	Stage-Critical Family Developmental Tasks
1. Married couple	Wife Husband	Establishing a mutually satisfying marriage Adjusting to pregnancy and the promise of parenthood Fitting into the kin network
2. Child-bearing	Wife-mother Husband-father Infant daughter or son or both	Having, adjusting to, and encouraging the development of infants Establishing a satisfying home for both parents and infant(s)
3. Preschool-aged	Wife-mother Husband-father Daughter-sister Son-brother	Adapting to the critical needs and interests of preschool children in stimulating growth-promoting ways Coping with energy depletion and lack of privacy as parents
4. School-aged	Wife-mother Husband-father Daughter-sister Son-brother	Fitting into the community of school-aged families in constructive ways Encouraging children's educational achievement
5. Teenage	Wife-mother Husband-father Daughter-sister Son-brother	Balancing freedom with responsibility as teenagers mature and emancipate themselves Establishing postparental interests and careers as growing parents
6. Launching center	Wife-mother-grandmother Husband-father-grandfather Daughter-sister-aunt Son-brother-uncle	Releasing young adults into work, military service, college, marriage, etc. with appropriate rituals and assistance Maintaining a supportive home base

(table continues on p. 190)

Table II–4. STAGE-CRITICAL FAMILY DEVELOPMENTAL TASKS THROUGH THE FAMILY LIFE CYCLE (*Continued*)

Stage of the Family Life Cycle	Positions in the Family	Stage-Critical Family Developmental Tasks
7. Middle-aged parents	Wife-mother-grandmother Husband-father-grandfather	Rebuilding the marriage relationship Maintaining kin ties with older and younger generations
8. Aging family members	Widow-widower Wife-mother-grandmother Husband-father-grandfather	Coping with bereavement and living alone Closing the family home or adapting it to aging Adjusting to retirement

➤ The family responding to crisis returns to precrisis functioning, develops improved functioning (adaptation), or develops destructive functioning (maladaptation).

➤ Constructive or functional coping mechanisms of families facing a stress crisis are as follows (Clemen-Stone et al., 2002):

Greater reliance on one another
Maintenance of a sense of humor
Increased sharing of feeling and thoughts
Promotion of each member's individuality
Accurate appraisal of the meaning of the problem
Search for knowledge and resources about the problem
Use of support systems

➤ Destructive or dysfunctional coping mechanisms of families facing a crisis are as follows (Smith-DiJulio, 1998):
Denial of a problem
Exploitation of one or more members (threats, violence, neglect, scapegoating)
Separation (hospitalization, institutionalization, divorce, abandonment)
Authoritarianism (no negotiation)
Preoccupation of family or members (who lack affection) with appearing to be close

➤ Parenthood is a crisis. Some common problems include the following:
Increased arguments in adults
Fatigue resulting from schedule
Disrupted social life
Disrupted sex life

Multiple losses, actual or perceived (e.g., independence, career, appearance, attention)
➤ Characteristics of families prone to crisis include the following (Fife, 1985; Smith-DiJulio, 1998):
Apathy (resignation to state in life)
Poor self-concept
Low income
Inability to manage money
Unrealistic preferences (materialistic)
Lack of skills and education
Unstable work history
Frequent relocations
History of repeated inadequate problem solving
Lack of adequate role models
Lack of participation in religious or community activities
Environmental isolation (no telephone, inadequate public transportation)
Interrupted Family Processes
➤ Successful outcomes of family efforts to achieve new adaptation after a crisis depend on the following (Nugent, Hughes, Ball & Davis, 1992):
Cohesiveness in response to past stressors
Interaction with others in support group
Belief that family can handle the crisis

TRANSCULTURAL CONSIDERATIONS

➤ The dominant US culture values two goals for families: (1) encouragement and nurturance of each individual and (2) cultivation of healthy autonomous children. Marital partners are expected to be supportive and share a sense of meaning. Each partner has the freedom for personality development. Children are encouraged to develop their own identity and life directions (Giger & Davidhizar, 2004).
➤ The family was found to be the principal source of support during illness in seven minority groups (Giger & Davidhizar, 2004).
➤ In Latin families, the needs of the family are more important than those of the individual. The father is provider, head of household and decision maker (Andrews & Boyle, 2003).
➤ Arab-American families are supposed to be supportive. A family is often criticized as a failure if a member is sent to the hospital for psychiatric care. Arab-American families may appear overindulgent and interfering to compensate for criticism (Giger & Davidhizar, 2004).
➤ Japanese Americans identify themselves by the generation in which they are born. First- and second-generation Japanese Americans see the family as one of the most important factors in their lives. They

manage problems within the family structure. The father and other male members are in the top position. Achievement or failure of one member reflects on the entire family. Caring for elderly parents, usually by the oldest son or an unmarried child, is expected. Adult children freely provide their parents with goods, money, and assistance (Andrews & Boyle, 2003).

➤ The nuclear family and the greater Jewish community are the center of Jewish culture. Families are close-knit and child-oriented. The commandments dictate expected behavior toward parents and within the community (Giger & Davidhizar, 2004).

➤ For the Vietnamese, family has been the chief source of cohesion and continuity for hundreds of years. Immediate family includes parents, unmarried children, and sometimes the husband's parents and sons with their wives and children. Individual behavior reflects on the whole family. A member is expected to give up personal wishes or ambitions if they disrupt family harmony. Family loyalty is "filial piety," which commands children to obey and honor their parents even after death (Giger & Davidhizar, 2004).

FOCUS ASSESSMENT CRITERIA

Assess for Defining Characteristics

Communication patterns

➤ Express feelings openly
➤ Straight messages
➤ No manipulation

Emotional/supportive pattern

➤ Constructive
   ➤ Appraise problem accurately
   ➤ Rely on one another
   ➤ Show optimism
   ➤ Seek knowledge and resources
   ➤ Share feelings, thoughts
   ➤ Deal with problems
   ➤ Use support systems
➤ Destructive
   ➤ Deny problems
   ➤ Use abandonment
   ➤ Show authoritarianism
   ➤ Exploit members (threats, violence, neglect, scapegoating)
   ➤ Show apathy

Socialization function

➤ Family members develop in a healthy pattern
➤ Family members negotiate roles and responsibilities

Parenting and marriage roles

➤ Satisfying
➤ Mutual agreement

Child behavior

➤ Home
➤ School

Assess for Related Factors

Addition of new family member

➤ Birth
➤ Adoption
➤ Marriage
➤ Elderly relative

Loss of family member

➤ Relocation
➤ Illness
➤ Death

Change in family roles

➤ Financial crisis
➤ Disaster
➤ Conflicts
➤ Family member with a coping problem
➤ Relocation history

If the family has a history or is demonstrative of maladaptive or destructive behavior, Interrupted Family Processes is not the appropriate diagnosis. Risk for Disabled Family Coping or Disabled Family Coping should be used. These diagnoses are too complex for a beginning student. Consult with your instructor on how you can refer this diagnosis to an expert, for example, a psychiatric clinical specialist or nurse practitioner.

GOAL

The family will maintain functional system of mutual support for another.

Indicators

Frequently verbalize feeling to professional nurse and one another.
Identify appropriate external resources available.

GENERAL INTERVENTIONS

1. Create a supportive environment.

➤ Keep client's door closed if desired.
➤ Provide family members with an alternative meeting place to the client's room.
➤ Make sure family members are oriented to visiting hours, bathrooms, vending machines, cafeteria, and so forth.
➤ If possible, provide pillows/blankets for family members spending the night.
➤ Promote positive family visits (Harkulich & Calamita, 1986).
  ➤ Relate a positive experience you've observed representing a strength or individuality of the person.
  ➤ Encourage the person to be well-dressed and groomed for visits.
  ➤ Encourage activities the person enjoys (e.g., walking, crafts, card games).
  ➤ If appropriate, share the weekly schedule of activities.
  ➤ Elicit suggestions from family for unmet needs.

Rationale: Approaching a family communicates a sense of caring and concern.

➤ Moderate or high anxiety impairs the ability to process information. Simple explanations impart useful information most effectively.

2. Facilitate family strengths.

➤ Acknowledge these strengths to family when appropriate.
  ➤ "I can tell you are a very close family."
  ➤ "You know just how to get your mother to eat."
  ➤ "Your brother means a great deal to you."
➤ Ask family members about care routine at home; determine how involved they want to be.
➤ Involve family members in client care conferences, when appropriate.
➤ Encourage family to find substitutes to care for the ill person to provide the family with time away.
➤ Promote self-esteem of individual members ("Your daughter may respond to your drawings if we place them in her crib"; see Disturbed Self-Concept).
➤ If appropriate, help ill member identify how to give support to caregiver (e.g., praise, listening).

➤ Mobilize ill person to accept responsibility for some activities that contribute to family functioning (e.g., create shopping list, phone inquiries, peel vegetables).

Rationale: The family unit is a system based on interdependent members and patterns that provide structure and support. Hospitalization can disrupt these patterns, leading to family dysfunction. These measures may help maintain an existing family structure, allowing it to function as a supportive unit.

3. Facilitate understanding, in other family members, of how ill person feels.

➤ Discuss stresses of hospitalization.
➤ Describe implications of "sick role" and how it will return to a "well role."
➤ Assist family members to have realistic expectations of the ill member.

Rationale: Evaluating family members' understanding can help identify any needs they may have.

4. Assist family to appraise the situation.

➤ Emphasize the importance of respites to prevent isolating behaviors that foster depression.
➤ Discuss with nonprimary caregivers their responsibilities in caring for the primary caregiver.

Rationale: Adequate support can eliminate or minimize family members feelings that they must "go it alone."

5. Provide anticipatory guidance as illness continues.

➤ Inform parents of effects of prolonged hospitalization on children (appropriate to developmental age).
➤ Prepare family members for signs of depression, anxiety, and dependency, which are a natural part of the illness experience.
➤ If the ill family member is an elderly parent undergoing surgery, inform children that the client may be confused or disoriented for a limited period after surgery.
➤ Refer to Caregiver Role Strain if indicated.

Rationale: Anticipatory guidance can alert family members to impending problems, enabling intervention to prevent the problems from occurring.

6. Discuss the implications of caring for ill family member.

➤ Available resources (financial, environmental)
➤ 24-hour responsibility
➤ Effects on other household members
➤ Likelihood of progressive deterioration

> ➤ Sharing of responsibilities (with other household members, siblings, neighbors)
> ➤ Likelihood of exacerbation of long-standing conflicts
> ➤ Effects on lifestyle
> ➤ Alternative or assistive options (e.g., community-based health care providers, life care centers, group living, nursing home)

Rationale: Illness of a family member may necessitate significant role changes, putting a family at high risk for maladaptation.

7. Identify any dysfunctional coping mechanisms.

> ➤ Substance abuse
> ➤ Continued denial
> ➤ Exploitation of one or more family members
> ➤ Separation or avoidance

Rationale: Families with a history of unsuccessful coping may need additional resources. Families with unresolved conflicts before a member's hospitalization are at high risk. Refer to a specialist.

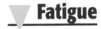 Fatigue

Definition

Fatigue: Self-recognized state in which a person experiences an overwhelming sustained sense of exhaustion and decreased capacity for physical and mental work that is not relieved by rest

Defining Characteristics

MAJOR (80% TO 100%)

Verbalization of an unremitting and overwhelming lack of energy (S)
Inability to maintain usual routines (S)
Verbalization of distress (S)

MINOR (50% TO 79%)

Perceived need for additional energy to accomplish routine tasks (S)
Impaired ability to concentrate (S)
Accident-prone (S)
Increased physical complaints (O)
Decreased performance (S)

Sleep disturbances (S)
Lethargy or listlessness (S)
Lack of interest in surroundings/introspection (S)
Decreased libido (S)
Depression (S)

Related Factors

Many factors can cause fatigue; combining related factors may be useful (e.g., Related to muscle weakness, accumulated waste products, inflammation, and infections secondary to hepatitis).

PATHOPHYSIOLOGIC

Related to hypermetabolic state secondary to

Viruses (e.g., Epstein-Barr)
Fever
Endocarditis

Related to inadequate tissue oxygenation secondary to

Chronic obstructive lung disease
Peripheral vascular disease
Congestive heart failure
Anemia

Related to biochemical changes secondary to

Diabetes mellitus
Hypothyroidism
Pituitary disorders
Addison's disease
AIDS

Related to muscular weakness secondary to

Myasthenia gravis
AIDS
Parkinson's disease
Amyotrophic lateral sclerosis
Multiple sclerosis

Related to hypermetabolic state, competition between body and tumor for nutrients, anemia, and stressors associated with cancer

Related to nutritional deficits or changes in nutrient metabolism secondary to

Nausea
Gastric surgery

Side effects of medications
Diarrhea
Vomiting
Diabetes mellitus

Related to chronic inflammatory process secondary to

Inflammatory bowel disease
Hepatitis
Cirrhosis
Lupus erythematosus
Lyme disease
Arthritis
Renal failure

TREATMENT-RELATED

Related to chemotherapy
Related to radiation therapy
Related to side effects of (specify)
Related to surgical damage to tissue and anesthesia
Related to increased energy expenditure secondary to

➤ Amputation
➤ Nausea/vomiting
➤ Pain
➤ Social isolation
➤ Diarrhea
➤ Fever
➤ Depression

Related to excessive role demands
Related to overwhelming emotional demands
Related to extreme stress
Related to sleep disturbance

Carp's Cue ▸ *Fatigue as a nursing diagnosis differs from acute tiredness. Tiredness is a transient temporary state (Rhoten, 1982) caused by lack of sleep, improper nutrition, increased stress, sedentary lifestyle, or temporarily increased work or social responsibilities. Fatigue is a pervasive, subjective, drained feeling that cannot be eliminated; however, the nurse can assist the person to adapt to it. Activity intolerance differs from fatigue in that the nurse will assist the person with activity intolerance to increase endurance and activity. The focus for the person with fatigue is not on increasing endurance. If the cause resolves or abates (e.g., acute infection, chemotherapy, radiation), Fatigue as a diagnosis is discontinued and Activity Intolerance can be initiated to focus on improving the deconditioned state.*

As a beginning nursing student, you will find Activity Intolerance a useful diagnosis with a client with an acute illness who now cannot tolerate his or her previous level of activity. If your client has a chronic fatigue problem, then Fatigue would be appropriate.

Key Concepts

GENERIC CONSIDERATIONS

➤ Fatigue is a subjective experience with physiologic, situational, and psychological components.

➤ Acute tiredness is an expected response to physical exertion, change in daily activities, additional stress, or inadequate sleep. Acute tiredness is not the same as fatigue.

➤ US society values energy, productivity, and vitality. It views those without energy as sluggish or lazy. It views fatigue and tiredness negatively.

➤ Fatigue can be physical, mental, and motivational. Causes of fatigue are multifactorial. Careful assessment of the causes and interventions to reduce them are critical (Adinolfi, 2001).

➤ Fatigue can be manifested in areas of cortical inhibition (Jiricka, 1994; Rhoten, 1982):
  ➤ Decreased attention
  ➤ Slowed or impaired perception
  ➤ Impaired thinking
  ➤ Decreased motivation
  ➤ Decreased performance in physical and mental activities
  ➤ Loss of fine coordination
  ➤ Poor judgment
  ➤ Indifference to surroundings

➤ People with rheumatoid arthritis reported that their fatigue was related to joint pain. In addition, clients with flare were observed to awaken more often and take longer to walk and perform activities than nonflare clients and the control group (Crosby, 1991).

➤ Cancer-related fatigue has been reported in 35% to 100% of cases and is reported to be the most distressing side effect (Badger et al., 2001). Stressors contributing to fatigue in clients with cancer are illustrated in Table II-5.

➤ Women receiving localized radiation to the breast reported that fatigue decreased in the second week but increased and reached a plateau after week 4 until 3 weeks after treatment ceased. Fatigue levels did not change significantly on weekends between treatments (Greenberg, Sawicka, Eisenthal & Ross, 1992).

Table II–5. CONTRIBUTING FACTORS TO FATIGUE IN CLIENTS WITH CANCER

Pathophysiologic

Hypermetabolic state associated with active tumor growth
Competition between the body and the tumor for nutrients
Chronic pain
Organ dysfunction (e.g., hepatic, respiratory, gastrointestinal)

Treatment-Related

Accumulation of toxic waste products secondary to radiation,
    chemotherapy
Inadequate nutritional intake secondary to nausea, vomiting
Anemia
Analgesics, antiemetics
Diagnostic tests
Surgery

Situational (personal, environmental)

Uncertainty about future
Fear of death, disfigurement
Social isolation
Losses (role responsibilities, occupational, body parts, function, appear-
    ance, economic)
Separation for treatments

➤ When fatigue is a side effect of treatment, it does not resolve when treatment ends but gradually lessens over months (Nail, 1997; Nail & Winningham, 1997).
➤ Depression slows thought processes and leads to decreased physical activities. Work output decreases, and endurance lessens. The effort to continue activity produces fatigue.

GERIATRIC CONSIDERATIONS

➤ The normal effects of aging do not in themselves increase the risk of or cause fatigue. Fatigue in older adults has basically the same etiologies as in younger adults. The difference is that older adults tend to experience more chronic diseases than younger adults. Thus, fatigue in older adults is not the result of age-related factors but is related to such risk factors as chronic diseases and medications.

➤ Depression is the most common psychosocial impairment in older adults. Depression-related affective disturbances affect 27% of adults in a community-living setting (Miller, 2004).

➤ Chronic fatigue and diminished energy are functional consequences of late-life depression (Miller, 2004).

FOCUS ASSESSMENT CRITERIA

Assess for subjective cues:

Onset of fatigue
Pattern: morning, evening, transient, unfading
Precipitated by what?
Relieved by rest?

Effects of fatigue on the following:

ADLs
Mood
Libido
Leisure activities
Concentration
Motivation

Assess for related factors:

Medical condition (acute, chronic; refer to Key Concepts)
Nutritional imbalances
Treatments

➤ Chemotherapy
➤ Medication side effects
➤ Radiation therapy

Stressors

➤ Excessive role demands
➤ Career
➤ Financial
➤ Family
➤ Depression

GOALS

The person will participate in activities that stimulate and balance physical, cognitive, affective, and social domains.

Indicators

Discuss the causes of fatigue
Share feelings regarding the effects of fatigue on life
Establish priorities for daily and weekly activities

GENERAL INTERVENTIONS

Nursing interventions for this diagnosis are for people with fatigue of etiology that cannot be eliminated. The focus is to assess the individual and family to adapt to the fatigue state.

1. Assess causative or contributing factors.

➤ Lack of sleep; refer to *Disturbed Sleep Pattern*
➤ Poor nutrition; refer to *Imbalanced Nutrition*
➤ Sedentary lifestyle; refer to *Health-Seeking Behaviors*
➤ Inadequate stress management; refer to *Health-Seeking Behaviors*
➤ Physiologic impairment
➤ Treatment (chemotherapy, radiation, medications)
➤ Chronic excessive role or social demands

Rationale: Every client experiences some emotional reaction to illness, hospitalization, or new events. The nature and degree of this reaction depends on how the client perceives his or her situation and its anticipated effects—physical, psychological, financial, social, occupational, and spiritual.

2. Explain the causes of Fatigue (see Key Concepts).

Rationale: Providing accurate information can help decrease the client's anxiety associated with the unknown and unfamiliar.

3. Allow expression of feelings regarding the effects of fatigue on life.

➤ Identify difficult activities.
➤ Help client verbalize how fatigue interferes with role responsibilities.
➤ Encourage client to convey how fatigue causes frustration.

Rationale: In many chronic diseases, fatigue is the most common, disruptive, and distressful symptom experienced because it interferes with self-care activities (Hart, Freel & Milde, 1990). Exploring with the client the effects of fatigue on his or her life will help both the nurse and client plan interventions.

4. Assist client to identify strengths, abilities, and interests.

➤ Identify values and interests.
➤ Identify areas of success and usefulness; emphasize past accomplishments.

➤ Use information to develop goals with the client.
➤ Assist client to identify sources of hope (e.g., relationships, faith, things to accomplish).
➤ Assist client to develop realistic short- and long-term goals (progress from simple to more complex; use a "goal poster" to indicate type and time for achieving specific goals).

Rationale: Support people and daily exercises are important tools in anxiety reduction.

5. Assist client to identify energy patterns.

➤ Instruct client to record fatigue levels every hour over 24 hours; select a usual day.
➤ Ask client to rate fatigue using the Rhoten fatigue scale (0 = not tired, 10 = total exhaustion).
  ➤ Record the activities during each activity.
➤ Analyze together the 24-hour fatigue levels.
  ➤ Times of peak energy
  ➤ Times of exhaustion
  ➤ Activities associated with increasing fatigue
➤ Explain benefits of exercise and what is realistic.

Rationale: Identifying times of peak energy and exhaustion can aid in planning activities to maximize energy conservation and productivity.

6. Assist client to identify tasks he or she can delegate.

➤ Explore what activities the client views as important to maintain self-esteem.
➤ Attempt to divide vital activities or tasks into components (e.g., preparing menus, shopping, storing, cooking, serving, cleaning up); client can delegate some parts and retain others.
➤ Plan important tasks during periods of high energy (e.g., prepare all meals in the morning).

Rationale: Such strategies can enable continuation of activities and contribute to positive self-esteem.

7. Explain the purpose of pacing and prioritization.

➤ Assist client to identify priorities and to eliminate nonessential activities.
➤ Plan each day to avoid energy- and time-consuming nonessential decision-making.
➤ Organize work with needed items within easy reach.
➤ Distribute difficult tasks throughout the week.
➤ Rest before difficult tasks and stop before fatigue ensues.

Rationale: The client requires rest periods before or after some activities. Planning can provide for adequate rest and reduce unnecessary energy expenditure. Such strategies can enable continuation of activities, contributing to positive self-esteem.

8. Teach energy conservation techniques.

➤ Modify the environment.
  ➤ Replace steps with ramps
  ➤ Install grab rails
  ➤ Elevate chairs to 3 to 4 inches
  ➤ Organize kitchen or work areas
  ➤ Reduce trips up and down stairs (e.g., put a commode on the first floor)
➤ Plan small frequent meals to decrease energy required for digestion.
➤ Use taxi instead of driving self.
➤ Delegate housework (e.g., employ a high school student for a few hours after school).

Rationale: Such strategies can enable continuation of activities and contribute to positive self-esteem.

9. Promote socialization with family and friends (Dzurec, 2000).

➤ Encourage client to participate in one social activity a week.
➤ Explain that feelings of correctedness decrease fatigue.

Rationale: Dzurec (2000) found that relatedness was linked to fatigue. People with fatigue who become disconnected from interpersonal relationships became more fatigued.

10. Explain effects of conflict and stress on energy levels.

➤ Teach the importance of mutuality in sharing concerns.
➤ Explain the benefits of distraction from negative events.
➤ Teach the value of confronting issues.
➤ Teach and assist with relaxation techniques before anticipated stressful events. Encourage mental imagery to promote positive thought processes.
➤ Allow client time to reminisce to gain insight into past experiences.
➤ Teach to maximize aesthetic experiences (e.g., smell of coffee, feeling warmth of the sun).
➤ Teach to anticipate experiences the client takes delight in each day (e.g., walking, reading favorite book, writing letter).

Rationale: In many chronic diseases, fatigue is the most common, disruptive, and distressing symptom because it interferes with self-care activities (Hart, Freel & Milde, 2001).

▼ Fear

Definition

Fear: State in which an individual or group experiences a feeling of physiologic or emotional disruption related to an identifiable source that is perceived as dangerous.

Defining Characteristics

Assess for subjective (S) and objective (O) cues:

MAJOR (MUST BE PRESENT, ONE OR MORE)

Feeling of dread, fright, apprehension and/or (S)
Behaviors of

➤ Avoidance (S)
➤ Narrowing of focus on danger (O)
➤ Deficits in attention, performance, and control (O)

MINOR (MAY BE PRESENT)

Verbal reports of panic, obsessions (S)
Behavioral acts (O)

➤ Crying
➤ Compulsive mannerisms
➤ Hypervigilance
➤ Dysfunctional immobility
➤ Escape
➤ Aggression
➤ Increased questioning/verbalization

Visceral-somatic activity (S,O)
Musculoskeletal
➤ Shortness of breath
➤ Muscle tightness
➤ Fatigue/limb weakness

Respiratory
➤ Increased rate
➤ Trembling

Cardiovascular
➤ Palpitations
➤ Rapid pulse
➤ Increased blood pressure

Skin

- ➤ Flush/pallor
- ➤ Sweating
- ➤ Paraesthesia

Gastrointestinal
- ➤ Anorexia
- ➤ Dry mouth/throat
- ➤ Nausea/vomiting
- ➤ Diarrhea/urge to defecate

CNS/perceptual
- ➤ Syncope
- ➤ Absentmindedness
- ➤ Pupil dilation
- ➤ Irritability
- ➤ Lack of concentration
- ➤ Insomnia
- ➤ Nightmares

Genitourinary
- ➤ Urinary frequency/urgency

Related Factors

Fear can be a response to various health problems, situations, or conflicts. Some common sources are indicated next.

PATHOPHYSIOLOGIC

Related to perceived immediate and long-term effects of the following:

Loss of body part
Terminal disease
Cognitive impairment
Permanent disability
Disabling illness
Loss of body function
Sensory impairment

TREATMENT-RELATED

Related to loss of control and unpredictable outcome secondary to

Hospitalization
Radiation
Invasive procedures

Anesthesia
Surgery and its outcome

SITUATIONAL (PERSONAL, ENVIRONMENTAL)

Related to loss of control and unpredictable outcome secondary to the following:

Change or loss of significant other
Divorce
Related to potential loss of income
Pain
Strangers
Lack of knowledge
Marriage
Aging
New environment
Success
Failure
Parenthood/pregnancy

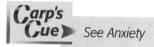 *See Anxiety*

Key Concepts

GENERIC CONSIDERATIONS

➤ Psychological defense mechanisms are distinctly individual and can be adaptive and maladaptive.
➤ Fear differs from anxiety in that fear is aroused by an identified threat (specific object); anxiety is aroused by a threat that cannot be easily identified (nonspecific or unknown).
➤ Both fear and anxiety lead to disequilibrium.
➤ Anger may be a response to certain fears.
➤ A sense of adequacy in confronting danger reduces fear. Awareness of factors that intensify fears enhances control and prevents heightened feelings. Confronting the safe reality of a situation reduces fear.
➤ Fear can become anxiety if it becomes internalized and serves to disorganize instead of becoming adaptive.
➤ Chronic physical reactions to stressors lead to susceptibility and chronic disease.
➤ People interpret the degree of danger from a threatening stimulus. The physiologic and psychological systems react with equal intensity (elevations in blood pressure and heart and respiratory rates).
➤ Fear is adaptive and a healthy response to danger.

➤ Fear differs from phobia, an irrational persistent fear of a circumscribed stimulus (object or situation) other than having a panic attack (panic disorder) or of humiliation or embarrassment in certain social situations (social phobia).

➤ Cesarone (1991) clustered the sources of fear in the elderly into five categories:

➤ Disease, suffering

➤ Dependence, abandonment

➤ Dying

➤ Illness or death of a loved one

➤ Miscellaneous reasons (crime, financial insecurity, diagnostic tests)

FOCUS ASSESSMENT CRITERIA

Assess for subjective (S) and objective (O) cues:

Subjective/Objective Data

Defining Characteristics

Onset

➤ Have the person tell you "story" about his or her fearfulness.

Thought process and content

➤ Are thoughts clear, coherent, logical, confused or forgetful?

➤ Can client concentrate or is he or she preoccupied?

Perception and judgment

➤ Does fear remain after stressor is eliminated?

➤ Is the fear a response to present stimulus or distorted by past influences?

Visceral-somatic activity

➤ (see Defining Characteristics)

GOALS

The adult will relate increased psychological and physiologic comfort.

Indicators

Show decreased visceral response (pulse, respirations)
Differentiate real from imagined situations.
Describe effective and ineffective coping patterns.
Identify own coping responses.

GENERAL INTERVENTIONS

Nursing interventions for *Fear* represent interventions for any person with fear regardless of the etiologic or contributing factors.

1. Assess possible contributing factors.

➤ Perception of threatening stimulus (realistic)
   ➢ Unfamiliar environment (new home, hospital admission, new people)
   ➢ Intrusion on personal space
   ➢ Lifestyle change (promotion, marriage/divorce, retirement)
   ➢ Biologic and physiologic change (dysfunction, disability, pain)
   ➢ Threat to self-esteem (abandonment, rejection)
   ➢ Distorted perceptions of dangerous stimulus

2. Reduce or eliminate contributing factors.

➤ Unfamiliar environment
   ➢ Orient client to environment using simple explanations
   ➢ Speak slowly and calmly
   ➢ Avoid surprises and painful stimuli
   ➢ Use soft lights and music
   ➢ Remove threatening stimulus
   ➢ Plan one-day-at-a-time, familiar routine
   ➢ Encourage gradual mastery of a situation
➤ Provide transitional object with symbolic safeness (security blanket, religious medals)

Rationale: Providing accurate information can help decrease the client's anxiety associated with the unknown and unfamiliar.

➤ Intrusion on personal space
   ➢ Allow personal space
   ➢ Move person away from stimulus
   ➢ Remain with person until fear subsides (listen, use silence)
➤ Later, establish frequent and consistent contacts; use family members and significant others to stay with person

➤ Use touch as tolerated (sometimes holding person firmly helps him or her maintain control)

Rationale: Feelings of being safe increase when a person identifies with another person who has successfully dealt with a similar fearful situation.

3. When intensity of feelings has increased, assist with insight and controlling response.

➤ Bring behavioral cues into client's awareness
➤ Teach signs that indicate increased fear (e.g., "Your face flushes and you clench your fists when we discuss your discharge.")
  ➤ Indicate adaptiveness of behavior
➤ Explain how expressed fear of one thing may hide fear of something else
➤ Teach how to solve problems
  ➤ What is the problem?
  ➤ Who or what is responsible?
  ➤ What are the options?
  ➤ What are the advantages and disadvantages of each option?
➤ Teach ways to enhance control
➤ Include client in treatment process (e.g., "Please raise your hand if the procedure causes pain.")
  ➤ Share test results when appropriate
  ➤ Inform ahead of time about tests (time interval depends on ability to cope)
  ➤ Identify activities that rechannel emotional energy to diffuse intensity
➤ Use nightlight or flashlight to diffuse fear (give child with fear of dark a flashlight to use as needed)
➤ Before tests or surgery, prepare client as to what to expect, especially sensations; define this role and how to participate in it (e.g., postoperative breathing exercises may distract from fears and dissipate physical reaction)

Rationale: Open honest dialogue may help initiate constructive problem solving and can instill hope.

4. Initiate health teaching and referrals as indicated.

➤ Recommend or instruct concerning methods that increase comfort or relaxation
  ➤ Progressive relaxation technique
  ➤ Desensitization, self-coaching
  ➤ Yoga, hypnosis, assertiveness training
  ➤ Reading, music, breathing exercises
  ➤ Thought stopping, guided fantasy

> ➤ Participate in community functions to teach parents age-related fears and constructive interventions (e.g., parent-school organizations, civic groups)

Rationale: Support people and daily exercises are important tools in anxiety reduction.

▼ Deficient Fluid Volume

Definition

Deficient Fluid Volume: State in which a person who can take fluids (not NPO) experiences or is at risk of experiencing vascular, interstitial, or intracellular dehydration.

MAJOR (MUST BE PRESENT, ONE OR MORE)

Insufficient oral fluid intake (O)
Negative balance of intake and output (O)
Dry skin/mucous membranes (O)
Weight loss (O)

MINOR (MAY BE PRESENT)

Increased serum sodium (O)
Concentrated urine and urinary frequency (O)
Thirst/nausea/anorexia (S)
Decreased urine output or excessive urine output (O)

Related Factors

PATHOPHYSIOLOGIC

Related to excessive urinary output secondary to, e.g.,

Uncontrolled diabetes
Diabetes insipidus (inadequate antidiuretic hormone)

Related to increased capillary permeability and evaporative loss from burn wound (nonacute)
Related to losses secondary to, e.g.,

Fever or increased metabolic rate
Abnormal drainage (wound, excessive menses)
Diarrhea

SITUATIONAL (PERSONAL, ENVIRONMENTAL)

Related to vomiting/nausea
Related to decreased motivation to drink liquids secondary to, e.g.,

Depression
Fatigue

Related to fad diets/fasting
Related to high-solute tube feedings
Related to difficulty swallowing or feeding self secondary to, e.g.,

Oral or throat pain
Fatigue

Related to extreme heat/sun/dryness
Related to excessive loss through

Indwelling catheters
Drains

Related to insufficient fluids for exercise effort or weather conditions
Related to excessive use of, e.g.,

Laxatives
Enemas

Related to increased vulnerability secondary to

Decreased fluid reserve and decreased sensation of thirst (older adult)

Deficient Fluid Volume is frequently used incorrectly in the clinical setting. This author recommends for you to differentiate between dehydration in those with insufficient oral fluid and those who are NPO and/or in shock. Those who can drink but are not drinking enough fluids, use Deficient Fluid Volume. Those who cannot drink or are at risk for fluid loss from bleeding or are in shock, refer to the appropriate collaborative problem as Fluid/Electrolyte Imbalance or Hypovolemia for medical and nursing interventions in Section III.

Key Concepts

GENERIC CONSIDERATIONS

➤ Table II-6 shows average intake and output over 24 hours for an adult. Ingested and excreted water and electrolytes (sodium, potassium, chloride) influence fluid balance.
➤ The two main causes of deficient fluid volume are inadequate fluid intake and increased fluid and electrolyte losses (e.g., GI, urinary, skin, third-space [edema]).

Table II–6. AVERAGE INTAKE AND OUTPUT IN AN ADULT FOR A 24-HOUR PERIOD

Intake		Output	
Oral liquids	1,300 ml	Urine	1500 ml
Water in food	1,000 ml	Stool	200 ml
Water produced by		Insensible	
Metabolism	300 ml	Lungs	300 ml
TOTAL	2,600 ml	Skin	600 ml
		TOTAL	2,600 ml

Metheny N. (2000). *Fluid and electrolyte balance: Nursing considerations* (4th ed.). Philadelphia: Lippincott Williams & Wilkins.

➤ Vomiting or gastric suctioning results in fluid, potassium, and hydrogen losses.
➤ The thirst sensation primarily regulates fluid intake. The kidneys' ability to concentrate urine primarily regulates fluid output.
➤ Urine specific gravity reflects the kidneys' ability to concentrate urine; the range of urine specific gravity varies with the state of hydration and the solids to be excreted. (Specific gravity is elevated with dehydration, signifying concentrated urine.) Normal values are 1.005 to 1.030. Diluted values are less than 1.005.
➤ People at high risk for fluid imbalance include the following:
 ➤ Those taking medication for fluid retention, high blood pressure, seizures, or "anxiety" (tranquilizers).
 ➤ Those with diabetes, cardiac disease, excessive alcohol intake, malnourishment, obesity, or GI distress.
 ➤ Adults older than 60 years, and children younger than 6 years.
 ➤ Those who are confused, depressed, comatose, or lethargic (no sensation of thirst)
 ➤ Athletes unaware of the need to replace electrolytes as well as fluids.
➤ Excessive fluid and electrolyte loss can be expected during the following:
 ➤ Fever or increased metabolic rate
 ➤ Extreme exercise or diaphoresis
 ➤ Climate extremes (heat/dryness)
 ➤ Excessive vomiting or diarrhea
➤ Fluid balance maintenance is a major concern for all athletes competing in hot climates. The following is true for both men and women (Maughan, Leiper & Shirreffs, 1997):
 ➤ Drinking large volumes of plain water will inhibit thirst and promote a diuretic response.
 ➤ To maintain hydration during extreme exercise, high levels of sodium (as much as 50 to 60 mmol) and possibly some potassium to replace losses in sweat are needed.

> ➤ Palatability of drinks is important to stimulate intake and ensure adequate volume replacement.
> ➤ Because adequate hydration greatly affects athletic performance, the goal should be to be hydrated at the beginning of exercise and to maintain hydration as well as possible thereafter, focusing on replacing salt loss as well as water.

GERIATRIC CONSIDERATIONS

> ➤ Older adults are more susceptible to fluid loss and dehydration because of the following (Miller, 2004)
>   > ➤ Decreased percentage of total body water
>   > ➤ Decreased renal blood flow and glomerular filtration
>   > ➤ Impaired ability to regulate temperature
>   > ➤ Decreased ability to concentrate urine
>   > ➤ Increased physical disabilities (decreased access to fluids)
>   > ➤ Self-limiting of fluids for fear of incontinence
>   > ➤ Diminished thirst sensation
> ➤ About 75% of fluid intake in older adults occurs between 6 am and 6 pm (Miller, 2004).
> ➤ Cognitive impairments can interfere with recognition of cues of thirst.
> ➤ Dehydration, defined as diminished total body water content, is the most common fluid and electrolyte disturbance among older adults. Because it is associated with morbidity rates, careful screening and prevention in primary care settings are essential.

FOCUS ASSESSMENT CRITERIA

Subjective Data

Assess for Defining Characteristics

> ➤ Fluid intake (amounts, type)
> ➤ Thirst
> ➤ Nausea, anorexia

Assess for related factors
Refer to Related Factors

Objective Data

Assess for Defining Characteristics

> ➤ Present weight/usual weight
> ➤ Intake (last 2 to 48 hours)

➤ Weight loss (How much? Since when?)
➤ Skin
➤ Mucosa (lips, gums) (dry)
➤ Tongue (furrowed/dry)
➤ Color (pale or flushed)
➤ Moisture (dry or diaphoretic)
➤ Fontanelles of infants (depressed)
➤ Eyeballs (sunken)
➤ Urine output
   ➤ Amount (varied; very large or minimal amount)
   ➤ Color (amber; very dark or very light; clear?; cloudy?)
   ➤ Specific gravity (increased or decreased)
   ➤ Odor?

Assess for Related Factors

➤ Abnormal or excessive fluid loss
   ➤ Liquid stools
   ➤ Diuresis or polyuria
   ➤ Fever
   ➤ Vomiting or gastric suction (e.g., fistulas, drains)
   ➤ Abnormal or excessive drainage
   ➤ Diaphoresis
   ➤ Loss of skin surfaces (e.g., healing burns)

Decreased fluid intake related to

➤ Fatigue
➤ Depression/disorientation
➤ Physical limitations (e.g., cannot hold a glass)
➤ Decreased level of consciousness
➤ Nausea or anorexia

For more information on Focus Assessment Criteria, visit http://connection.lww.com.

GOAL

The person will maintain urine specific gravity within normal range.

Indicators

Increase fluid intake to a specified amount according to age and metabolic needs.

Identify risk factors for fluid deficit and relate need for increased fluid intake as indicated.

Demonstrate no signs and symptoms of dehydration.

GENERAL INTERVENTIONS

1. Assess causative factors.

➤ Inability to feed self
➤ Dislike of available fluids
➤ Sore throat/mouth
➤ Extreme fatigue or weakness
➤ Lack of knowledge (of the need for increased fluid or electrolyte intake)
➤ Difficulty swallowing (see *Impaired Swallowing*)
➤ Inadequate fluid intake before and during exercise (usually in athletes)
➤ Vomiting
➤ Fever
➤ Wound drainage
➤ Diarrhea

2. Reduce or eliminate causative factors.

➤ Inability to feed self (see *Deficient Self-Care*)
➤ Dislike of available liquids
  ➤ Assess likes and dislikes; provide favorite fluids with dietary restrictions
➤ Plan an intake goal for each shift (e.g., 1,000 ml during the day; 800 ml during afternoon; 300 ml at night)
➤ Set a schedule for supplementary liquids
➤ Sore throat/mouth
  ➤ Offer warm or cold fluids; consider ices
  ➤ Consider warm saline gargle or anesthetic lozenges before fluids
➤ Extreme fatigue or weakness
  ➤ Give small amounts of fluids frequently
  ➤ Provide for rest periods before meals

Rationale: Identifying the specific cause of decreased fluid intake can help with individualizing the plan.

➤ Lack of knowledge
➤ Assess client's understanding of reasons to maintain adequate hydration and methods to reach fluid intake goal
  ➤ Include significant others
  ➤ Proceed with teaching
➤ Vomiting
➤ Encourage small frequent ice chips or clear fluids; see *Diarrhea* for replacement therapy.

Rationale: The focus of treatment is replacing both water and electrolytes lost (Porth, 2002). Careful daily monitoring of weight and intake and output is needed.

➤ Diarrhea/loose stools
  ➤ See *Diarrhea*
➤ Wound drainage
  ➤ Keep careful records of amount and type of drainage
➤ Weigh dressings, if necessary, to estimate fluid loss (weigh a wet dressing; weigh the dry dressing of the same type; compare the difference)
➤ Weigh client daily if drainage is excessive and difficult to measure (e.g., soaked sheets)
➤ Replace fluid loss (may be contraindicated in cardiac failure, renal failure, or head trauma)

Rationale: The focus of treatment is replacing both water and electrolytes lost (Porth, 2002). Careful monitoring of weight and intake and output is needed.

3. Prevent dehydration

➤ Monitor intake; ensure at least 2,000 ml of oral fluids every 24 hours
➤ Monitor output; ensure at least 1,000 to 1,500 ml every 24 hours
➤ Monitor serum electrolyte studies as needed
➤ Offer fluids in large glasses, 120 to 240 ml
➤ Weigh daily in same clothes, at same time. A 2% to 4% weight loss indicates mild dehydration; 5% to 9% weight loss indicates moderate dehydration
➤ Monitor urine and serum electrolytes, blood urea nitrogen, osmolality, creatinine, hematocrit, and hemoglobin
➤ For people scheduled to fast before diagnostic studies, advise them to increase fluid intake 8 hours before fasting
➤ Review client's medications: Do they contribute to dehydration (e.g., diuretics)? Do they require increased fluid intake (e.g., lithium)?
➤ Teach that coffee, tea, and grapefruit juice are diuretics and can contribute to fluid loss
➤ Consider the additional fluid losses associated with vomiting, diarrhea, and fever

Rationale: Output may exceed intake, which already may be inadequate to compensate for insensible losses. Dehydration may increase glomerular filtration rate, making output inadequate to clear wastes properly and leading to elevated blood urea nitrogen and electrolyte levels. Accurate daily weights can detect fluid loss. To monitor weight effectively, weights should be measured at the same time on the same scale with the same clothes.

4. Initiate health teaching, as indicated.

➤ Give verbal and written directions for desired fluids and amounts
➤ Include the person/family in keeping a written record of fluid intake, output, and daily weights
➤ Provide a list of alternative fluids (e.g., ice cream, pudding)

> ➤ Explain the need to increase fluids during exercise, fever, infection, and hot weather
> ➤ Seek medical consultation for continued dehydration

Rationale: Specific interventions can help reduce dehydration after discharge.

5. For athletes, stress the need to hydrate before and during exercise, preferably with a high-sodium-content beverage (refer to *Hyperthermia* for additional interventions).

▼ Excess Fluid Volume

Definition

Excess Fluid Volume: State in which a person experiences or is at high risk of experiencing intracellular or interstitial fluid overload.

Defining Characteristics

MAJOR (MUST BE PRESENT, ONE OR MORE)

Edema (peripheral, sacral)
Taut shiny skin

MINOR (MAY BE PRESENT)

Intake greater than output
Shortness of breath
Weight gain

Related Factors

PATHOPHYSIOLOGIC

Related to compromised regulatory mechanisms secondary to

Renal failure (acute or chronic)
Endocrine dysfunction
Systemic and metabolic abnormalities
Lymphedema

Related to portal hypertension, lower plasma colloidal osmotic pressure, and sodium retention secondary to

Liver disease
Cancer

Cirrhosis
Ascites

Related to venous and arterial abnormalities secondary to

Varicose veins
Peripheral vascular disease
Phlebitis
Thrombus
Immobility
Lymphedema
Infection
Trauma
Neoplasms

TREATMENT-RELATED

Related to sodium and water retention secondary to, e.g.,

Corticosteroid

Related to inadequate lymphatic drainage secondary to

Mastectomy

SITUATIONAL (PERSONAL, ENVIRONMENTAL)

Related to excessive sodium intake/fluid intake
Related to low protein intake

Fad diets
Malnutrition

Related to dependent venous pooling/venostasis secondary to

Standing or sitting for long periods of time
Immobility
Obesity
Tight cast or bandage

Related to venous compression from pregnant uterus

Excess Fluid Volume *frequently is used to describe pulmonary edema, ascites, or renal failure. These are all collaborative problems that should not be renamed as* Excess Fluid Volume. *This diagnosis represents a situation for which nurses can prescribe if the focus is on peripheral edema. Nursing interventions center on teaching the client or family how to minimize edema and on protecting tissue.*

Key Concepts

GENERIC CONSIDERATIONS

➤ See *Deficient Fluid Volume.*

➤ Edema results from the accumulation of fluid in the interstitial compartment of the extravascular space. Without intervention, edema can progress to further tissue damage and permanent swelling.

➤ Determining the underlying cause is essential to identifying specific interventions.

➤ Peripheral edema should be classified as unilateral or bilateral. Unilateral usually results from venous and arterial abnormalities, lymphedema, infection, trauma, and neoplasms. Bilateral usually results from congestive heart failure, systemic and metabolic abnormalities, endocrine dysfunction, lipedema, and pregnancy (Terry, O'Brien & Kerstein, 1998).

➤ Distribution of peripheral edema is important to differentiating its etiology (Powell & Armstrong, 1997).

➤ People with cardiac pump failure are at high risk for excesses in both vascular and tissue fluids (i.e., pulmonary and peripheral edema). Pulmonary edema is a medical emergency.

➤ The most frequent vascular cause of tissue edema is increased venous pressure, which leads to increased capillary blood pressure. Obesity is one cause.

➤ Older adults are more prone to stasis edema of the feet and ankles as a result of increased vein tortuosity and dilatation and decreased valve efficiency (Miller, 2004).

FOCUS ASSESSMENT CRITERIA

Subjective Data

Assess for subjective (S) and objective (O) cues.
History of symptoms
Complaints of

➤ Shortness of breath (S)

➤ Edema (O)

➤ Weakness/fatigue (S)

➤ Weight gain (O)

Assess for related factors
See Related Factors

Objective Data

Assess for defining characteristics

➤ Signs of fluid overload (O)
  ➤ Pulse (bounding or dysrhythmic)
➤ Respirations (Rate [tachypnea], lung sounds [rales or ronchi], quality [labored or shallow])
  ➤ Blood pressure (elevated)
  ➤ Edema
  ➤ Press thumb for at least 5 seconds into the skin and note any remaining indentations.
➤ Rate edema according to the following scale:
  ➤ None = 0
  ➤ Trace = +1
  ➤ Moderate = +2
  ➤ Deep = +3
  ➤ Very deep = +4
➤ Note degree and location (feet, ankles, legs, arms, sacral, generalized).
➤ Weight gain (weigh daily on the same scale at the same time)
➤ Neck vein distention (distended neck veins at 45-degree elevation of head may indicate fluid overload or decreased cardiac output).

GOALS

The person will exhibit decreased edema (specify site).

Indicators

Relate causative factors
Relate methods of preventing edema

GENERAL INTERVENTIONS

1. Identify contributing and causative factors.

➤ Improper diet (inadequate protein intake, excessive sodium intake)
➤ Dependent venous pooling/venostasis
➤ Inadequate lymphatic drainage

2. Reduce or eliminate causative and contributing factors.

Improper diet

➤ Assess dietary intake and habits that may contribute to fluid retention
   ➤ Be specific; record daily and weekly intake of food and fluids
➤ Assess weekly diet for inadequate protein or excessive sodium intake
➤ Discuss likes and dislikes of foods that provide protein
➤ Teach client to plan weekly menu that provides protein at an affordable price
➤ Teach client to decrease salt intake
   ➤ Read labels for sodium content
   ➤ Avoid convenience, canned, and frozen foods
➤ Cook without salt; use spices (lemon, basil, tarragon, mint) to add flavor
➤ Use vinegar in place of salt to flavor soups, stews, etc. (e.g., 2 to 3 teaspoons of vinegar to 4 to 6 quarts, according to taste)
➤ Ascertain whether client may use salt substitute (caution that he or she must use the exact substitute prescribed)

Rationale: Identifying the specific cause of decreased fluid intake can help with individualizing the plan.

Dependent venous pooling

➤ Assess for evidence of dependent venous pooling or venostasis
➤ Encourage altering periods of horizontal rest (legs elevated) with vertical activity (standing); this may be contraindicated in congestive heart failure
➤ Keep edematous extremity elevated above level of the heart whenever possible (unless contraindicated by heart failure)
➤ Elevate legs whenever possible, using pillows under legs (avoid pressure points, especially behind knees)
➤ Keep edematous arms elevated on two pillows or with IV pole sling
➤ Discourage leg and ankle crossing
➤ Reduce constriction of vessels
   ➤ Assess clothing for proper fit and constrictive areas
➤ Instruct client to avoid panty girdles/garters, knee-highs, and leg crossing and to practice elevating legs when possible
➤ Consider using antiembolism stockings or Ace bandages
   ➤ Apply stockings while lying down (e.g., in the morning before arising)
➤ Check extremities frequently for adequate circulation and evidence of constrictive areas

Rationale: Compression stockings promote venous return and reduce chronic leg edema.

Inadequate lymphatic drainage

- Keep extremity elevated on pillows
- If edema is present, the arm should be elevated, but not in adduction (this position may constrict the axilla)
  - The elbow should be higher than the shoulder
  - The hand should be higher than the elbow
- Measure blood pressure in the unaffected arm
- Do not give injections or start IV fluids in affected arm
- Protect affected limb from injury
- Teach client to avoid using strong detergents, carrying heavy bags, holding cigarettes, injuring cuticles or hangnails, reaching into hot ovens, wearing jewelry or wristwatch, or using Ace bandages
- Advise client to apply lanolin or similar cream often daily to prevent dry flaky skin
- Encourage client to wear a Medic-Alert tag engraved with *Caution: lymphedema arm—no tests—no needle injections*
- Caution client to visit a doctor if arm becomes red, swollen, or unusually hard
- After a mastectomy, encourage ROM exercises and use of affected arm to facilitate development of collateral lymphatic drainage system (explain that lymphedema often decreases within 1 month but that she should continue massaging, exercising, and elevating the arm for 3 to 4 months after surgery).

Rationale: Elevation facilitates lymphatic drainage and prevents pooling. Lymphedema causes tissue compression, decreased circulation, and decreased sensation which all increase the risk of injury (Chapman & Goodman, 2000).

3. Protect edematous skin from injury.

- Inspect skin for redness and blanching
- Reduce pressure on skin areas; pad chairs, knee-high stockings, and footstools
- Prevent dry skin
  - Use soap sparingly
  - Rinse off soap completely
  - Use a lotion to moisten skin

Rationale: Edema inhibits blood flow to the tissue, resulting in poor cellular nutrition and increased susceptibility to injury.

4. Initiate health teaching and referrals, as indicated.

- Give clear verbal and written instructions for all medications: what, when, why, how often, side effects; pay special attention to drugs that directly influence fluid balance (e.g., diuretics, steroids)

➤ Write down instructions for diet, activity, use of Ace bandages, stockings, and so forth
➤ Have client demonstrate the instructions
➤ Have client keep a written record of intake/output
➤ With severe fluctuations in edema, have client weigh himself or herself every morning and before bedtime daily; instruct client to keep a written record of weights. For less severe illness, the client may need to weigh himself or herself daily only and record.
➤ Consider home care or visiting nurses referral to follow at home
➤ Provide literature concerning low-salt diets; consult with a dietitian if necessary

Rationale: Specific instructions can help to prevent edema after discharge.

▼ Ineffective Health Maintenance

Definition

Ineffective Health Maintenance: State in which a person or group experiences or is at risk of experiencing a disruption in health because of an unhealthy lifestyle or lack of knowledge to manage a condition.

Defining Characteristics (In the Absence of Disease)

MAJOR (MUST BE PRESENT, ONE OR MORE)

Reports or demonstrates an unhealthy practice or lifestyle:

Reckless driving
Overeating
Substance abuse
High-fat diet

MINOR (MAY BE PRESENT)

Reports or demonstrates the following:

Skin and nails

➤ Malodorous
➤ Skin lesions (pustules, rashes, dry or scaly skin)
➤ Unexplained scars
➤ Sunburn
➤ Unusual color, pallor

Respiratory system

➤ Frequent infections
➤ Dyspnea with exertion
➤ Chronic cough

Oral cavity

➤ Frequent sores (on tongue, buccal, mucosa)
➤ Loss of teeth at early age
➤ Lesions associated with lack of oral care or substance abuse (leukoplakia, fistulas)

GI system and nutrition

➤ Obesity
➤ Chronic bowel irregularity
➤ Chronic anemia
➤ Chronic dyspepsia
➤ Anorexia
➤ Cachexia

Musculoskeletal system

➤ Frequent muscle strain, backaches, neck pain
➤ Diminished flexibility and muscle strength

Genitourinary system

➤ Frequent sexually transmitted infections
➤ Frequent use of potentially unhealthy over-the-counter products (e.g., chemical douches, perfumed vaginal products, nasal sprays)

Constitutional

➤ Chronic fatigue

Neurosensory

➤ Facial tics (nonconvulsant)

Psychoemotional

➤ Emotional fragility
➤ Behavior disorders (compulsiveness, belligerence)
➤ Frequent feelings of being overwhelmed

Related Factors

Various factors can produce Ineffective Health Maintenance. Common causes are listed next.

SITUATIONAL (PERSONAL, ENVIRONMENTAL)

Related to the following:

Information misinterpretation
Lack of access to adequate health care services
Lack of motivation
Inadequate health teaching
Lack of education or readiness
Impaired ability to understand secondary to (specify)

MATURATIONAL

Table II-7 lists age-related conditions.
Related to lack of education or to age-related factors. Examples include the following:

Child

➤ Sexuality and sexual development
➤ Inactivity
➤ Substance abuse
➤ Poor nutrition
➤ Safety hazards

Adolescent

➤ Same as children
➤ Substance abuse
➤ Vehicle safety practices

Adult

➤ Parenthood
➤ Safety practices
➤ Sexual function

Older adult

➤ Effects of aging
➤ Sensory deficits

Carp's Cue▶ *The nursing diagnosis Ineffective Health Maintenance applies to both well and ill populations. Health is a dynamic ever-changing state defined by the individual based on his or her perception of highest level of functioning (e.g., a marathon runner's definition of health will differ from a paraplegic person's). Because clients are responsible for their own health, Ineffective Health Maintenance represents a diagnosis that the person is motivated to treat. An important associated nursing responsibility involves raising client consciousness that better health is possible.*

Table II–7. PRIMARY AND SECONDARY PREVENTION FOR AGE-RELATED CONDITIONS

Developmental Level	Primary Prevention	Secondary Prevention

Infancy (0–1 year)	Parent education
	  Infant safety
	  Nutrition
	  Breast feeding
	Sensory stimulation
	  Infant massage and touch
	  Visual stimulation
	    Activity
	    Colors
	  Auditory stimulation
	    Verbal
	    Music
	Immunizations
	  DPT or DTaP
	  tOPV or IPV, Hib } at 2, 4, and
	  Hepatitis B 6 months
	  H. influenzae (2, 4 months)
	Oral hygiene
	  Teething biscuits
	  Fluoride (if needed > 6 months)
	  Avoid sugared food and drink
		Complete physical examination
		  every 2–3 months
		Screening at birth
		  Congenital hip dysplasia
		  PKU
		  G-6-PD deficiency in blacks,
		    Mediterranean, and Far
		    Eastern origin children
		  Sickle cell
		  Hemoglobin or hematocrit
		    (for anemia)
		  Cystic fibrosis
		  Vision (startle reflex)
		  Hearing (response to and
		    localization of sounds)
		  TB test at 12 months
		  Developmental assessments
		Screen and intervene for high risk
		  Low birth weight
		  Maternal substance abuse
		    during pregnancy
		      Alcohol: fetal alcohol syndrome
		      Cigarettes: SIDS
		      Drugs: addicted neonate, AIDS
		  Maternal infections during
		    pregnancy

Preschool (1–5 years)	Parent education
	  Teething
	  Discipline
	  Nutrition
	  Accident prevention
	  Normal growth and
	    development
	Child education
	  Dental self-care
	  Dressing
	  Bathing with assistance
	  Feeding self-care
		Complete physical examination
		  between 2 and 3 years and
		  preschool (UA, CBC)
		TB test at 3 years
		Development assessments (annual)
		  Speech development
		  Hearing
		  Vision
		Screen and intervene
		  Lead poisoning
		  Developmental lag
		  Neglect or abuse

(table continues on p. 228)

**Table II–7. PRIMARY AND SECONDARY PREVENTION
FOR AGE-RELATED CONDITIONS (*Continued*)**

Developmental Level	Primary Prevention	Secondary Prevention

Preschool (1–5 years)	Immunizations
	  DTaP ⎫
	  TOPV ⎬ at 18 months
	  MMR at 12–15 months
	  HIB at 24 months
	  H. influenzae (for high risk)
	Dental/oral hygiene
	  Fluoride treatments
	  Fluoridated water
		Strong family history of arteriosclerotic diseases (e.g., MI, CVA, peripheral vascular disease), diabetes, hypertension, gout, or hyper-lipidemia—fasting serum cholesterol at age 2 years, then every 3–5 years if normal
		Strabismus
		Hearing deficit
		Vision deficit

School age (6–11 years)	Health education of child
	  "Basic 4" nutrition
	  Accident prevention
	  Outdoor safety
	  Substance abuse counsel
	  Anticipatory guidance for physical changes at puberty
	Immunizations
	  Tetanus age 10
	  MMR ⎫
	  DTaP ⎬ boosters between 4 and 6 years
	  TOPV ⎭
	  Varicella (at age 11–12 if no history of infection)
	Dental hygiene every 6–12 months
	  Continue fluoridation
	  Complete physical examination
		Complete physical examination
		TB test every 3 years (at ages 6 and 9)
		Developmental assessments
		  Language
		  Vision: Snellen charts at school 6–8 years, use "E" chart Over 8 years, use alphabet chart
		  Hearing: audiogram
		Cholesterol profile, if high risk, every 3–5 years
		Serum cholesterol one time (not high risk)

Adolescence (12–19 years)	Health education
	  Proper nutrition and healthful diets
	  Sex education
	    Choices
	    Risks
	    Precautions
	  Sexually transmitted diseases
		Complete physical exam (prepuberty or age 13)
		Blood pressure
		Cholesterol profile
		PPD test at 12 years and yearly if high risk
		RPR, CBC, U/A
		Female: breast self-exam (BSE)

Table II–7. PRIMARY AND SECONDARY PREVENTION FOR AGE-RELATED CONDITIONS (*Continued*)

Developmental Level	Primary Prevention	Secondary Prevention

Adolescence (12–19 years)	Safe driving skills
	Adult challenges
	  Seeking employment and career choices
	  Dating and marriage
	  Confrontation with substance abuse
	Safety in athletics, water
	Skin care
	Dental hygiene every 6–12 months
	Immunizations
	  Hepatitis B series if needed
	  tOPV booster at 12–14 years
		Male: testicular self-exam (TSE)
		Female, if sexually active: Pap and pelvic exam yearly (cervical gonorrhea and chlamydia culture and wet mount with pelvic)
		Screening and interventions if high risk
		  Depression
		  Suicide
		  Substance abuse
		  Pregnancy
		  Family history of alcoholism or domestic violence

Young adult (20–39 years)	Health education
	  Weight management with good nutrition as BMR changes
	  Low-cholesterol diet
	Lifestyle counseling
	  Stress management skills
	  Safe driving
	  Family planning
	  Divorce
	  Sexual practices
	  Parenting skills
	  Regular exercise
	  Environmental health choices
	  Alcohol, drug use
	  Use of hearing protection devices
	Dental hygiene every 6–12 months
	Immunizations
	  Tetanus at 20 years and every 10 years
		Complete physical exam at about 20 years, then every 5–6 years
		Cancer checkup every 3 years
		Female: BSE monthly, Pap yearly
		Male: TSE monthly
		All females: baseline mammography between ages 35 and 40
		Parents-to-be: high-risk screening for Down syndrome, Tay-Sachs
		Female pregnant: RPR, rubella titer, Rh factor, amniocentesis for women 35 years or older (if desired)
		Screening and interventions if high risk
		  Female with previous breast cancer: annual mammography at 35 years and after
		  Female with mother or sister who has had breast cancer, same as above

(table continues on p. 230)

Table II–7. PRIMARY AND SECONDARY PREVENTION FOR AGE-RELATED CONDITIONS (*Continued*)

Developmental Level	Primary Prevention	Secondary Prevention
Young adult (20–39 years)	Female: rubella, if serum negative for antibodies Hepatitis B for high-risk people	Family history colorectal cancer or high risk: annual stool guaiac, digital rectal, and sigmoidoscopy PPD if high risk Glaucoma screening at 35 years and along with routine physical exams Cholesterol profile every 5 years, if normal Cholesterol profile every 1–2 years if borderline
Middle-aged adult (40–59 years)	Health education: continue with young adult Midlife changes, male and female counseling (see also Young adult) "Empty nest syndrome" Anticipatory guidance for retirement Grandparenting Dental hygiene every 6–12 months Immunizations Tetanus every 10 years Influenza—annual if high risk (ie, major chronic disease [COPD, CAD]) Pneumococcal—every 5–6 years	Complete physical exam every 5–6 years with complete laboratory evaluation (serum/urine tests, x-ray, ECG) Cancer checkup every year Female: BSE monthly Male: TSE monthly All females: mammogram every 1–2 years (40–49 years) then annual mammography 50 years and over Schiotz's tonometry (glaucoma) every 3–5 years Sigmoidoscopy at 50 and 51, then every 4 years if negative Stool guaiac annually at 50 and yearly after Screening yearly if high risk Endometrial cancer: have endometrial sampling at menopause Oral cancer: screen more often if substance abuser
Older adult (60–74 years)	Health education: continue with previous counseling Home safety	Complete physical exam every 2 years with laboratory assessments

Table II–7. PRIMARY AND SECONDARY PREVENTION FOR AGE-RELATED CONDITIONS (*Continued*)

Developmental Level	Primary Prevention	Secondary Prevention

Older adult (60–74 years)	Retirement
	Loss of spouse, relatives, friends
	Special health needs
	  Nutritional changes
	  Changes in hearing or vision
	Dental/oral hygiene every 6–12 months
	Immunizations
	  Tetanus every 10 years
	  Influenza—annual if high risk
	  Pneumococcal—every 5–6 years
		Annual cancer checkup
		Blood pressure annually
		Female: BSE monthly, Pap every 1–3 years for high risk
		Male: TSE monthly, PSA yearly
		Female: annual mammogram
		Annual stool guaiac
		Sigmoidoscopy every 4 years
		Schiotz's tonometry every 3–5 years
		Podiatric evaluation with foot care PRN
		Screen for high risk
		  Depression
		  Suicide
		  Alcohol/drug abuse
		  "Elder abuse"

Old-age adult (75 years and over)	Health education: continue counseling
	Anticipatory guidance
	  Dying and death
	  Loss of spouse, relatives, friends
	  Increasing dependency on others
	Dental/oral hygiene every 6–12 months
	Immunizations
	  Tetanus every 10 years
	  Influenza—annual
	  Pneumococcal—if not already received
		Complete physical exam annually
		  Laboratory assessments
		  Cancer checkup
		  Blood pressure
		  Stool guaiac
		Female: annual mammogram, sigmoidoscopy every 4 years
		Schiotz's tonometry every 3–5 years
		Podiatrist PRN

This diagnosis is appropriate for a person expressing a desire to change an unhealthy lifestyle. Examples are excessive dissatisfaction with occupation; lack of exercise; failure to be refreshed after rest; diet high in fat, salt, and simple carbohydrates; tobacco use; obesity; excessive alcohol use; and insufficient leisure time.

The nursing diagnosis Risk for Ineffective Health Maintenance is useful to describe a person who needs teaching or referrals before discharge from an acute care center to prevent problems with health maintenance after discharge.

The diagnosis of Health-Seeking Behaviors is used to describe a person or group desiring health teaching related to the promotion and maintenance of high-level wellness (e.g., preventive behavior, age-related screening, optimal nutrition) or, according to NANDA, "seeking ways to alter personal health habits in order to move to a higher level of health." In most cases, this diagnosis describes an asymptomatic person. It also can be used in cases of chronic disease to help that person attain higher wellness in a particular area. Different from good health, high-level wellness is defined as an integrated method of functioning oriented toward maximizing potential (Dunn, 1959). For example, a woman with multiple sclerosis and many physical problems could learn breast self-examination or relaxation exercises using Health-Seeking Behaviors: Breast self-examination.

Health-Seeking Behaviors is best written as a one-part diagnostic statement with the sought-after health practice specified (e.g., Health-Seeking Behaviors: Breast self-examination).

Using "related to" is unnecessary; it is understood that all people with Health-Seeking Behaviors are motivated to achieve a higher level of health. Related factors could not represent causative or contributing factors, unless the nurse wants to repeat the same factors for each client (e.g., Health-Seeking Behaviors: Breast self-examination related to desire to maximize health).

As focus shifts from an illness/treatment-oriented to a health-oriented health care system, Ineffective Health Maintenance and Health-Seeking Behaviors are becoming increasingly significant. These diagnoses are difficult to use in the hospital. The increasingly high acuity and shortened lengths of stay in hospitals require nurses to be creative in addressing health promotion by using printed materials, television instruction, and community-based programs.

Key Concepts

GENERIC CONSIDERATIONS

➤ Many people view health as the absence of disease. Rather, health can be viewed as a return (or recovery) to a previous state or to a heightened awareness of full potential and life meaning (Allen & Phillips, 1997).

➤ Control of major health problems in the United States depends directly on modification of individual behavior and habits of living (Allen & Phillips, 1997).

➤ The goals of prevention are as follows:
  ➤ Avoidance of disease through healthy lifestyles
  ➤ Decrease mortality from disease through early detection and intervention
  ➤ Improved quality of life

➤ The three levels of prevention are primary, secondary, and tertiary.
  ➤ Primary prevention involves actions that prevent disease and accidents and promote well-being. Key Concepts are as follows:

Concept	Examples
Wellness	Diet low in salt, sugar, and fat
A lifestyle that incorporates the principles of health promotion and is directed by self-responsibility	Regular exercise and stress management; elimination of smoking; minimal alcohol intake
Self-help	Reading self-help books
Mutual sharing with others who have similar needs	LaLeche League; childbirth education; assertiveness training; specific written resources (books, pamphlets, magazines); public media
Safety	Adherence to speed limits; use of seat belts and car seats; proper storage of household poisons
Immunizations	Children: varicella
	Nonpregnant women of childbearing age: rubella if antibody titer is negative
	Elderly: influenza, pneumonia

➤ Secondary prevention concerns actions that promote early detection of disease and subsequent intervention: regular examination by a health professional and self-examination.
➤ Tasks of screening are as follows:
  ➤ Identify major disabling conditions (e.g., hypertension, diabetes mellitus)
  ➤ Identify those at high risk for specific conditions through personal health history (e.g., concurrent disease such as diabetes mellitus means higher risk for hypertension), family health history (e.g., substance abuse, cancer, heart disease; sexually transmitted disease; domestic violence, person abuse).
  ➤ Identify tests and procedures that accurately detect the condition: Who will do them? How often are they done? Who bears the cost?
  ➤ Plan a strategy for disseminating screening information to health care professionals and the public.
  ➤ Plan evaluation of screening effectiveness.
➤ Types of screening include the following:
  ➤ Physical findings (periodic examinations by health care professionals and self-examinations of breasts, testicles, and skin)

> ➤ Survey of risk factors (smoking, alcohol abuse)
> ➤ Laboratory tests (serum, e.g., tuberculin skin tests, sickle cell in African Americans, phenylketonuria in newborns; urine, e.g., renal disease in older adults)

➤ Tertiary prevention involves actions that restore and rehabilitate and prevent complications in cases of illness. Examples for a person with coronary artery disease are as follows:

> ➤ Restorative (surgery, such as coronary artery bypass, angioplasty, and medications)
> ➤ Rehabilitative (weight loss, exercise program, stop smoking)

Nutrition

See Key Concepts for Imbalanced Nutrition.

Exercise

➤ Regular exercise can increase the following:

> ➤ Cardiovascular—respiratory endurance
> ➤ Muscle strength
> ➤ Muscle endurance
> ➤ Flexibility
> ➤ Delivery of nutrients to tissue
> ➤ Tolerance for psychological stress
> ➤ Ability to reduce body fat content

➤ Vigorous exercise sessions should include a warm-up phase (10 minutes at a slow pace), endurance exercises, and a cool-down phase (5 to 10 minutes of a slow pace and stretching).

➤ Current beliefs regarding optimal exercise are as follows:

> ➤ Emphasize physical activity over "exercise."
> ➤ Moderate physical activity is very beneficial.
> ➤ Intermittent physical activity that accumulates to 30 or more minutes is beneficial.

➤ To enhance long-term exercise, the person should (Moore & Charvat, 2002)

> ➤ Respond to relapses with a plan to prevent recurrences.
> ➤ Set realistic goals.
> ➤ Keep an exercise log.
> ➤ Exercise with a friend.

Weight Reduction

➤ Overeating is a complex problem with physical, social, and psychological components.

➤ Eighty percent of children of two obese parents will become obese, as opposed to 40% with one obese parent and 7% with no obese parent (Buiten & Metzger, 2000).

➤ Body mass index (BMI) is a ratio of weight and height that estimates total body fat (Dudek, 2001). According to the third National Health and Nutrition Examination Survey (NHANES III), 54.9 million Americans 20 years and older are overweight (BMI 25 to 29.9) or obese (BMI > 30; Dudek, 2001).

➤ Excess weight contributes to hypertension, type 2 diabetes, heart disease, sleep apnea, osteoarthritis, gallstones, stress incontinence, and high low-density-lipoprotein and low high-density-lipoprotein levels (Dudek, 2001).

➤ To maintain ideal body weight, food consumed must equal physical activity daily (Roberts, 2000). Dieting without exercise decreases resting metabolic rate. Exercise, even without dieting, produces the best long-term effects (Roberts, 2000).

➤ Fluctuations in body weight are common, especially in women. Daily weight can be misleading and disheartening. Body measurements are a better gauge of losses.

➤ Regular exercise causes lean muscle mass to increase. Because muscle weighs more than fat, the scale may reflect a weight gain.

➤ Restrictive diets usually do not last and fail to establish healthy eating patterns. A better approach is modifying existing eating habits (Wierenga & Oldham, 2002).

Smoking

➤ Cigarette smoke causes more than 4,000 chemicals to be absorbed in the blood and swallowed into the GI tract to act directly in the oral cavity and respiratory system (Andrews, 1998).

➤ Smokers have a chronic cough, increased sputum production, dyspnea, and decreased lung capacity (Andrews, 1998).

➤ Women who smoke have fertility problems and impaired uteroplacental function when pregnant. Tobacco use during pregnancy can adversely affect a child's physical growth and intellectual development. Women who smoke are at risk for early menopause, decreased bone density, and osteoporosis (Andrews, 1998).

➤ Smoking has immediate and long-term effects on the cardiovascular system. Immediate effects are vasoconstriction and decreased oxygenation of the blood, elevated blood pressure, increased heart rate and possible dysrhythmias, and increased work of the heart. Long-term effects are an increased risk for coronary artery disease, stroke, hyperlipidemia, and myocardial infarction. Smoking also contributes to hypertension, peripheral vascular disease (e.g., leg ulcers), and chronically abnormal arterial blood gases (low oxygen, or Po_2, and high carbon dioxide, or Pco_2 (USDHHS, 2000).

➤ Use of smokeless tobacco (snuff, chewing tobacco) is associated with oral leukoplakia (premalignant lesions), oral cancer, and nicotine addiction. At least 12 million Americans are at risk, mostly male teens and male adults (USDHHS, 2000).

➤ Tobacco use is a significant risk factor for cancers of the tongue and oral mucosa, larynx, lungs, bladder, and cervix. Combined with other carcinogens (e.g., alcohol, asbestos, coal dust, radon), the health risk intensifies. The rate of cancer recurrence increases in clients who continue tobacco use during and after treatment (USDHHS, 2000).

➤ Nicotine is the primary addicting substance in tobacco smoke and juice. Clients with tobacco addiction need special assistance with short-term withdrawal and long-term maintenance of a tobacco-free life.

➤ Passive smoking, the inhalation of tobacco smoke by nonsmokers, has been shown to have negative health effects (Andrews, 1998; Pletsch, 2002):

  ➤ People with angina experience more discomfort in a smoke-filled room.

  ➤ Bronchospasm increases when a person with asthma is exposed to tobacco smoke.

  ➤ Children living with smoking parents have more upper respiratory and ear infections than those living with nonsmokers.

  ➤ Passive smoking causes lung cancer in nonsmokers.

  ➤ Sudden infant death syndrome is two to four times more common in infants whose mothers smoked during pregnancy.

➤ In the last 25 years, most health professions have seen a significant decline in the smoking behavior of its members—but not nursing. Estimates show that 25% to 29% of nurses still smoke. Studies on nurses link occupational stress and social influences with tobacco use (Cinelli & Glover, 1988). A nurse who smokes sends the wrong signals to clients.

Osteoporosis

➤ Of all hip and vertebral fractures, 30% of hip fractures and 20% of vertebral fractures occur in men with osteoporosis (Eastell et al., 1998).

➤ Loss of trabecular bone begins in the fourth decade and progresses at 6% to 8% per decade. This rate accelerates in women after menopause (Woodhead & Moss, 1998).

➤ Osteoporosis is classified as primary (associated with age- and menopause-related changes) or secondary (caused by medications or diseases; Miller, 2004).

➤ Contributing factors to osteoporosis include loss of female hormones after menopause; hypogonadism; low calcium or vitamin D intake; insufficient exercise; small stature; fair skin; family history; cigarette smoking; excessive consumption of alcohol, caffeine, or protein; excessive use of aluminum-type antacids; long-term use of corticosteroids; therapy for chronic illness (bowel, kidney, liver); excessive thyroid replacement; and excessive thyroid function (Woodhead & Moss, 1998).

GERIATRIC CONSIDERATIONS

➤ According to Miller (2004), health is the ability of older adults to function at their highest capacity, despite age-related changes and risk factors. Of all age-related changes, osteoporosis is most likely to have serious negative functional consequences, even without additional risk factors.

➤ About 70% of people older than 65 years rate their health as excellent (Miller, 2004).

➤ Differentiating between age-related changes and risk factors that affect the functioning of older people is important. Such risk factors as inadequate nutrition, fluid intake, exercise, and socialization can have more influence on functioning than can most age-related changes.

➤ Maximal aerobic capacity and maximal heart rate decline with age. For aerobic conditioning, an older person must exercise to reach target heart rate for at least 20 to 30 minutes three times a week. The following formula will obtain target heart rate: 220–Person's Age × 60% to 70% = Target Training Heart Rate. Older adults must learn to monitor carotid pulse for rate and rhythm. The time to return to baseline heart rate, blood pressure, and respiratory rate after exercise is greater for older people (Allison & Keller, 1997).

➤ Older adults have decreased thermoregulation and diminished ability to cool the body through perspiration, affecting tolerance of physical activity (Allison & Keller, 1997).

➤ There is an age-related increase in systolic blood pressure at rest and at submaximal workloads. Sensitivity of the cardiovascular system to the chronotropic, inotropic, and vasodilatory effects of catecholamines diminishes. Studies have shown that catecholamines or β-adrenergic stimulation, when administered during exercise, had greater effects on young people as opposed to those of advanced age (Miller, 2004).

➤ Regular exercise has been shown to correlate positively with increased self-esteem. Adult learning principles support encouraging exercise or regular activity that has meaning to the older person if compliance is expected. When exercising, the older adult should exercise to the point of mild intolerance and then cut back by 25% (Allison & Keller, 1997).

TRANSCULTURAL CONSIDERATIONS

➤ Health and illness are culturally prescribed. One culture may view an obese person as strong and healthy, whereas another culture views that same person as weak and unhealthy. Nurses must remember that treatment strategies consistent with a person's cultural beliefs may have a better chance of success (Andrews & Boyle, 2003).

➤ A future orientation to illness, disease, and health care is necessary for prevention. The dominant US culture is oriented to the future, whereas other cultures have a present-oriented perception (e.g., African American, Hispanic, Southern Appalachian, traditional Chinese). Some members of these cultures, however, are future-oriented.

➤ Some cultures believe that fate depends of God or other supernatural forces. Humans are at the mercy of these forces despite their behavior (Andrews & Boyle, 2003).

➤ Some Asian cultures believe in balance and harmony for health. They emphasize moderation and avoid excesses. In the yin/yang theory, the yin force in the universe represents female aspects of nature: fullness, light, and warmth. An imbalance of yin and yang creates illness.

➤ In Hispanic and black cultures, health is maintained by the hot/cold humoral theory. This ancient Greek concept describes four body humors: yellow bile, black bile, phlegm, and blood. When these humors are balanced, health is present. Treatment of illness consists of restoring humoral balance by adding or deleting substances (e.g., foods, beverages, herbs, drugs) that are either hot or cold. For example, an earache is classified as cold and thus needs hot substances for treatment (Andrews & Boyle, 2003).

FOCUS ASSESSMENT CRITERIA

Assess for subjective (s) and objective (O) cues.

Defining Characteristics

Health status

➤ General appearance, weight, height
➤ Client's description of health
➤ Immediate health concerns

Frequency of

➤ Bowel irregularity (S)
➤ Urinary tract infections (O)
➤ Mouth lesions (O)
➤ Respiratory infections (O)
➤ Headaches (S)
➤ Skin rashes (O)
➤ Influenza (S)
➤ Fatigue (S)
➤ Feeling overwhelmed (S)

Related Factors

INFLUENCING FACTORS: HEALTH MANAGEMENT AND ADHERENCE BEHAVIOR

What factors make it difficult to follow health advice?
What daily health management activities are practiced?

RISK FACTORS

Family incidence of

➤ Cardiovascular disease
➤ Drug or alcohol abuse
➤ Diabetes mellitus
➤ Abuse or violence
➤ Cancer
➤ Psychiatric illness
➤ Hypertension
➤ Genetic disorders
➤ Other (specify)

Health habits

➤ Smoking (how much)
➤ Alcohol
➤ Drug use (prescribed, over the counter)
➤ Dietary consumption of fat/salt/sugar
➤ Exercise program

ENVIRONMENTAL RISK FACTORS

Do you use seat belts or child restraints?
Is home child-proofed? (If appropriate, determine measures taken.)
Could any factors in the home or at work cause falls or accidents?
Could any other factors potentially threaten your health or cause injury?
Ineffective Health Maintenance

PREVENTIVE HEALTH SCREENING ACTIVITIES

Self-examination (breasts, testicles, blood pressure): indicate frequency and perceived problems
Last professional examination (dental, pelvic, rectal, vision, hearing, complete physical)
Last laboratory or other diagnostic testing (electrocardiogram, CBC, cholesterol, stool for occult blood, Pap, chest x-ray, prostate-specific antigen)

GOAL

The person or caregiver will verbalize intent to engage in health maintenance behaviors.

Indicators

Identify barriers to health maintenance
Commit to eating a balanced diet
Commit to an exercise program

GENERAL INTERVENTIONS

1. Assess for barriers to health maintenance.

➤ Lack of knowledge
➤ Lack of access or finance
➤ Low priority
➤ Family lifestyle patterns

Rationale: Low-income families usually focus on meeting basic needs (food, shelter, and safety) and seeking help with curing illness, not preventing it (Hanson & Boyd, 1996). Providing information and resources can help foster a sense that change is possible.

2. Explain primary and secondary prevention measures for age (Table II-7).

Rationale: Many of the most serious disorders can be prevented or postponed by immunizations, chemoprophylaxis, and healthy lifestyles or detected early with screening and treated effectively (USDHHS, 2002).

3. Teach basics of balanced nutritional intake.

➤ Choose a plan that encourages high intake of complex carbohydrates and limited intake of fat.
➤ Know what you are eating. The "basic four" label is misleading (e.g., a chicken-fried steak is a protein converted to high fat content through its preparation [frying]).
➤ Obtain more calories from fruits and vegetables than from meat and dairy products. Also, eat more chicken and fish, which contain less fat and fewer total calories than beef, removing the fat and skin.
➤ Avoid salad dressings with mayonnaise (216 to 308 calories per 2-oz serving).
➤ Avoid fast foods (they have high fat and total caloric content).

➤ Dine in or make special requests in restaurants for food selection/ preparation (e.g., salad dressing on side, no sauce on entrée).

➤ Plan meals in advance. If attending a party or restaurant, decide what to eat ahead of time and stick to it.

➤ Adhere to grocery list.

➤ Involve family in meal planning for better nutrition.

➤ Buy the highest quality beef (ground round = 10% fat; hamburger = 25% fat).

➤ Choose a variety of foods.

➤ Avoid serving family style.

➤ Drink eight to ten 8-oz glasses of water daily.

➤ Measure foods and count calories; keep records.

➤ Read labels on foods, noting composition and calories per serving.

➤ Eat slowly.

➤ Experiment with spices, substitutes, and low calorie recipes.

Rationale: The US diet currently consists of 42% fat, 12% protein, 22% complex carbohydrates, and 24% simple carbohydrates. Recommended dietary goals are 30% fat, 12% protein, 48% complex carbohydrates, and 10% simple carbohydrates (USDHHS, 2002).

4. Discuss benefits of exercise.

➤ Reduces caloric absorption

➤ Suppresses appetite

➤ Improves self-esteem

➤ Preserves lean muscle mass

➤ Increases oxygen uptake

➤ Increases restful sleep

➤ Reduces depression, anxiety, stress

➤ Increases caloric expenditure

➤ Increases resistance to age

➤ Maintains weight loss

➤ Reduces degeneration

➤ Improves body posture

➤ Increases metabolic rate

➤ Provides fun, recreation, diversion

Rationale: Any increase in activity also increases energy output, caloric deficits, and increased flexibility and endurance.

5. Assist client to identify realistic exercise program.

➤ Personality

➤ Lifestyle

➤ Time of factor

➤ Time of day

➤ Season

➤ Occupation

➤ Safety

➤ Costs

➤ Age

➤ Physical size

➤ Physical conditions

Rationale: The safest activities for the unconditioned obese person are walking, water aerobics, swimming, and cycling.

6. Discuss aspects of starting the exercise program.

➤ Start easy and slow. Obtain clearance from physician.
➤ Choose an activity that uses many body parts and is vigorous enough to cause "healthful fatigue."
➤ Read, consult experts, and talk with friends/coworkers who exercise.
➤ Plan a daily walking program.
> Start at 5 to 10 blocks for 0.5 to 1 mile/day; increase 1 block or 0.1 mile/week.
> Gradually increase rate and length of walk; remember to progress slowly.
> Avoid straining or pushing too hard and becoming overly fatigued.
> Stop immediately if any of the following occur:
Lightness or pain in chest
Severe breathlessness
Lightheadedness
Dizziness
Loss of muscle control
Nausea
> If pulse is 120 beats/min (bpm) at 5 minutes or 100 bpm at 10 minutes after stopping exercise or if shortness of breath occurs 10 minutes after exercise, slow down either the rate or the distance of walking.
> If client cannot walk 5 blocks or 0.5 mile without signs of overexertion, decrease length of walking for 1 week to point before signs appear and then start to add 1 block/0.1 mile each week.
> Walk at same rate; time with stopwatch or second hand on watch; after reaching 10 blocks (1 mile), try to increase speed.
> Remember, increase only the rate or the distance of walking at one time.
> Establish a regular time for exercise, with the goal of three to five times a week for 15 to 45 minutes and a heart rate of 80% of stress test or gross calculation (170 bpm for 20 to 29 years of age; decrease 10 bpm for each additional decade [e.g., 160 bpm for 30 to 39 years of age, 150 bpm for 40 to 49 years of age]).
➤ Encourage significant others also to engage in walking program.
➤ Add supplemental activity (e.g., parking far from destination, gardening, using stairs, spending weekends at activities that require walking).
➤ Work up to 1 hour of exercise per day at least 4 days per week.
➤ Avoid lapses of more than 2 days between exercise sessions.

Rationale: A regular exercise program should be enjoyable, use a minimum of 400 calories in each session, sustain a heart rate of approximately 120 to 150 bpm, involve rhythmic alternating contracting and relaxing of muscles, and be integrated into the person's lifestyle 4 to 5 days/week for at least 30 to 60 minutes.

7. Teach about the risks of obesity.

➤ Vascular insufficiency
➤ Arteriosclerosis
➤ Heart disease
➤ Hypertension
➤ Left ventricular hypertrophy
➤ Diabetes mellitus
➤ Gallbladder disease
➤ Complications of surgery
➤ Respiratory diseases
➤ Joint degeneration
➤ Cancer (e.g., breast)
➤ Risk of accident/injury
➤ Increased low-density lipoprotein cholesterol
➤ Decreased high-density lipoprotein cholesterol

Rationale: Obesity affects all body systems negatively.

▼ Health-Seeking Behaviors

Definition

Health-Seeking Behaviors: State in which a person in stable health actively seeks ways to alter personal health habits and/or the environment to move toward a higher level of wellness.

Defining Characteristics

MAJOR (MUST BE PRESENT)

Expressed or observed desire to seek information for health promotion

MINOR (MAY BE PRESENT)

Expressed or observed desire for increased control of health

Expression of concern about current environmental conditions on
   health status
Stated or observed unfamiliarity with wellness community resources
Demonstrated or observed lack of knowledge of health-promotion
   behaviors

Related Factors

No related factors are needed.

 Carp's Cue ▶ *As discussed earlier, the nursing diagnosis Health-Seeking Behaviors does not need related factors. When you use Health-Seeking Behaviors you have a person who is healthy but desires to be healthier.*

You can write Health-Seeking Behaviors: Enhanced Nutrition with less
carbohydrates.

Key Concepts

GENERIC CONSIDERATIONS

➤ A major focus of nursing care is to promote effective health-seeking
   behaviors in clients. Activities that do so include nurturing, encouraging, teaching, communicating, and providing
➤ According to Nyamathi (1989), "The health goals of the client and
   desired goals of the nurse are mutually concerned with enhancing
   the individual's motivation to attain and maintain health and function, to avoid disease and disability, and to attain or retain the highest possible level of health, function or productivity."
➤ The NHANES III found that of Americans 20 years and older, 32.6%
   are overweight (BMI 25 to 29.5) and 22.3% are obese (BMI > 30;
   Dudek, 2001).
➤ Adequate dietary intake of complex carbohydrates, found in grains,
   fruits, legumes, and vegetables, improves human health in many
   ways (e.g., decreases obesity, cardiovascular disease, cancer, malnutrition, diabetes, and dental caries). Current recommendations
   advise an increase in total dietary carbohydrates to 55% of daily
   calories and a decrease in fat to less than 30% of total calories
   (Dudek, 2001).
➤ Recent studies prove that decreasing serum cholesterol through
   diet and drugs (if necessary) can reduce the risk of heart disease

(Woodhead, 2003). Recommended dietary changes to prevent or reduce serum cholesterol level include the following:

➤ Decreased total fats, saturated fats, and cholesterol
➤ In overweight people, reduced daily caloric intake to attain desired body weight
➤ Increased intake of nutrients that may help decrease the risk of cardiovascular disease (e.g., oat bran and other water-soluble fibers, fruit gums, vegetables, garlic, polyunsaturated fats, olive oil, legumes, fatty fish)

➤ Many people find it difficult to maintain health-seeking diets even when they have been successful. Examples of helpful approaches include designing behavioral contracts, engaging in positive self-talk, and strengthening family supports.

➤ Risk factors for cardiovascular disease include the following (Woodhead, 2003):

➤ Male gender
➤ Family history (parent or sibling) of myocardial infarction or sudden death younger than 55 years
➤ Smoking more than 10 cigarettes per day
➤ Hypertension
➤ High-density-lipoprotein level less than 35 mg/dl
➤ History of definite occlusive vascular disease (peripheral or cerebral)
➤ Morbid obesity (more than 30% overweight)

➤ Dietary recommendations for children older than 2 years are as follows (Wong, 1999):

➤ Provide a variety of foods daily
➤ Maintain desirable body weight
➤ Limit total dietary fat to 30% of calories
➤ Limit total daily cholesterol to 100 mg/1,000 calories and not more than 300 mg/day
➤ Limit daily protein intake to 15% of calories
➤ Limit daily carbohydrate intake to 55% of calories
➤ Limit sodium intake by reducing processed foods and keeping salt off the table

➤ Research on both animals and humans has suggested a link between nutrition and cancer (Dudek, 2001). To reduce the risk of diet-related cancers:

➤ Eat five or more servings of fruits and vegetables daily
➤ Add grain products to every meal (e.g., whole grains over refined)
➤ Add soy-based foods to daily intake (e.g., one glass of soy milk)
➤ Substitute dried peas and beans for meat at some meals
➤ Limit intake of high-fat foods and animal fat
➤ Avoid high intake of alcohol (>14 drinks a week for men, >drinks a week for women).

➤ Avoid excessive intake of nitrite-containing foods (e.g., bacon, cured foods).

➤ The exact relationship between dietary sodium and essential hypertension has yet to be described unequivocally. Studies show, however, that blood pressure in many (not all) clients with hypertension decreases when they restrict dietary sodium. Thus, all people with hypertension should try a reduced sodium diet (2 g sodium/day).

FOCUS ASSESSMENT CRITERIA

Does the person/family report good or excellent health?
Does the person/family desire to adopt a behavior to maximize health?

GOAL

The person will assume responsibility for own wellness (physical, dental, safety, nutritional).

Indicators

Describe screening appropriate for age and risk factors.
Perform self-screening for cancer.
Participate in a regular exercise program.
State an intent to use positive coping mechanisms and constructive stress management.
State an intent to evaluate daily nutrition and to identify areas for improvement.

GENERAL INTERVENTIONS

1. Assess for factors that contribute to health promotion and maintenance.

➤ Knowledge of disease and preventive behavior
➤ Appropriate screening practices for age and risk
➤ Good nutrition and weight control
➤ Regular exercise program
➤ Constructive stress management
➤ Supportive social networks

Rationale: As a person strives to improve health, he or she moves through a process of introspection, planning new healthier activities, coping with barriers and setbacks, and ultimately absorbing these new behaviors into everyday life.

2. Promote health behaviors in client and family.
   a. Determine Knowledge or Perception of

➤ Specific diseases (e.g., heart disease, cancer, respiratory disease, childhood diseases, infections, dental disease)
➤ Susceptibility (e.g., risk factors, family history)
➤ Seriousness
➤ Value of early detection

   b. Determine past patterns of health care.

➤ Expectations
➤ Interactions with health care system or providers
➤ Influences of family, cultural group, peer group, and mass media

   c. Provide specific information about screening for age-related conditions (Table II-7).
   d. Discuss the role of nutrition in health maintenance and illness prevention (see Key Concepts for Imbalanced Nutrition for specific explanations).

➤ Basic food groups
➤ Nutrient needs for age, level of physical activity, pregnancy, and lactation
➤ Prudent use of
   ➤ Salt (see Excess Fluid Volume)
   ➤ Fried foods
   ➤ Fats (butter, margarines)
   ➤ Snack foods (potato chips, candy, soda)
   ➤ Foods containing nitrosamines (smoked meats, preservatives)
   ➤ Canned vegetables
   ➤ Red meats
   ➤ High-calorie desserts
   ➤ Refined sugar
➤ Generous use of health-promoting foods
   ➤ Cruciferous vegetables (broccoli, cabbage, cauliflower, Brussels sprouts)—protect against colorectal cancer
   ➤ High-fiber foods—protect against colorectal cancer
   ➤ Calcium-containing foods (e.g., dairy, dark leafy vegetables)—protect against osteoporosis
   ➤ Soy products—may reduce the risk of hormone-related cancers (e.g., breast, prostate)
➤ See Ineffective Health Maintenance for specific information concerning weight control.

e. Discuss the benefits of a regular exercise program.

➤ See Key Concepts for Ineffective Health Maintenance for positive effects of regular exercise.

➤ Determine optimal exercise for the client, considering physical limitations, preferences, and lifestyle:

Walking briskly	Aerobic dancing
Jogging	Swimming
Running	Bicycling
Skipping rope	

➤ Stress the importance of beginning any physical activity slowly.

f. Discuss the elements of constructive stress management (Lyon, 2002).

➤ Maintain realistic expectations of self.
➤ Set clear realistic goals and subgoals.
➤ Allow for interruptions.
➤ Be aware of toxic thinking.
➤ Acknowledge personal strengths.
➤ Let go of unrealistic expectations of others.
➤ Plan to manage time.

g. Discuss strategies to develop positive social networks.

➤ Relate the functions of a support system.
  ➤ Provide love and affection.
  ➤ Provide dependable assistance (emotional, economic, if appropriate).
  ➤ Serve as buffers against life's stressors.
  ➤ Share common social concerns.
  ➤ Respect mutual pursuits of members.
  ➤ Prevent isolation.
  ➤ Cooperate for a common purpose.
➤ Suggest methods to strengthen this system:
  ➤ Be supportive of others.
  ➤ Practice active listening.
    ➤ Don't interrupt the person.
    ➤ Allow a few seconds to lapse between dialogue to provide time to gather thoughts and to reduce the "rush to speak."
➤ Provide others with opportunities to share their concerns without judgment. Refrain from giving solutions; rather, discuss options (e.g., "You have several options: You can quit your job, request a transfer, discuss the problem with your boss, or do nothing").
➤ When confronted with a relationship problem, review the situation.
  ➤ What is the problem?
  ➤ Who/what is responsible?
  ➤ What are the options?

> ➤ What are the advantages and disadvantages of each option?
➤ Show love and mutual respect to significant others.
>> ➤ Show unconditional love to own children.
>> ➤ Provide encouragement to significant others facing challenges.
>> ➤ Avoid criticism, punishment, excessive praise, or pampering.
>> ➤ Demonstrate genuine warmth and affection.
➤ Practice mutual goal setting to direct common efforts; reevaluate them periodically.
➤ Offer sincere assistance to others to promote trust.
➤ Build relationships with people and families who share common interests and values.
➤ Recognize when additional assistance is needed.
Marital counseling
Self-help group
Health professional
Religious affiliation

Allow self and each family member (children, spouse, parents) to enhance personal identity by pursuing individual interests (refer to Delayed Growth and Development for age-related needs of children).

Rationale: Health-seeking and coping behaviors are closely intertwined; nurses assist clients to maximize their abilities to handle stress throughout life. Healthy eating can prevent disease and decrease complications. Regular exercise improves cardiovascular endurance, increases muscle strength and endurance, and lowers low-density-lipoprotein cholesterol and triglyceride levels, blood pressure, and body fat. Social support helps maintain health and prevent disequilibrium (Clemen-Stone et al., 2002).

3. Initiate health teaching and referrals, as indicated.
   a. Review client's daily health practices.

➤ Dental care
➤ Food and fluid intake
➤ Exercise regimen, leisure activities
➤ Responsibilities in the family (e.g., chores)
➤ Use of
Tobacco
Salt, sugar, fat products
Alcohol
Drugs, (over-the-counter, prescribed)
➤ Knowledge of safety practices
Fire prevention
Bicycle
Car (maintenance, seat belts, car seats, air bags)
Water safety
Poison control

b. Suggest selective disease-preventing behaviors when appropriate.

Skin cancer

➤ Avoid frequent sun exposure.
➤ Avoid tanning salons.
➤ Wear effective sunscreens and protective clothing.
➤ Plan outdoor activities for before 10 am and after 2 pm. During these hours, wear a hat and sunscreen.

Sexually transmitted diseases

➤ Use barrier contraceptive methods.
➤ Avoid casual sex.
➤ Avoid high-risk partners (e.g., history of multiple partners, no use of condoms).

AIDS/hepatitis B/hepatitis C

➤ Use condoms.
➤ Avoid high-risk sexual practices.
➤ Avoid use of contaminated needles.
➤ Get hepatitis A and B vaccine.

Hearing loss

➤ Use ear protection routinely (e.g., mowing lawn, using machinery).
➤ Avoid loud music (e.g., headphones).
➤ Avoid prolonged exposure to loud noises.
➤ Treat infections promptly.

Congenital deformities

➤ Avoid use of alcohol and drugs during pregnancy.

Oral cancer

➤ Avoid tobacco chewing.
➤ Avoid concurrent heavy use of alcohol and tobacco.

Lung cancers, COPD

➤ Avoid tobacco smoking.
➤ Avoid chronic exposure to known inhalable carcinogens (e.g., asbestos).
➤ Include carotene-rich foods in diet (e.g., yellow vegetables and fruits).
➤ Avoid smoke-filled rooms; discourage smoking in your living and work spaces.
➤ Routinely test home for radon.

Coronary artery disease

➤ Avoid obesity.
➤ Avoid tobacco use.

➤ Practice stress management.
➤ Exercise regularly.
➤ Avoid dietary cholesterol and saturated fats; reduce total dietary fats.
➤ Maintain normal blood pressure.
➤ Increase daily intake of water-soluble fibers in diet (e.g., oat bran, fruit pectins, psyllium).

Stroke

➤ Avoid tobacco use, especially if taking oral contraceptives.
➤ Maintain normal blood pressure.
➤ Avoid dietary cholesterol and saturated fats, and reduce total dietary fats.

Reye's syndrome

➤ Avoid aspirin products in children with viral infections.

Osteoarthritis

➤ Avoid obesity.
➤ Avoid repeated trauma to joints.

Osteoporosis for high-risk women and men

➤ Refer to Ineffective Health Maintenance.

Colorectal cancer

➤ Avoid chronic constipation.
➤ Avoid foods prepared containing nitrites (cured and smoked meats); consume orange juice or other products rich in vitamin C with same meal when including nitrites in diet.
➤ Include generous amounts of cruciferous vegetables and other sources of fiber in diet.

Breast cancer

➤ Avoid high-fat diet.
➤ Add soy products to daily intake.

Gastroenteritis from contaminated food

➤ Avoid foods prepared with raw egg.
➤ Avoid raw or incompletely cooked seafood, poultry, or meats.
➤ Avoid shellfish from polluted waters.

Hematologic cancers

➤ Avoid consumption of fish from dangerously polluted waters (mercury, polychlorinated biphenyl).

Lyme disease

➤ Avoid tick-infested wooded or grassy areas during peak seasons (late spring, summer, early fall).

> ➤ If entering hazardous areas, wear long sleeves, hat, and long pants with socks pulled over cuffs of pants.
> ➤ Light colors make ticks more visible.
> ➤ Use effective insect repellent (adults only).
> ➤ Search clothes, body, and pets for ticks after hiking in hazardous areas.
> ➤ Because deer ticks are the size of a dot, inspect all skin areas for reddened dots or rash. Have a physician or nurse evaluate bites or rashes.

Rationale: The client is responsible for choosing a healthy pattern of living. The nurse is responsible for explaining the choices.

 Risk for Imbalanced Fluid Volume

Definition

Risk for Imbalanced Fluid Volume: State in which a person is at risk to experience a decrease, increase, or rapid shift from one to the other of intravascular, interstitial, and/or intracellular fluid.

Risk Factors

Major invasive procedures scheduled
Others needed to be developed (NANDA, 2002)

This diagnosis can represent several clinical conditions, such as edema, hemorrhage, dehydration, and compartmental syndrome. If the nurse is monitoring a person for imbalanced fluid volume, labeling the specific imbalance as a collaborative problem, such as hypovolemia, compartmental syndrome, increased intracranial pressure, GI bleeding, or postpartum hemorrhage, would be more useful clinically. For example, most intraoperative clients would be monitored for hypovolemia. If the procedure were neurosurgery, then cranial pressure also would be monitored. If the procedure were orthopedic, compartmental syndrome would be addressed. Refer to Section III for the specific collaborative problems and interventions. If a person is vulnerable to Deficient Fluid Volume, use Risk for Deficient Fluid Volume. Review the related factors under Deficient Fluid Volume, if they are relevant to your client, write them as the related to's as risk factors. Follow the same for Excess Fluid Volume. If a person is vulnerable to both, then use Risk for Imbalanced Fluid Volume.

▼ Bowel Incontinence

Definition

Bowel Incontinence: A state in which an individual experiences a change in normal bowel habits characterized by involuntary passage of stool.

Defining Characteristics

Assess for involuntary passage of stool (S,O).

Related Factors

PATHOPHYSIOLOGIC

Related to impaired rectal sphincter secondary to

Anal or rectal surgery
Anal or rectal injury
Obstetric injuries
Peripheral neuropathy

Related to overdistention of rectum secondary to chronic constipation
Related to lack of voluntary sphincter control secondary to

Progressive neuromuscular disorder
Spinal cord compression
Cerebral vascular accident
Spinal cord injury
Multiple sclerosis

Related to impaired reservoir capacity secondary to

Colectomy
Radiation proctitis

SITUATIONAL (PERSONAL, ENVIRONMENTAL)

Related to inability to recognize, interpret, or respond to rectal cues secondary to

Depression
Cognitive impairment

Key Concepts

GENERIC CONSIDERATIONS

➤ Bowel incontinence has three major causes: underlying disease of the colon, rectum, or anus; long-standing constipation or fecal impaction; and neurogenic rectal changes (McLane & McShane, 1992).

➤ Complete spinal cord injury, spinal cord lesions, neurologic disease, or congenital defects that interrupt the sacral reflex arc (at the sacral segments S2, S3, S4) result in a flaccid bowel. Flaccid paralysis at this level, known as an LMN lesion, results in loss of the defecation reflex, loss of sphincter control (flaccid anal sphincter), and no bulbocavernosus reflex (Demata, 2000).

GERIATRIC CONSIDERATIONS

➤ The sensation of rectal fullness, which produces the urge to defecate, may be diminished in older adults (Demata, 2000).

FOCUS ASSESSMENT CRITERIA

Refer to Constipation

GOAL

The person will evacuate soft, formed stool every other day or every third day.

Indicators

Relate bowel elimination techniques
Describe fluid and dietary requirements

GENERAL INTERVENTIONS

1. Assess contributing factors.

➤ Lack of routine evacuation schedule
➤ Insufficient fluid and fiber intake

➤ Constipation
➤ Lack of knowledge of bowel elimination techniques
➤ Insufficient physical activity
➤ Use of elimination aids (e.g., laxatives)
➤ Inability to recognize rectal cues

Rationale: To maintain bowel continence, a person must be motivated, have intact anorectal sensation, be able to store feces consciously, be able to contract puborectalis and external anal sphincter muscles, and have access to a toileting facility (McLane & McShane, 1991).

2. Assess person's ability to participate.

➤ Neurologic status
➤ Functional ability

Rationale: Bowel incontinence is common in institutionalized older adults and those with chronic illnesses. Cognitive impairments can impede recognition of bowel cues. Long-standing constipation can cause leaking around the impaction. Another cause of bowel incontinence is rectal sphincter abnormalities.

3. Plan a consistent appropriate time for elimination.

➤ Institute a daily bowel program for 5 days or until a pattern develops, and then move to an alternate-day program (morning or evening).
➤ Provide privacy and a nonstressful environment.
➤ Give reassurance and protect from embarrassment while establishing the bowel program.

Rationale: A routine will gradually become a pattern.

4. Teach effective bowel elimination techniques.

➤ Position a functionally able person upright or sitting. If he or she is not functionally able (e.g., quadriplegic), place in left side-lying position.
➤ For a functionally able person, use assistive devices (e.g., dil stick, digital stimulator, raised commode seat, lubricant and gloves), as appropriate.
➤ For a person with upper extremity mobility and abdominal musculature innervation, teach bowel elimination facilitation techniques as appropriate:
    ➤ Valsalva maneuver
    ➤ Sitting push-ups
    ➤ Pelvic floor exercises
    ➤ Forward bends
    ➤ Abdominal massage

5. Assist with or provide equipment needed for hygiene measures, as necessary.

➤ Maintain an elimination record or flow sheet of bowel schedule that includes time, stool characteristics, assistive methods used, and number of voluntary stools, if any.

Rationale: Pelvic floor exercises can increase the strength of the puborectalis and external anal sphincter muscles.

Rationale: Digital stimulation results in reflex peristalsis and evacuation.

6. Explain fluid and dietary requirements for good bowel movements.

➤ Ensure client drinks 8 to 10 glasses of water daily.
➤ Design a diet high in bulk and fiber.

Rationale: Stool consistency and volume are important for continence. Large volumes of loose stool overwhelm the continence mechanism. Small hard stools that do not distend or stimulate the rectum do not alert the person to the need to defecate (McLane & McShane, 1991). Dietary fiber increases stool volume.

7. Explain the effects of activity on peristalsis.

➤ Assist in determining the appropriate exercises for person's functional ability.

Rationale: Exercise increases GI motility and hastens bowel function.

8. Initiate health teaching, as indicated.

➤ Explain the hazards of using stool softeners, laxatives, suppositories, and enemas.
➤ Explain the signs and symptoms of fecal impaction and constipation.
➤ Initiate teaching of a bowel program before discharge. If the client is functionally able, encourage independence with bowel program; if not, incorporate assistive devices or attendant care, as needed.

Rationale: Laxatives cause unscheduled bowel movements, loss of colon tone, and inconsistent stool consistency. Enemas can overstretch the bowel and decrease tone. Stool softeners are not needed with adequate food or fluid intake (Alterman, 1995).

Rationale: Long-standing constipation or fecal impaction causes overdistention of the rectum by feces. Subsequent continuous reflex stimulation reduces sphincter tone. Incontinence will be either diarrhea leaking around the impaction or leaking of feces from a full rectum (Chassagne et al., 2000).

▼ Functional Incontinence

Definition

Functional Incontinence: state in which a person experiences incontinence because of a difficulty or inability to reach the toilet in time.

Defining Characteristics

MAJOR (MUST BE PRESENT)

Incontinence before or during an attempt to reach the toilet

Related Factors

PATHOPHYSIOLOGIC

Related to diminished bladder cues and impaired ability to recognize bladder cues secondary to

Brain injury/tumor/infection
Parkinsonism
Multiple sclerosis
Alcohol neuropathy
Demyelinating disease
Diabetes mellitus
Cerebrovascular accident
Progressive dementia

TREATMENT-RELATED

Related to decreased bladder tone secondary to

Antihistamines
Diuretics
Sedatives
Immunosuppressant therapy
Anticholinergics
Muscle relaxants
Epinephrine
Tranquilizers

SITUATIONAL (PERSONAL, ENVIRONMENTAL)

Related to impaired mobility

Related to decreased attention to bladder cues:

Depression
Confusion

Related to environmental barriers to bathroom:

Distant toilets
Siderails
Bed too high
Unfamiliar surroundings
Poor light

MATURATIONAL

Older Adult

Related to motor and sensory losses

Key Concepts

➤ Functional incontinence is the inability or unwillingness of the person with a normal bladder and sphincter to reach the toilet in time.
➤ Functional incontinence may be caused by conditions affecting physical and emotional ability to manage the act of urination.
➤ Underlying psychological problems can be a functional etiology of incontinence.
➤ Approximately 45% of all nursing home residents are incontinent. Of those with bladder incontinence, 82% have limited mobility (Miller, 2004).

FOCUS ASSESSMENT CRITERIA

See Impaired Urinary Elimination

GOAL

The person will report no or decreased episodes of incontinence

Indicators

Remove or minimize environmental barriers of incontinence

Use proper adaptive equipment to assist with voiding, transfers, and
   dressing
Describe causative factors for incontinence

GENERAL INTERVENTIONS

1. Assess environment barriers to the client's access to the bathroom.

Rationale: Barriers can delay access to the toilet and cause incontinence if
client cannot delay urination.

2. Provide grab rails and a raised toilet seat if necessary.

Rationale: These devices can promote independence and reduce toileting
difficulties.

3. If client requires assistance, provide ready access to a call bell and
   respond promptly when summoned.

Rationale: A few seconds' delay in reaching the bathroom can make the difference between continence and incontinence.

4. Encourage client to wear pajamas or ordinary clothes.

Rationale: Wearing normal clothing or nightwear helps to simulate the home
environment, where incontinence may not occur. A hospital gown may reinforce incontinence.

5. For a client with cognitive deficits, do the following:
   ➤ Offer toileting reminders every 2 hours after meals and before
      bedtime
   ➤ Provide verbal instructions for toileting activities
   ➤ Praise success and good attempts

Rationale: A client with a cognitive deficit needs constant verbal cues and
reminders to establish a routine and reduce incontinence.

6. Maintain optimal hydration (2,000 to 2,500 ml/day unless contraindicated). Space fluids every 2 hours.

Rationale: Dehydration can prevent the sensation of a full bladder and can
contribute to loss of bladder tone. Spacing fluids helps to promote regular
bladder filling and emptying.

7. Minimize intake of coffee, tea, colas, and grapefruit juice.

Rationale: These beverages acts as diuretics, which can cause urgency.

8. Teach prevention of urinary tract infection.

Rationale: Bacteria multiply rapidly in stagnant urine retained in the bladder. Moreover, overdistention hinders blood flow to the bladder wall, increasing the susceptibility to infection from bacterial growth. Regular complete bladder emptying greatly reduces the risk of infection. Dilute urine helps to prevent infection.

9. Teach client to monitor signs and symptoms of infection.

Rationale: Bacteria can act as a pyrogen by raising the hypothalamic thermostat through the production of endogenous pyrogen that may mediate though prostaglandins. Chills can occur when the temperature set point of the hypothalamus changes rapidly. Lower back pain results from distension of the renal capsule. Bacteria change the odor and pH of urine and irritate bladder tissue, causing spasm and frequency.

10. For geriatric clients:

➤ Emphasize that incontinence is not an inevitable age-related event.
➤ Explain not to restrict fluid intake for fear of incontinence.
➤ Explain not to rely on thirst as a signal to drink fluids.
➤ Teach the need to have easy access to bathroom at night, If needed, consider commode chair or urinal.

Rationale: Explaining the cause can motivate the person to participate. Dehydration can cause incontinence by eliminating the sensation of full bladder (the signal to urinate) and also by reducing the person's alertness to the sensation. The older adult has an age-related decrease in thirst (Miller, 2004).

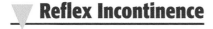

▼ Reflex Incontinence

Definition

Reflex Incontinence: State in which a person experiences predictable involuntary loss of urine with no sensation of urge, voiding, or bladder fullness.

Defining Characteristics

MAJOR (MUST BE PRESENT)

Uninhibited bladder contractions
Involuntary reflexes producing spontaneous voiding
Partial or complete loss of sensation of bladder fullness or urge to void

Related Factors

PATHOPHYSIOLOGIC

Related to impaired conduction of impulses above the reflex arc level secondary to

Cord injury/tumor/infection

 Reflex incontinence is usually caused by a spinal cord injury or tumor. The care for this client is complex and specialized and probably beyond the preparation of a beginning student. Consult with your instructor for assistance with this diagnosis.

▼ Stress Incontinence

Definition

Stress Incontinence: State in which a person experiences an immediate involuntary loss of urine with an increase in intraabdominal pressure.

Defining Characteristics

MAJOR (MUST BE PRESENT)

The person reports loss of urine (usually <50 ml) occurring with increased abdominal pressure from standing, sneezing, coughing, running, or lifting heavy objects

Related Factors

PATHOPHYSIOLOGIC

Related to incompetent bladder outlet secondary to congenital urinary tract anomalies
Related to degenerative changes in pelvic muscles and structural supports secondary to estrogen deficiency

SITUATIONAL (PERSONAL, ENVIRONMENTAL)

Related to high intraabdominal pressure and weak pelvic muscles secondary to

Obesity
Poor personal hygiene

Sex
Pregnancy

Related to weak pelvic muscles and structural supports secondary to

Recent substantial weight loss
Childbirth

MATURATIONAL

Older Adult

Related to loss of muscle tone

Key Concepts

GENERIC CONSIDERATIONS

➤ Urinary continence is maintained by the junction of the bladder and the urethra, support from the perineal floor, and the muscle around the urethra.
➤ Stress incontinence is the leakage of small amounts of urine when the outlet cannot control passage of urine in the presence of increased intraabdominal pressure.
➤ Menopausal decreases in elasticity usually worsen stress incontinence.
➤ A trial of vaginal estrogen cream in the postmenopausal woman who exhibits a pale atrophic vaginal vault may help to reduce the incidence of incontinence.
➤ The client with pure stress incontinence has a normal cystometrogram.
➤ The degrees of stress incontinence are as follows:
   Grade 1: urine is lost with sudden increase in abdominal pressure, but never at night
   Grade 2: lesser degrees of physical stress, such as walking, standing erect from a sitting position, or sitting up in bed, produce incontinence
   Grade 3: there is total incontinence, and urine is lost without any relation to physical activity or to position

FOCUS ASSESSMENT CRITERIA

See Impaired Urinary Elimination

GOAL

The person will report a reduction or elimination of stress incontinence.

Indicator

Be able to explain the causes of incontinence and rationale for treatments

GENERAL INTERVENTIONS

1. Determine contributing factors.

Loss of tissue or muscle tone from

➤ Childbirth
➤ Recent weight loss
➤ Atrophic vaginitis or urethritis
➤ Obesity
➤ Prolapsed uterus
➤ Aging
➤ History of surgery of the bladder and urethra with adhesions to the vaginal wall
➤ Increased intraabdominal pressure from overdistention between voidings, pregnancy, and obesity

Rationale: In stress incontinence, childbirth, trauma, menopausal atrophy, or obesity have weakened or stretched the pelvic floor muscles (pubococcygeus) and levator ani muscles.

2. Explain the effect of incompetent muscles on incontinence (see Key Concepts).
3. Teach pelvic muscle exercise (Dougherty, 1998).

➤ Teach how to self-assess whether exercises are being done correctly.
   ➤ Stand with one foot elevated on a stool, insert finger in vagina, and feel the strength of the contraction. Evaluate the strength of the contraction on a scale of 0 to 5 (Sampselle & DeLancey, 1998):
     0 = no palpable contraction
     1 = very weak, barely felt
     2 = weak, but clearly felt
     3 = good but not maintained when moderate finger pressure is applied
     4 = good but not maintained when intense finger pressure is applied
     5 = maximum strength with strong resistance
➤ Use a mirror to observe whether the clitoris has downward movement and the anus tightens with contraction.
➤ Consult an incontinence specialist for use of vaginal weights for pelvic floor strengthening (Perkins, 1998).

➤ Provide instructions for pelvic muscle exercises.

   ➤ For anterior pelvic floor muscles, imagine you are trying to stop the passage of urine, tighten the muscles (back and front) for 10 seconds, and then release them. Wait 10 seconds before the next contraction. Repeat 10 times a day. Stop and start the urine stream several times during voiding.

➤ Use the urine stop test to measure the effectiveness of a contraction by the time it takes to stop voiding. Advise not to perform the urine stop test more than once a day.

➤ Explain the pelvic muscle exercises are effective within 6 to 8 weeks with a 50% to 100% reduction in urine loss (Dougherty, 1998).

➤ Advise that exercises should continue at least three times a week after optimal results are achieved (usually within 16 weeks; Dougherty, 1998).

Rationale: Pelvic muscle exercises strengthen and tone the muscles of the pelvic floor. They may provide enough augmentation or urethral pressure to prevent mild stress incontinence. They should be taught to all women as a preventative measure. Studies have shown that pelvic muscle exercises improve or completely control stress incontinence (Dougherty, 1998).

4. Initiate health teaching for people who continue to remain incontinent after attempts at bladder reconditioning or muscle retraining.

➤ Promote personal integrity (see *Total Incontinence*).

➤ Promote skin integrity (see *Total Incontinence*).

➤ Schedule intermittent catheterization program (ICP), if appropriate (see *Total Incontinence*).

Rationale: When exercises are not enough, other control methods may be indicated.

▼ Total Incontinence

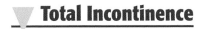

Definition

Total Incontinence: State in which a person experiences continuous unpredictable loss of urine without distention or awareness of bladder fullness.

Defining Characteristics

MAJOR (MUST BE PRESENT, ONE OR MORE)

Constant flow of urine with distention
Nocturia more than two times during sleep
Incontinence refractory to other treatments

MINOR (MAY BE PRESENT)

Unaware of bladder cues to void
Unaware of incontinence

Related Factors

Refer to *Impaired Urinary Elimination*.

Total incontinence *is a nursing diagnosis that is used after a thorough assessment. If a person is incontinent, initially use* Impaired Urinary Incontinence related to Unknown Etiology as evident by <u>specify signs/symptoms.</u> *If after careful assessment and selected interventions the person has continuous unpredictable loss of urine without distention or has no awareness of bladder fullness (cues), then use* Total Incontinence.

Key Concepts

See *Impaired Urinary Elimination*.

FOCUS ASSESSMENT CRITERIA

See *Impaired Urinary Elimination*.

GOAL

The person will be continent (specify during day, night, 24 hours).

Indicators

Identify the cause of incontinence and rationale for treatments
Identify daily goal for fluid intake

GENERAL INTERVENTIONS

1. Develop a bladder retraining or reconditioning program, which should include communication, assessment of voiding pattern, scheduled fluid intake, and scheduled voiding times.

   ➤ Promote communication among all staff members and among individual, family, and staff.

➤ Assess the person's potential for participation in a bladder-retraining program.
➤ Provide rationale for a plan and acquire client's informed consent.
➤ Encourage person to continue program by providing accurate information concerning reasons for success or failure.
➤ Assess voiding pattern.
➤ Monitor and record:
  ➤ Intake and output
  ➤ Time and amount of fluid intake
  ➤ Type of fluid
  ➤ Amount of incontinence
  ➤ Amount of void
  ➤ Presence of sensation of need to void
  ➤ Amount of retention
  ➤ Amount of residual
  ➤ Amount of triggered urine
  ➤ Record in appropriate column
➤ Schedule fluid intake and voiding times.
  ➤ Provide fluid intake of 2,000 ml each day unless contraindicated
  ➤ Discourage fluids after 7 pm

Rationale: Continence training programs are either self-directed or caregiver-directed. Self-directed programs of bladder training, retraining, and exercises are for motivated cognitively intact clients. Caregiver-directed programs of scheduled toileting or habit training are appropriate for motivated caregivers of clients with cognitive impairment (Miller, 2004). The essential components of any continence training program (self-directed or caregiver-directed) include motivation, assessment of voiding and incontinence patterns, a regular fluid intake of 2,000 to 3,000 ml/day, timed voiding of 2- to 4-hour intervals in an appropriate place, and ongoing assessment (Miller, 2004).

➤ Reduce incontinence-related irritant dermatitis (Scardillo, 1999).
➤ Decrease the alkalizing effect of urine on the skin.
  ➤ Use a no-rinse perineal cleanser
➤ Decrease injury with washing.
  ➤ Do not try to remove all the ointment with cleaning
  ➤ Gently wash skin

Rationale: Increased alkalinity of skin, moisture, friction, occlusive clothing, and heat cause incontinence-related irritant dermatitides (Scardillo, 1999).

2. Schedule ICP, if indicated.

➤ Monitor input and output
➤ Fluid intake should be at least 2,000 ml/day
➤ Use sterile catheterization technique in the hospital and clean technique at home.

➤ Desired catheter volumes are less than 500 ml
➤ Encourage client to attempt to void before scheduled catheterization time
➤ Initially obtain postvoid residuals at least every 6 hours
➤ Terminate ICP when the bladder is consistently emptied voluntarily or by triggering with less than 50 ml residual urine after each void

Rationale: Intermittent self-catheterization, periodic drainage of urine through the use of a catheter in the bladder, is indicated when neurologic impairment alters bladder emptying. Intermittent catheterization, when performed in a health care facility, should follow aseptic technique, because of the organisms found in the environment. People at home can practice clean technique because of the lack of virulent organisms in the home environment.

3. Teach ICP to person and family for long-term management of bladder (see Key Concepts)

➤ Explain the reasons for catheterization program
➤ Explain the relation of fluid intake and the frequency of catheterization
➤ Explain the importance of emptying the bladder at the prescribed time

Rationale: Dehydration can cause incontinence by eliminating the sensation of a full bladder (the signal to urinate) and also by reducing the person's alertness to the sensation. An overdistended bladder reduces blood flow to the bladder wall, making it more susceptible to infection from bacterial growth. Intermittent catheterization provides a decrease in morbidity associated with long-term use of indwelling catheters, increased independence, a more positive self-concept, and more normal sexual relations.

4. Teach the client/family about the bladder reconditioning program.

➤ Explain rationale and treatments (see Key Concepts)
➤ Explain the schedule of fluid intake, voiding attempts, manual triggering, and catheterization to control incontinence.
➤ Teach person and family the importance of positive reinforcement
➤ Refer to community nurses for assistance in bladder reconditioning if necessary

Rationale: Continence training programs are either self-directed or caregiver-directed. Self-directed programs of bladder training, retraining, and exercises are for motivated cognitively intact clients. Caregiver-directed programs of scheduled toileting or habit training are appropriate for motivated caregivers of clients with cognitive impairment (Miller, 2004).

5. If bladder retraining fails, consider use of indwelling catheter.

➤ For men, use a catheter no larger than 16F
➤ For women, use up to 18F for routine use

➤ Teach care of indwelling catheter
➤ Do not lift collection bag above the level of the bladder without pinching off the tube to prevent backflow
➤ Connect the catheter to a leg bag drainage system during the day

Rationale: The indwelling catheter provides direct access to the bladder and care is needed to prevent infection.

▾ Urge Incontinence

Definition

Urge Incontinence: State in which person experiences an involuntary loss of urine associated with a strong sudden desire to void.

Defining Characteristics

MAJOR (MUST BE PRESENT)

Urgency followed by incontinence

Related Factors

PATHOPHYSIOLOGIC

Related to decreased bladder capacity secondary to

Infection
Demyelinating diseases
Neurogenic disorders or injury
Parkinsonism
Cerebrovascular accident
Urethritis
Trauma
Diabetic neuropathy
Alcoholic neuropathy
Brain injury/tumor/infection

TREATMENT RELATED

Related to decreased bladder capacity secondary to

Abdominal surgery
Postindwelling catheters

SITUATIONAL (PERSONAL, ENVIRONMENTAL)

Related to irritation of bladder stretch receptors secondary to

Alcohol
Caffeine
Excess fluid intake

Related to decreased bladder capacity secondary to frequent voiding

MATURATIONAL
Older Adult

Related to decreased bladder capacity

Key Concepts

> ➤ Urge incontinence is an involuntary loss of urine associated with a strong desire to void. It is characterized by loss of large volumes of urine and may be triggered by emotional factors, body position changes, or the sight and sound of running water. This type of incontinence is commonly called bladder detrusor instability or vesical instability.
> ➤ Detrusor instability is characterized by uninhibited detrusor contractions sufficient to cause urinary incontinence.
> ➤ A person with an uninhibited neurogenic bladder has damage to the cerebral cortex (e.g., cerebrovascular accident, Parkinson's disease, brain injury/tumor) affecting the ability to inhibit urination.
> ➤ Warning time is the time a person can delay urination after feeling the urge to void. Diminished warning time can cause incontinence if the person cannot reach the toilet in time.

FOCUS ASSESSMENT CRITERIA

See *Impaired Urinary Elimination.*

GOAL

The person will report no or decreased episodes of incontinence (specify).

Indicators

Explain causes of incontinence
Describe bladder irritants

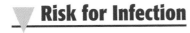

▼ Risk for Infection

Definition

Risk for Infection: State in which a person is at risk to be invaded by an opportunistic or pathogenic agent (virus, fungus, bacteria, protozoa, or other parasite) from endogenous or exogenous sources.

Risk Factors

See Related Factors

Related Factors

Various health problems and situations can create favorable conditions that would encourage the development of infections. Some common factors follow.

PATHOPHYSIOLOGIC

Related to compromised host defenses secondary to

Chronic diseases

➤ Cancer
➤ Hepatic disorders
➤ Renal failure
➤ Respiratory disorders
➤ Arthritis
➤ Hematologic disorders
➤ Diabetes mellitus
➤ AIDS
➤ Alcoholism
➤ Immunosuppression
➤ Immunodeficiency
➤ Altered or insufficient leukocytes

Blood dyscrasias
Skin disorder
Periodontal disease

Related to compromised circulation secondary to

Lymphedema
Obesity
Peripheral vascular disease

TREATMENT-RELATED

Related to a site for organism invasion secondary to

Surgical incision
Tracheotomy
Total parenteral nutrition
Dialysis
Urinary catheter
Enteral feedings
Intravenous line

Related to compromised host defenses secondary to

Radiation therapy
Chemotherapy
Organ transplant
Steroid therapy

SITUATIONAL (PERSONAL, ENVIRONMENTAL)

Related to compromised host defenses secondary to

History of infections
Stress
Malnutrition
Increased hospital stay
Prolonged immobility
Smoking

Related to a site for organism invasion secondary to

Trauma
Postpartum trauma
Bites (animal, insect, human)
Thermal injuries
Warm, moist, dark environment (skin folds, casts)

Related to contact with contagious agents (nosocomial or community acquired, e.g., measles, hepatitis B)

MATURATIONAL
Older Adult

Related to increased vulnerability secondary to

Debilitated condition
Chronic diseases
Diminished immune response

All people are at the risk for infection. Body fluid control, environmental control, and handwashing before and after client care reduce the risk of transmission of organisms.

As a beginning student you will routinely use Risk for Infection with most of your hospitalized clients. Foley catheters, surgical wounds, and intravenous lines are risk factors. The interventions to prevent infection for all hospitalized clients will become routine. At some point, your instructor may no longer expect Risk for Infection on all your care plans. Instead, you will use High Risk for Infection for clients that are more vulnerable to infection than the usual hospitalized client.

High Risk for Infection describes a person whose host defenses are compromised, thus increasing susceptibility to environmental pathogens or his or her own endogenous flora (e.g., a person with chronic liver dysfunction or with an invasive line). Nursing interventions for such a person focus on minimizing introduction of organisms and increasing resistance to infection (e.g., improving nutritional status). For a person with an infection, the situation is best described by the collaborative problem PC: Sepsis.

Key Concepts

GENERIC CONSIDERATIONS

➤ Resistance to infection depends on the person's immune response (susceptibility) the amount of the infecting agent, and strength of the organism. Factors influencing the host's immune response include the following:
   ➤ Anatomic barriers—each system has specific lines of defenses
   ➤ Therapies—pose a threat to normal lines of defense by either invasiveness or alteration of body function
   ➤ Developmental and heritable factors—factors that negatively affect the person's immune system function (e.g., newborn status; agammaglobulinemia)
   ➤ Hormonal factors—males are more vulnerable to infection than are females; pregnancy increases the female's vulnerability; steroid therapy increases vulnerability in both sexes
   ➤ Age—includes both extremes (immaturity or degeneration of immune system)
   ➤ Nutrition—influences protein synthesis and phagocytosis, decreasing the body's vulnerability to infection
   ➤ Fever—hyperthermia may inhibit the growth of organisms
   ➤ Secretions such as mucus, saliva, and skin secretions—contain substances that are bactericidal, decreasing the risk of infection and colonization

Host Defenses

Specific host defenses of each system that influence the immune response include the following:

CNS

Because the most common route for both bacterial and viral infections of the CNS is through the blood route, blood host defenses play an important primary role.

Cutaneous

➤ Skin provides a first line of defense against organisms, both anatomically and chemically.
➤ Sweat glands and sebaceous glands do not allow overgrowth of bacteria.
➤ The acid pH of the skin does not allow pathogenic organisms to grow or survive on the skin for any length of time.
➤ The flushing and lysozyme actions of tears control eye infections. The lacrimal duct flushes out organisms and deposits them in the nasopharynx.

Blood

➤ Circulating blood is the major vehicle for transporting internal defense mechanisms.
➤ The febrile response is associated with the circulation of pyrogens to the hypothalamus.

Genitourinary Tract

➤ Anatomic structure eliminates easy ascent of perineal microorganisms into the bladder.
➤ Mucous layer allows entrapment of organisms and engulfment by bladder cells.
➤ The pH and osmolarity of urine prevent bacterial multiplication.
➤ The ability to empty the bladder completely eliminates stasis of invading organisms and allows continual flushing.

Respiratory Tract

➤ The nares entrap most foreign matter on the mucous membranes as a result of turbulence caused by the turbinates and hairs.
➤ The mucociliary transport system consists of cilia and mucus, which remove additional matter passing to the upper and lower bronchi.
➤ Lysozymes and immunoglobulin A, a secretion of phagocytes, are found in nasal secretions and assist in the prevention of colonization.
➤ Particles reaching as far as the alveoli can be removed through the expulsive action of sneezing and coughing and the gag reflex.

➤ Phagocytosis occurs in the alveoli, with the macrophages used as a major defense mechanism.

GI Tract

➤ A mucous layer traps ingested microbes in the epithelium of the GI tract.
➤ Gastric acids kill most organisms.
➤ Peristalsis aids in the removal of organisms.
➤ Intestinal secretions contain antibody (immunoglobulin A), bile salts, lysozyme, glycolipids, and glycoproteins that prevent proliferation and adherence.
➤ Normal gut floras interact to restrict overproliferation.

Wounds

➤ Skin provides a first line of defense; the opening of the skin, either surgically or traumatically, increases the risk of infection.
➤ A wound essentially closes within 24 hours, eliminating the risk of direct entry of organisms.
➤ Wound infections rely on the capabilities of other host defenses to assist in healing.
➤ Wounds are at risk for infection due to the following factors:
  ➢ Sutures and staples, unlike tape, create their own wounds, act like drains, and cause their own inflammatory response.
  ➢ Drains provide a site for microorganism entry.
  ➢ The incidence of infection in clients who are not shaved or clipped is 0.9%. It increases to 1.4% with electric shaving, 1.7% with clipping, and 2.5% with razor shaving (Kovach, 1990).

GERIATRIC CONSIDERATIONS

➤ A slower rate of epidermal proliferation causes injured skin to take twice as long to heal in older adults.
➤ Studies have shown 5% to 20% of residents in long-term care facilities to have infections. The most frequent are those of the urinary tract, respiratory system, and skin and soft tissues (usually pressure ulcers; Miller, 2004).
➤ The increased susceptibility of older adults to infections is multifactorial (either host factors or environmental). Host factors include underlying diseases, invasive treatment modalities, indiscriminate use of antibiotics, malnutrition, dehydration, impaired mobility, and incontinence. Environmental factors in institutions include limited surveillance for infection, crowded areas, cross-contamination, and delay in early detection.
➤ Skin and urinary tract colonization is a greater problem in older than in younger clients. Changes in immune competence with aging

increase susceptibility to fungal, viral, and mycobacterial pathogens (Miller, 2004).

➤ Older adults do not exhibit the usual signs of infection (fever, chills, tachypnea, tachycardia, leukocytosis) but instead present with anorexia, weakness, change in mental status, normothermia, or hypothermia (Miller, 2004).

FOCUS ASSESSMENT CRITERIA

Assess for subjective (S) and objective (O) cues.

Risk Factors

Does the person complain of (S)

➤ Previous infections
➤ Pain or swelling (generalized, localized)
➤ Hemoptysis
➤ Productive prolonged cough
➤ Chest pain associated with other criteria
➤ Systemic symptoms
    ➤ Fever, continuous or intermittent
    ➤ Loss of appetite
    ➤ Easy fatigability
    ➤ Night sweats
    ➤ Chills
    ➤ Weight loss

History of recent travel (S)

➤ Within United States
➤ Outside United States

History of exposure to infectious diseases (S)

➤ Air-borne (most childhood infections result from communicable diseases, e.g., chickenpox, tuberculosis)
➤ Vector-borne and other vector-associated infections (malaria, plague)
➤ Vehicle-borne and other food- and water-borne infections (hepatitis A, salmonellas)
➤ Contact spread (most common type of exposure)
    ➤ Direct (person to person)
    ➤ Indirect (e.g., by instruments, clothing, and so forth)
➤ Contact droplet (e.g., pneumonias, colds)

Presence of wounds (O)

➤ Surgical
➤ Burns

➤ Invasive devices (tracheostomy, intravenous (IV), drains)
➤ Self-induced

Temperature, abnormal (O)
Nutritional deficiency (O)

GOAL

The person will report risk factors associated with infection and precautions needed.

Indicators

Demonstrate meticulous handwashing technique by time of discharge
Describe methods of transmission of infection
Describe the influence of nutrition on prevention of infection

GENERAL INTERVENTIONS

1. Identify clients at high risk for nosocomial infections.
   a. Consider a person with one or more factors to be at high risk for infection.

➤ Abdominal or thoracic surgery
➤ Surgical procedure longer than 2 hours
➤ Genitourinary procedure
➤ Instrumentation (ventilator, suction, catheters, nebulizers, tracheostomy, invasive monitoring)
➤ Anesthesia
➤ Age younger than 1 year or older than 65 years
➤ Obesity
➤ Underlying disease conditions (COPD, diabetes, cardiovascular, blood dyscrasias)
➤ Substance abuse
➤ Medications (steroids, chemotherapy, antibiotic therapy) that modify immune response
➤ Nutritional status (intake less than minimum daily requirements)
➤ Smoking

   b. Consider those with the following factors at risk for delayed wound healing:

➤ Malnourishment
➤ Anemia

➤ Corticosteroid therapy
➤ Hypoxia
➤ Smoking
➤ Diabetes
➤ Renal insufficiency
➤ Surgery > 3 hours
➤ Obesity
➤ Cancer
➤ Hypovolemia
➤ Night or emergency surgery
➤ Immune system compromise
➤ Zinc, copper, magnesium deficiency

Rationale: Intervention can be implemented to control or influence the degree of vulnerability associated with risk factors.

2. For surgical wounds, teach client about factors that can delay wound healing.

➤ Dehydrated wound tissue

Rationale: Studies report that epithelial migration is impeded under dry crust; movement is three times faster over moist tissue.

➤ Wound infection

Rationale: The exudates in infected wounds impair epithelialization and wound closure.

➤ Inadequate nutrition and hydration

Rationale: To repair tissue, the body needs increased protection and carbohydrate intake and adequate hydration for vascular transport of oxygen and wastes.

3. Monitor for signs and symptoms of wound infection

➤ Increased swelling redness
➤ Wound separation
➤ Increased or purulent drainage
➤ Prolonged subnormal temperature or significantly elevated temperature

Rationale: Tissue responds to pathogen infiltration with increased blood and lymph flow (manifested by edema, redness, and increased drainage) and reduced epithelialization (marked by wound separation). Circulating pathogens trigger the hypothalamus to elevate the body temperature; certain pathogens cannot survive at higher temperatures.

4. Monitor wound healing by nothing the following:

> ➤ Evidence of intact, approximated wound edges (primary intention)
> ➤ Evidence of granulation tissue (secondary and tertiary intention)

Rationale: A surgical wound with edges approximated by sutures usually heals by primary intention. Granulation tissue is not visible, and scar formation is minimal. In contrast, a surgical wound with a drain or an abscess heals by secondary intention or granulation and has more distinct scar formation. A restructured wound heals by third intention and results in a wider and deeper scar.

5. Take steps to prevent infection.

> ➤ Wash hands before and after dressing changes.
> ➤ Wear gloves until wound is sealed.
> ➤ Keep tubing away from incision.
> ➤ Discard unused irrigation solutions after 24 hours.

Rationale: These measures help to prevent introduction of microorganisms into the wound; they also reduce the risk of transmitting infection to others.

6. Initiate measures to prevent urinary tract infection.

> ➤ Assess for abdominal signs and symptoms after any urologic procedure, including frequency, urgency, burning, and abnormal color and odor.
> ➤ Monitor client's temperature at least every 24 hours for elevation; notify physician if temperature is greater than 100.8°F.
> ➤ Encourage fluids when appropriate.
> ➤ Instruct client and family as to risk for development of urinary tract infections.
> ➤ Use universal precautions with all fluids from client.
> ➤ Use aseptic technique when emptying any urinary drainage device; keep bag off the floor but below bladder or clamped during transport.
> ➤ Teach client undergoing IV therapy not to bump or disturb the IV catheterization site.
> ➤ Teach a client with an indwelling catheter in place to do the following:
>> ➤ Avoid pressure on the catheter.
>> ➤ Wipe from front to back after a bowel movement.

Rationale: Nosocomial infections occur in hospitalized clients. Early detection enables prompt intervention to prevent serious complications and a prolonged hospital stay. Catheter movement can cause tissue trauma, predisposing to inflammation. Feces can readily contaminate an indwelling catheter.

7. Prevent infection at invasive site lines.

➤ Assess all invasive lines every 24 hours for redness, inflammation, drainage, and tenderness.
➤ Monitor client's temperature at least every 24 hours; notify physician if greater than 100.8°F.
➤ Maintain aseptic technique for all invasive devices, changing sites, dressings, tubing, and solutions per policy schedule.

Rationale: Intravenous lines permit direct exposure to circulatory system. Movement of the device can cause tissue trauma and possible inflammation.

8. Prevent respiratory tract infection.

➤ Evaluate risk for infection after any instrumentation of the respiratory tract for at least 48 hours after procedure.
➤ Monitor temperature at least every 8 hours and notify physician if greater than 100.8°F.
➤ Evaluate sputum characteristics for frequency, purulence, blood, and odor.
➤ Evaluate sputum and blood cultures, if done, for significant findings.
➤ Evaluate CBC for significant shift in white blood cell counts.
➤ Assess lung sounds every 8 hours or PRN.
➤ If client has abdominal/thoracic surgery, instruct before surgery on importance of coughing, turning, and deep breathing.
➤ Evaluate need for suctioning if client cannot clear secretions adequately.
➤ Assess for risk of aspiration, keeping head of bed elevated 30 degrees unless otherwise contraindicated.
➤ Instruct on principles of cough and deep breathing and prevention of infection.

Rationale: Hypoventilation, decreased sensorium immobility, and pain can cause retained secretions.

9. Protect the client with immune deficiency from infection.

➤ Place client in private room.
➤ Instruct client to ask all visitors and personnel to wash their hands before approaching.
➤ Limit visitors when appropriate.
➤ Screen all visitors for known infections or exposure to infection.
➤ Teach client and family members signs and symptoms of infection.
➤ Evaluate client's personal hygiene habits.
➤ Nurses must practice precautions with blood and body fluids from all clients to protect themselves from exposure to all potentially infectious organisms (CDC, 2000).
    ➤ Wash hands before and after all client or specimen contact.
    ➤ Handle the blood of all clients as potentially infectious.

➤ Wear gloves for potential contact with blood and body fluids.
➤ Place used syringes immediately in nearby impermeable container; avoid recapping or manipulating needle. Recapping or needle removal must be accomplished through the use of a mechanical device or a one-handed technique.
➤ Wear protective eyewear and mask if splatter with blood or body fluids is possible (e.g., bronchoscopy, oral surgery).
➤ Wear gowns when splash with blood or body fluids is anticipated.
➤ Handle all linen soiled with blood or body secretions as potentially infectious.
➤ Process all laboratory specimens as potentially infectious.
➤ Wear mask for tuberculosis and other respiratory organisms (human immunodeficiency virus [HIV] is not air-borne).
➤ Place resuscitation equipment where respiratory arrest is predictable.
➤ Wear shoe covers or surgical caps or hoods when gross contamination can reasonably be anticipated (e.g., autopsy, orthopedic surgery, obstetrics).

Rationale: Persons with compromised immune systems need additional protection from infection from others.

▼ Risk for Infection Transmission

Definition

Risk for Infection Transmission: The state in which an individual is at risk for transferring an opportunistic or pathogenic agent to others.

Risk Factors

Presence of risk factors (see Related Factors)

Related Factors

PATHOPHYSIOLOGIC

Related to

Airborne transmission exposure
Contact transmission exposure (direct, indirect, contact droplet)
Vehicle transmission exposure
Vector-borne transmission exposure

TREATMENT-RELATED

Related to contaminated wound
Related to devices with contaminated drainage:

Urinary, chest, endotracheal tubes
Suction equipment

SITUATIONAL (PERSONAL, ENVIRONMENTAL)

Related to

Unsanitary living conditions (sewage, personal hygiene)
Areas considered high risk for vector-borne diseases (malaria, rabies, bubonic plague)
Areas considered high risk for vehicle-borne disease (hepatitis A, Shigella, Salmonella)
Lack of knowledge of sources or prevention of infection
Intravenous drug use
Multiple sex partners
Natural disaster (e.g., flood, hurricane)
Disaster with hazardous infectious material

Risk for infection transmission describes a person at risk for transmitting an infectious agent to others such as HIV or tuberculosis. This diagnosis is very important to protect staff and visitors.

Key Concepts

GENERIC CONSIDERATIONS

➤ To spread an infection, three elements are required:
  ➤ A source of infecting organism
  ➤ A susceptible host
  ➤ A means of transmission for the organism
➤ Sources of infecting organisms include the following:
  ➤ Clients, personnel, and visitors with acute disease, incubating infection, or colonized organisms without apparent disease.
  ➤ Person's own endogenous flora (autogenous infection)
  ➤ Inanimate environment, including equipment and medications
➤ Susceptibility of the host varies according to
  ➤ Immune status
  ➤ Ability to develop a commensal relationship with the infecting organism and become an asymptomatic carrier
  ➤ Preexisting diseases

➤ Means of transmission for the organism include one or more of the following:

   ➤ Contact transmission, the most frequent method of transferring organisms into the conjunctiva, nose, or mouth of a susceptible host by coughing, sneezing, or talking. Droplets travel no more than 3 feet.

   ➤ Vehicle route transmission infections are spread through means such as
      ➢ Food (e.g., hepatitis A, Salmonella)
      ➢ Water (e.g., Legionella)
      ➢ Drugs (e.g., IV-contaminated products)
      ➢ Blood (e.g., hepatitis B, hepatitis C, HIV)

   ➤ Airborne infections are disseminated by droplet nuclei (residue of evaporated droplets that may remain suspended in the air for long periods) or dust particles in the air containing the infectious agent.

   ➤ Vector-borne infections are spread through vectors such as animals or insects.

➤ Universal body substance precautions require safety measures with all blood and body fluids. Those clients with a suspected or confirmed medical diagnosis indicative of an infectious disease process, however, need documentation with a comprehensive plan of care for that infection or potential infection. The nursing diagnosis Risk for Infection Transmission can be used to document specific universal precaution practices.

➤ The cause of AIDS is a retrovirus labeled HIV. Transmission is by exposure to contaminated semen, vaginal fluids, or blood.

➤ AIDS has a latency or incubation period of 18 months to 5 years. During this period, the person transmits disease through sexual activity or contaminated blood.

FOCUS ASSESSMENT CRITERIA

Refer to *Risk for Infection*

GOAL

The person will describe the mode of transmission of disease by the time of discharge.

Indicators

Relate the need to be isolated until noninfectious
Demonstrate meticulous handwashing during hospitalization

GENERAL INTERVENTIONS

1. Identify people who are susceptible hosts based on focus assessment for risk for infection and history of exposure.
2. Identify the mode of transmission based on infecting agent.

- ➤ Airborne
- ➤ Contact
  - ➤ Direct
  - ➤ Indirect
  - ➤ Contact droplet
- ➤ Vehicle-borne
- ➤ Vector-borne

Rationale: To prevent transmission of infection, the mode of transmission (i.e., air-borne, contact, vehicle-borne, or vector-borne) must be known.

3. Reduce the transfer of pathogens.

- ➤ Isolate clients with air-borne communicable infections.
- ➤ Secure appropriate room assignment depending on the type of infection and hygienic practices of the infected person.
- ➤ Use universal precautions to prevent transmission to self or other susceptible host.
  - ➤ Wash hands before and after all client or specimen contact.
  - ➤ Handle the blood of all clients as potentially infectious.
  - ➤ Wear gloves for potential contact with blood and body fluids.
  - ➤ Place used syringes immediately in nearby impermeable container; avoid recapping or manipulating needle. Recapping or needle removal must be accomplished through the use of a mechanical device or a one-handed technique.
  - ➤ Wear protective eyewear and mask if splatter with blood or body fluids is possible (e.g., bronchoscopy, oral surgery).
  - ➤ Wear gowns when splash with blood or body fluids is anticipated.
  - ➤ Handle all linen soiled with blood or body secretions as potentially infectious.
  - ➤ Process all laboratory specimens as potentially infectious.
  - ➤ Wear mask for tuberculosis and other respiratory organisms (HIV is not air-borne).
- ➤ Place resuscitation equipment where respiratory arrest is predictable.
- ➤ Wear shoe covers or surgical caps or hoods when gross contamination can reasonably be anticipated (e.g., autopsy, orthopedic surgery, obstetrics).

Rationale: Nurses must use precautions with blood fluids from all clients to protect themselves from exposure to HIV and hepatitis B and C.

4. Discuss the mode of transmission of infection with client, family, and significant others.

➤ Evaluate client for secondary sites of infection (e.g., urine, respiratory, wound).

Rationale: Prevention of infection transmission must continued after discharge.

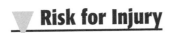

Risk for Injury

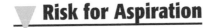

Risk for Aspiration

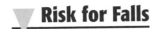

Risk for Falls

Definition

Risk for Injury: State in which a person is at risk for harm because of a perceptual or physiologic deficit, a lack of awareness of hazards, or maturational age.

Risk Factors

Presence of risk factor (see Related Factors)

Related Factors

PATHOPHYSIOLOGIC

Related to altered cerebral function secondary to

Tissue hypoxia
Syncope
Vertigo

Related to altered mobility secondary to

Unsteady gait
Loss of limb
Amputation
Cerebrovascular accident
Arthritis
Parkinsonism

Related to impaired sensory function (specify)

Vision
Thermal/touch
Hearing
Smell

Related to fatigue
Related to orthostatic hypotension
Related to vertebrobasilar insufficiency
Related to vestibular disorders
Related to lack of awareness of environmental hazards secondary to

Confusion
Depression
Hypoglycemia
Electrolyte imbalance

Related to tonic-clonic movements secondary to

Seizures

Related to carotid sinus syncope

TREATMENT-RELATED

Related to effects of (specify) on mobility or sensorium:

Medications
Sedatives
Diuretics
Vasodilators
Phenothiazine
Antihypertensives
Psychotropics
Hypoglycemics

Related to use of casts/crutches, canes, walkers

SITUATIONAL (PERSONAL, ENVIRONMENTAL)

Related to decrease in or loss of short-term memory
Related to faulty judgment secondary to

Stress
Alcohol, drugs
Dehydration

Related to prolonged bed rest
Related to vasovagal reflex

Related to household hazards (specify)

Unsafe walkways
Stairs
Unsafe toys
Slippery floors
Inadequate lighting
Faulty electric wires
Bathrooms (tubs, toilets)
Improperly stored poisons

Related to automotive hazards

Lack of use of seat belts or child seats
Mechanically unsafe vehicle

Related to fire hazards
Related to unfamiliar setting (hospital, nursing home)
Related to improper footwear
Related to inattentive caretaker
Related to improper use of aids (crutches, canes, walkers, wheelchairs)
Related to history of accidents

MATURATIONAL

Older Adult

Related to faulty judgments secondary to motor and sensory deficits, medication (accidental overdose), cognitive deficits

This diagnosis has five subcategories: Risk for Aspiration, Poisoning, Suffocation, Trauma, and Falls. Interventions to prevent falling, poisoning, suffocation, and trauma are included under the general category Risk for Injury. Should you choose to isolate interventions only for prevention of poisoning, suffocation, or trauma, then the diagnosis Risk for Poisoning, Risk for Suffocation, Risk for Falls, or Risk for Trauma would be useful.

Nursing interventions related to Risk for Injury focus on protecting a person from and teaching precautions to reduce the risk of injury. When the nurse is teaching a client or family safety measures to prevent injury but is not providing on-site protection (as in the community or outpatient department or for discharge planning), the diagnosis Risk for Injury related to insufficient knowledge of safety precautions may be more appropriate.

Risk for Injury should not be used to describe clinical situations of hemorrhage or electrolyte imbalance; instead, refer to the collaborative problem section.

Key Concepts

GENERIC CONSIDERATIONS

➤ Injury is the fourth leading cause of death in the general population (40.1 deaths per 100,000) and the leading of death in children and young adults (US Public Health Services, 1998).

➤ Health education activities that focus on fire safety, home safety, water safety, seat belt use, motor vehicle safety, cardiopulmonary resuscitation (i.e., CPR) training, poison control, and first aid can reduce the rate of accidents (Clemen-Stone, Eigasti & McGuire, 2002).

➤ Table II.8 lists common sources of poisoning in the home.

Table II–8. POISONOUS SUBSTANCES AROUND THE HOUSE

Drugs

Aspirin	Cough medicines	Laxatives
Tranquilizers	Vitamins	Oral contraceptives
Barbiturates	Acetaminophen	

Petroleum Products

Cleaning Agents

Soaps and polishes	Disinfectants	Drain cleaners

Poisonous Plants

Amaryllis	Iris	Philodendron
Azalea	Jack-in-the-pulpit	Poinsettia
Baneberry	Jerusalem cherry	Poison hemlock
Belladonna	Jimsonweed	Poison ivy
Bittersweet	Lily of the valley	Pokeweed
Bloodroot	Marijuana	Potato leaves
Castor-bean plant	Mistletoe	Rhododendron
Climbing nightshade	Morning glory	Rhubarb leaves
Daffodil	Mountain laurel	Schefflera
Devil's ivy	Mushrooms	Tomato leaves
Dieffenbachia	Oleander	Wisteria
Foxglove	Peacelily	Yew
Holly		

Miscellaneous

Baby powder	Cosmetics	Lead paint

Orthostatic Hypotension

➤ Postural hypotension refers to a sudden drop in blood pressure of 20 mm Hg or more for at least 1 minute when standing.

➤ Studies have shown that postprandial hypotension occurs in about one third of healthy adults 1 hour after eating breakfast and lunch (Miller, 2004).

➤ Postural hypotension can affect quality of life if it contributes to falls or fear of falling. It also can precipitate stroke and myocardial infarction (Porth, 2002).

GERIATRIC CONSIDERATIONS

➤ Falls are more frequent in older adults, and the mortality, dysfunction, disability, and need for medical services that result are greater than in younger age groups. Unintentional injury, a category including falls, motor vehicle collisions, and burns, is the seventh leading cause of death in older adults, and the incidence of falls represents more than 60% of that category.

➤ Approximately 25% of hospital admissions for older adults are directly related to falling; 47% of these people are admitted to long-term care facilities (Miller, 2004)

➤ "Fallophobia" refers to fears related to a person's loss of confidence to perform activities without falling. These fears actually increase the risk for falling, and the person eventually becomes housebound (Miller, 2004).

➤ A fall-free existence is not always possible for some people. Increased independence and mobility may be an important and valuable trade-off for increased risk of falling. Collaboration among client, family, and team members helps arrive at the decision of a less restricted environment.

➤ With age comes some loss of the postural control system. To not fall, a person must be able to keep his or her center of gravity over an adequate base and be able to rapidly process and respond to sensory information (Baumann, 1999).

➤ Older adults frequently lack muscle strength in lower extremities and have insufficient torque in their ankles (Baumann, 1999)

➤ Regular walking, as little as 60 minutes twice a week, can improve sensory function, balance, stability, hip flexion strength, hip extension, and dorsiflexion, all of which can reduce falls (Schoenfelder, 2000).

➤ The following factors increase the risk for falls in older adults (Miller, 2004):
  ➤ History of falls
  ➤ Sensory-motor deficits (e.g., vision, hearing, hemianopia [loss of half of visual field], paresis, aphasia)
  ➤ Gait instability

➤ Improper footwear or foot problems (corns, bunions, calluses)
➤ Postural hypotension, especially with complaints of dizziness
➤ Confusion (persistent or acute)
➤ Incontinence, urinary urgency
➤ Cardiovascular disease affecting cerebral perfusion and oxygenation: dysrhythmias, syncopal episodes, congestive heart failure, fibrillation
➤ Neurologic disease affecting movement or judgement: cerebrovascular accident with impulsivity, parkinsonism, moderate Alzheimer's disease, seizure disorder, vertigo
➤ Orthopedic disorders or devices affecting movement or balance: casts, splints, slings, prostheses, recent surgery, severe arthritis
➤ Medications affecting blood pressure or level of consciousness: psychotropics, sedatives, analgesics, diuretics, antihypertensives, medication change, more than five drugs
➤ Agitation, increased anxiety, emotional lability
➤ Willfulness, uncooperativeness
➤ Situational factors: new admission, room change, roommate change

FOCUS ASSESSMENT CRITERIA

This entire assessment is indicated only when the client is at high risk for injury because of personal deficits, alterations (e.g., mobility problems), or maturational age. In households without such a family member, the functional assessment of the individual can be deleted.

Subjective Data

These consist of the person's physical capabilities (as reported by person or caretaker).
Assess for subjective (S) and objective (O) cues:

Vision (S,O)

➤ Corrected (date of last prescription)
➤ Complaints of
   ➤ Blurriness
   ➤ Difficulty focusing
   ➤ Loss of side vision
   ➤ Inability to adjust to darkness

Hearing (S,O)

➤ Need to read lips
➤ Inadequate
➤ Use of hearing aid (condition, batteries)

Thermal/tactile (S)

➤ Decreased ability to sense of hot/cold

Mental status

➤ Drowsy (O)
➤ Confused (O)
➤ Oriented to time, place, events (O)
➤ Complaints of (S)
   ➤ Vertigo
   ➤ Orthostatic hypotension
➤ Altered sense of balance (S)

Mobility

➤ Reports of (S)
   ➤ Feeling lightheaded, dizzy
   ➤ Losing balance
   ➤ Difficulty standing, sitting
   ➤ Wandering
   ➤ Falling or almost falling
➤ Ability to ambulate (S,O)
   ➤ Around room
   ➤ Around house
   ➤ Up and down stairs
   ➤ Outside house
➤ Ability to travel (S)
   ➤ Drive car (date of last reevaluation)
   ➤ Use public transportation
➤ Use of devices
   ➤ Cane
   ➤ Walker
   ➤ Condition of devices
   ➤ Wheelchair
   ➤ Prosthesis
   ➤ Competence in their use
➤ Shoes/slippers (O)
   ➤ Condition
   ➤ Nonskid soles
   ➤ Fit

Assess for objective cues:

Blood pressure (left, right, sitting/lying more than 5 min, 1 min after standing)

➤ Gait
   ➤ Steady
   ➤ Requires aids
   ➤ Unsteady

➤ Strength
  ➤ Can stand on one leg
  ➤ Can sit, stand, sit

Cognitive processes

➤ Can communicate needs
➤ Can interact
➤ History of wandering
➤ Can understand cause and effect (witnessed and reported by others)

Presence of

➤ Anger
➤ Withdrawal
➤ Depression
➤ Faulty judgment

Ability for self-care activities

➤ Dress and undress
➤ Bathe
➤ Groom self
➤ Feed self
➤ Reach toilet

GOAL

The person will relate fewer falls and less fear of falling.

Indicators

Identify factors that increase risk for injury
Relate intent to use safety measures to prevent injury (e.g., remove or
    anchor throw rugs)
Relate intent to practice selected prevention measures (e.g., wear sun-
    glasses to reduce glare)
Increase daily activity, if feasible

GENERAL INTERVENTIONS

1. Assess for causative or contributing factors.

➤ Unfamiliar surroundings
➤ Impaired vision
  ➤ Altered spatial judgment
  ➤ Blurred vision

> ➤ Diplopia
> ➤ Blind spots
> ➤ Cataracts
> ➤ Altered peripheral vision
> ➤ Hemianopia
> ➤ Increased susceptibility to visual glare
> ➤ Decreased ability to tell object from background
➤ Decreased hearing acuity
➤ Decreased tactile sensitivity (touch)
➤ Orthostatic hypotension
➤ Decreased strength/flexibility
➤ Unstable gait
➤ Pain
➤ Fatigue
➤ Improper shoes or slippers
➤ Improper use of crutches, canes, walkers
➤ Joint immobility
➤ Side effects of medication (e.g., tranquilizers, diuretics)
➤ Hazardous environmental factors

Rationale: The nurse can reduce or eliminate factors that increase the risk of injury.

2. Reduce or eliminate causative or contributing factors, if possible.

Unfamiliar surroundings

➤ Orient each client to surroundings on admission; explain the call system, and assess client's ability to use it.
➤ Closely supervise client during the first few nights to assess safety.
➤ Use nightlight.
➤ Encourage person to request assistance during the night.
➤ Teach about side effects of certain drugs (e.g., dizziness, fatigue).
➤ Keep bed at lowest level during the night.
➤ Consider use of a movement detection monitor, if needed.

Rationale: An unfamiliar environment and problems with vision, orientation, mobility, and fatigue can increase risk of falling.

Impaired vision

➤ Provide safe illumination and teach client to
> ➤ Ensure adequate lighting in all rooms, with soft light at night.
> ➤ Have light switch easily accessible, next to bed.
> ➤ Provide background light that is soft.
➤ Teach client how to reduce glare.
> ➤ Avoid glossy surfaces (e.g., glass, highly polished floors).
> ➤ Use diffuse rather than direct light; use shades that darken the room.

> ➤ Turn head away when switching on a bright light.
> ➤ Wear sunglasses or hats with brims or carry umbrellas to reduce glare outside.
> ➤ Avoid looking directly at bright lights (e.g., headlights).

➤ Teach person or family to provide sufficient color contrast for visual discrimination and to avoid green and blue.

> ➤ Color-code edges of steps (e.g., with colored tape).
> ➤ Avoid white walls, dishes, and counters.
> ➤ Choose objects colored black on white (e.g., black phone)
> ➤ Avoid colors that merge (e.g., beige switches on beige walls).
> ➤ Paint doorknobs bright colors.

Rationale: Identifying the types of visual disturbances and options available allows the client to take the necessary precautions. A client with mobility problems needs to have safety devices installed and hazards eliminated to aid in ADLs.

3. Teach client technique to reduce orthostatic hypotension.

➤ Change positions slowly.
> ➤ Move from lying to an upright position in stages.

➤ Sit up in bed.
> ➤ Dangle first one leg and then the other over the side of the bed.
> ➤ Allow a few minutes before going on to each step.
> ➤ Gradually pull oneself from a sitting to a standing position.
> ➤ Place a chair, walker, cane, or other assistive device nearby to use to steady oneself when getting out of bed.

➤ Sleep with head of bed elevated up to 30 degrees.
➤ During the day, rest in a recliner rather than in bed.
➤ Avoid prolonged standing.
➤ Avoid stooping to pick something up from the floor; use an assistive device available from an orthotics department or a self-help store.
➤ Evaluate the possible effectiveness of waist-high stockings.
> ➤ Wrap legs from below toes to top of thigh with elastic compression bandages. Check compression effectiveness before purchase.
> ➤ Put stocking on in morning before getting out of bed if compression is advised.
> ➤ Avoid sitting for long periods.
> ➤ Remove stockings when supine.

Rationale: The client's understanding of orthostatic hypotension may help him or her modify behavior to reduce the frequency and severity of episodes. Prolonged bed rest increases venous pooling. Gradual position change allows the body to compensate for venous pooling (Porth, 2002).

4. Teach client to avoid dehydration and vasodilation.

➤ Replace fluids during periods of excess fluid loss (e.g., hot weather).
➤ Minimize diuretic fluids (e.g., coffee, tea, cola).

> ➤ Minimize alcohol consumption.
> ➤ Avoid sources of intense heat (e.g., direct sun, hot showers, baths, electric blankets).
> ➤ Avoid taking nitroglycerin while standing.

Rationale: Adequate hydration is necessary to prevent decreased circulation volume. Alcohol, heat, and certain medications (e.g., vasodilators, antihistamines) can cause vasodilatation.

5. Describe and document falls, injuries, previous falls, medications, and measures taken.

Rationale: Falls in hospitals must be carefully documented according to protocol.

6. Decreased strength/flexibility.

> ➤ Perform ankle-strengthening exercises daily (Schoenfelder, 2000).
> ➤ Stand behind a straight chair, with feet slightly apart.
> ➤ Slowly raise both heels until body weight is on balls of feet, hold for count of 3 (e.g., 1 Mississippi, 2 Mississippi, 3 Mississippi).
> ➤ Do 5 to 10 repetitions; increase repetitions as strength increases.
> ➤ Walk at least two or three times a week.
> ➤ Use ankle exercises as a warm-up before walking.
> ➤ Begin walking with someone at side, if needed, for 10 minutes.
> ➤ Increase time and speed according to capabilities.

Rationale: Ankle strengthening and a walking program can improve balance, increase ankle strength, improve walking speed, decrease falls and fear of falling, and increase confidence in performing ADLs (Schoenfelder, 2000).

7. Use assistive devices.

Crutches

> ➤ Teach exercises to strengthen arm and shoulder muscles to facilitate use of crutches; use weights and parallel bars.
> ➤ Measure and fit crutches to each person (2 to 3 inches between top of crutch and armpit); improper length of crutches may cause nerve damage or falls.
> ➤ Instruct person to wear shoes that fit properly and have nonskid sole.
> ➤ Assess ability to walk and climb up and down stairs.
> ➤ Consult with physical therapist for proper gait training.

Canes

> ➤ Teach person to hold cane in hand opposite affected leg and move cane and impaired limb together.

➤ Cane should be proper length to allow person to extend elbow and bear weight on hand.
➤ Cane should be fitted with rubber tip.
➤ Consult with physical therapist for proper gait training.

Walkers

➤ Teach person exercises to strengthen triceps muscles used in proper crutch walking.
➤ See that floors are clean, dry, and free of obstacle and that rugs are anchored.
➤ Instruct person to wear properly fitted shoes with nonslip soles.
➤ Consult with physical therapist for proper gait training.

Prosthesis

➤ Teach person to bathe and inspect stump daily.
➤ Instruct him or her to put on prosthesis soon after rising to minimize stump swelling.
➤ Prepare person for crutch walking with triceps exercises using weights and parallel bars.
➤ Consult with physical therapist for proper gait training.

Rationale: Incorrect use of assistive devices can cause falls and injury.

8. Assess for any side effects of drugs that may cause vertigo.

➤ Hypotension
➤ Vasodilation
➤ Sedation
➤ Vasoconstriction
➤ Hypokalemia

Rationale: Vertigo will contribute to falls.

▼ Risk for Aspiration

Definition

Risk for Aspiration: State in which a person is at risk for entry of secretions, solids, or fluids into the tracheobronchial passages.

Risk Factors

Presence of favorable conditions for aspiration (see Related Factors)

Related Factors

PATHOPHYSIOLOGIC

Related to reduced level of consciousness secondary to

Presenile dementia
Parkinson's disease
Seizures
Head injury
Alcohol/drug induced
Anesthesia
Cerebrovascular accident (CVA)
Coma

Related to depressed cough/gag reflexes
Related to delayed gastric emptying secondary to

Intestinal obstruction
Gastric outlet syndrome
Ileus

Related to increased intragastric pressure secondary to

Lithotomy position
Obesity
Enlarged uterus

Related to impaired swallowing or decreased laryngeal and glottic reflexes secondary to

Achalasia
Muscular dystrophy
Scleroderma
CVA
Esophageal strictures
Parkinson's disease
Myasthenia gravis
Debilitating conditions
Guillain-Barré syndrome

Related to tracheoesophageal fistula
Related to impaired protective reflexes secondary to

Facial/oral/neck surgery or trauma
Paraplegia or hemiplegia

TREATMENT-RELATED

Related to depressed laryngeal and glottic reflexes secondary to

Tracheostomy/endotracheal tube
Sedation
Tube feeding

Related to impaired ability to cough secondary to

Wired jaw
Imposed prone position

SITUATIONAL (PERSONAL, ENVIRONMENTAL)

Related to inability/impaired ability to elevate upper body
Related to eating when intoxicated

MATURATIONAL

Premature

Related to impaired sucking/swallowing reflexes

Neonate

Related to decreased muscle tone of inferior esophageal sphincter

Older Adult

Related to poor dentition

Risk for Aspiration is a clinically useful diagnosis for people at high risk for aspiration because of reduced level of consciousness, structural deficits, mechanical devices, and neurologic and GI disorders. People with swallowing difficulties often are at risk for aspiration; the nursing diagnosis Impaired Swallowing should be used to describe a client with difficulty swallowing who also is at risk for aspiration. Risk for Aspiration should be used to describe people who require nursing interventions to prevent aspiration but not to improve swallowing for nutritional purposes.

Key Concepts

GENERIC CONSIDERATIONS

➤ Swallowing is a complicated mechanism with three stages:
  ➤ The voluntary stage is the moving of the food from the palate to the pharynx.
  ➤ The pharyngeal stage is automatic:
    ➢ The soft palate is pulled up to close the posterior nares.
    ➢ Palatopharyngeal folds on the sides of the pharynx constrict to permit passage of properly masticated food.
    ➢ The epiglottis swings backward over the larynx opening to prevent aspiration into the trachea.

➤   Relaxation of hypopharyngeal sphincter stretches the opening of the esophagus.

➤   Rapid peristaltic wave forces food into the upper esophagus.

➤   The esophageal stage moves the food from the pharynx to the stomach by peristaltic movements controlled by vagal reflexes.

➤   CNS depression interferes with the protective mechanism of the sphincters.

➤   Nasogastric and endotracheal tubes cause incomplete closure of the esophageal sphincters and depress the gag and cough reflexes.

➤   Clients with debilitating conditions who aspirate are at high risk for aspiration pneumonia.

➤   The volume and characteristics of the aspirated contents influence morbidity and mortality. Good particles can cause mechanical blockage. Gastric juice erodes alveoli and capillaries causes chemical pneumonitis.

FOCUS ASSESSMENT CRITERIA

Assess for subjective (S) and objective (O) data:

History of problem of swallowing or aspiration (S)
Presence or history of (see Pathophysiologic Related Factors) (S)

➤   Ability to swallow, chew, feed self (O)
➤   Neuromuscular impairment (O)
    ➤   Decreased/absent gag reflex
    ➤   Decreased strength on excursion of muscles involved in mastication
    ➤   Perceptual impairment
    ➤   Facial paralysis
➤   Mechanical obstruction (O)
    ➤   Edema
    ➤   Tracheotomy tube
    ➤   Tumor
➤   Perceptual patterns/awareness (O)
➤   Level of consciousness (O)
➤   Hoarseness
➤   Coughing 1 or 2 times after swallowing (O)

GOAL

The person will not experience aspiration.

Indicators

Relate measures to prevent aspiration.
Name foods or fluids that are high risk for causing aspiration.

GENERAL INTERVENTIONS

1. Assess causative or contributing factors.

➤ Susceptible individual
➤ Reduced level of consciousness
➤ Autonomic disorders
➤ Debilitated
➤ Newborn
➤ Tracheostomy/endotracheal tubes
➤ GI tubes/feedings

2. Reduce the risk of aspiration in the following.

Clients with decreased strength, decreased sensorium, or autonomic disorders

➤ Maintain a side-lying position if not contraindicated by injury.
➤ If the person cannot be positioned on the side, open oropharyngeal airway by lifting the mandible up and forward and tilting the head backward (for a small infant, hyperextension of the neck may not be effective).
➤ Assess for position of the tongue, ensuring it has not dropped backward, occluding the airway.
➤ Keep the head of the bed elevated, if not contraindicated by hypertension injury.
➤ Maintain good oral hygiene. Clean teeth and use mouthwash on cotton swab; apply petroleum jelly to lips, removing encrustation gently.
➤ Clear secretions from mouth and throat with a tissue or gentle suction.
➤ Reassess frequently for obstructive material in mouth and throat.
➤ Reevaluate frequently for good anatomic positioning.
➤ Maintain side-lying position after feedings.

Rationale: Regurgitation is often silent in people with decreased sensorium or depressed mental states. Increased intragastric pressure can contribute to regurgitation and aspiration. Causes include bolus tube feedings, obstructions, obesity, pregnancy, and autonomic dysfunction.

Tracheotomy or endotracheal tubes

➤ Inflate cuff:
  ➢ During continuous mechanical ventilation
  ➢ During and after eating
  ➢ During and 1 hour after tube feedings
  ➢ During intermittent positive-pressure breathing treatments
➤ Suction every 1 to 2 hours and as needed.

Rationale: Tracheotomy tubes interfere with the synchrony of the glottis closure. Inadequate cuff inflation provides a path for aspirate.

GI tube feedings

➤ Confirm that tube placement has been verified by radiography or aspiration of greenish fluid.
➤ Confirm that tube position has not changed since it was inserted and verified.
➤ Elevate head of bed 30 to 45 minutes during feeding periods and 1 hour after to prevent reflux by use of reverse gravity.
➤ Aspirate for residual contents before each feeding for tubes positioned gastrically.
➤ Administer feeding if residual contents are less than 150 ml at 10% to 20% of hourly rate (continuous).
➤ Regulate gastric feedings using an intermittent schedule, allowing periods for stomach emptying between feeding intervals.

Rationale: Verifying correct placement of feeding tubes is done most reliably by radiography. Aspiration of green-colored fluid or gastric aspirant with a pH of 6.5 or lower is also reliable. Verifying placement by instilling air and simultaneously auscultating or by aspirating nongreen fluid has proved inaccurate. Such regulation is necessary to prevent overfeeding and increased risk of reflux and aspiration. Gastric feedings should be administered intermittently when the potential for aspiration is high. Continuous feedings increase the risk of aspiration because the stomach contains a constant supply formula.

3. Initiate health teaching and referrals, as indicated.

➤ Instruct person and family on causes and prevention of aspiration.
➤ Have family demonstrate tube-feeding technique.
➤ Refer family to community nursing agency for assistance at home.
➤ Teach client about the danger of eating when under the influence of alcohol.
➤ Teach the Heimlich or abdominal thrust maneuver to remove aspirated foreign bodies.

▼ Risk for Falls

Definition

Risk for Falls: State in which a person has increased susceptibility to falling.

Risk Factors

Presence of risk factors (see Related Factors under Risk for Injury)

 This nursing diagnosis can be used to specify a person at risk for falls. If the person is at risk for various types of injuries (e.g., a cognitively impaired person), the broader diagnosis Risk for Injury is more useful.

Key Concepts

Refer to Risk for Injuries

GENERAL INTERVENTIONS

Refer to Risk for Injuries

▼ Deficient Knowledge

Definition

Deficient Knowledge: State in which a person or group experiences a deficiency in cognitive knowledge or psychomotor skills concerning the condition or treatment plan.

Defining Characteristics

MAJOR (MUST BE PRESENT, ONE OR MORE)

Verbalizes a deficiency in knowledge or skill/request for information
Expresses "inaccurate" perception of health status
Does not correctly perform a desired or prescribed health behavior

MINOR (MAY BE PRESENT)

Lack of integration of treatment plan into daily activities

Exhibits or expresses psychological alteration (e.g., anxiety, depression) resulting from misinformation or lack of information

Deficient knowledge does not represent a human response, alteration, or pattern of dysfunction but a related factor. All people have knowledge deficits. It is when this lack of knowledge causes or could cause a problem that the nurse acts on a nursing diagnosis. Lack of knowledge can contribute to various responses (e.g., anxiety, self-care deficits, noncompliance). All nursing diagnoses have related client/family teaching as part of nursing interventions (e.g., Impaired Verbal Communication). When lack of or insufficient knowledge is the primary cause of a diagnosis or a risk factor for a potential diagnosis, the nurse lists lack of knowledge as a "Related to." For example, when specific teaching is indicated before a procedure, the nurse can use Anxiety Related to Unfamiliar Environment and Procedures. When information giving is directed to assist a person or family with a decision, Decisional Conflict may be indicated. Consult with your instructor about the use of this diagnosis. If Deficient Knowledge is required for you to use, write Deficient Knowledge: (specify), for example, Deficient Knowledge: wound care; Deficient Knowledge: ostomy care.

▼ Ineffective Therapeutic Regimen Management

Definition

Ineffective Therapeutic Regimen Management: Pattern in which a person experiences or is at risk to experience difficulty integrating into daily living a program for treatment of illness and the sequelae of illness that meets specific health goals.

Defining Characteristics

MAJOR (MUST BE PRESENT, ONE OR MORE)

Verbalized desire to manage the treatment of illness and prevention of sequelae

Verbalized difficulty with regulation/integration of one or more prescribed regimens for treatment of illness and its effects or prevention of complications

MINOR (MAY BE PRESENT)

Acceleration (expected or unexpected) of illness symptoms
Verbalized to include treatment regimens in daily routines
Verbalized to reduce risk factors for progression of illness and sequelae

Related Factors

TREATMENT-RELATED

Related to

Complexity of therapeutic regimen
Financial costs of regimen
Complexity of health care system
Side effects of therapy

SITUATIONAL (PERSONAL, ENVIRONMENTAL)

Related to

Previous unsuccessful experiences
Questions seriousness of problem
Questions benefits of regimen
Mistrust of health care personnel
Insufficient knowledge
Family conflicts
Insufficient social support
Health belief conflicts
Questions susceptibility
Mistrust of regimen
Insufficient confidence
Decisional conflicts

Related to barriers to comprehension secondary to

Cognitive deficits
Fatigue
Hearing impairments
Motivation
Anxiety
Memory problems

MATURATIONAL
Child/Adolescent

Related to fear of being different

Carp's Cue ▶ *Ineffective Therapeutic Regimen Management is a very useful diagnosis for nurses in most settings. Individuals and families experiencing various health problems, acute or chronic, usually face treatment programs that require changes in previous functioning or lifestyle. These changes or adaptations can be instrumental in influencing positive outcomes.*

The diagnosis describes individuals or families experiencing difficulty achieving positive outcomes. The nurse is the primary professional who, with the client, determines available choices and how to achieve success. The primary nursing interventions are exploring the options available and teaching the client how to implement the selected option.

When a person faces a complex regimen or has compromised functioning that impedes successful management, the diagnosis Risk for Ineffective Therapeutic Regimen Management would be appropriate. In addition to teaching how to manage the regimen, the nurse also must assist the client to identify the adjustments needed because of a functional deficit.

Key Concepts

GENERIC CONSIDERATIONS

➤ Self-efficacy is a theory that describes a person's evaluation of his or her capacity to manage or to change behaviors to manage stressful situations. Successful management depends on the person believing that the behavior change will improve the situation (outcome expectancy) and that he or she can make the behavior change (self-efficacy expectancy; Bandura, 1982).

➤ Health education is the teaching–learning process of influencing client and family behavior through changes in knowledge, attitudes, and beliefs and by acquiring psychomotor skills. The goal of client teaching is to help the client assume responsibility for self-care.

➤ Physical factors that affect learning or the learner include the following (Redman & Thomas, 1999):
  ➢ Acute illness
  ➢ Fluid and electrolyte imbalance
  ➢ Nutritional status
  ➢ Illness or treatments that interfere with mental alertness (pain, medications)
  ➢ Illness or treatments that interfere with motor abilities (fatigue, equipment)
  ➢ Activity tolerance (endurance)

➤ Personal factors that affect learning or the learner include the following:

> - Age
> - Past experiences or knowledge
> - Intelligence
> - Locus of control
> - Reading ability
> - Perceived seriousness of condition
> - Level of motivation
> - Level of anxiety
> - Denial of disease process
> - Perceived susceptibility to complications
> - Prognosis
> - Depression
> - Stage of adaptation to illness
> - Ability to control progression or to cure condition
> - Factors resulting in ineffective teaching include the following (Redman & Thomas, 1999):
>   - Inadequate or no assessment before teaching
>   - Assessment data not communicated or not considered when teaching (the most influential assessment factors are psychological status, physical stability, educational level, cultural background, socioeconomic status)
>   - Teaching not individualized
>   - Information not presented at a level consistent with the client's ability
>   - Tendency to talk down to client
>   - Use of misunderstood terms
>   - Fragmented presentation of information
>   - Too much information given, with important information hidden or lost among irrelevant information
>   - No repetition of information
>   - No feedback given in relation to process (or client is punished for not learning)
>   - No evaluation made of client learning.

GERIATRIC CONSIDERATIONS

> - The ability to manage one's therapeutic regimen profoundly influences self-esteem and independence. Using education to increase the self-care capacity of older adults can be an effective way to meet their self-esteem needs.
> - It is a myth that older adults cannot learn new concepts and skills. Some changes during aging may deter learning, such as decreased visual acuity, decreased hearing, slowing of information processing, decreased attention span, difficulty in unlearning habits, fear of uncertainty or failure, decreased problem solving, and the need for a longer time and more repetition to retain learning.

TRANSCULTURAL CONSIDERATIONS

➤ Because the dominant US culture is future-oriented, it values a lifestyle that promotes health and prevents disease. This value is challenged when a client or family of another culture is oriented to the present (Andrews & Boyle, 2003).

➤ Clients with an external locus of control believe that outside factors or forces determine health. This belief challenges the entire concept of health promotion (Andrews & Boyle, 2003).

➤ Folk remedies are treatments or practices that cultural groups use to stay healthy or to treat illnesses.

➤ Folk remedies are used to treat many illnesses, such as headaches, colds, rashes, coughs, sore throats, constipation, fever, warts, and menstrual cramps. Examples of folk remedies for headaches include lying down and resting in complete darkness (Canadian); boiling a beef bone, breaking up toast in the broth, and drinking (German); applying a cold or hot face cloth to the forehead and resting (Irish); putting a kerchief with ice around the head (Italian); and taking aspirin and hot liquids (Andrews & Boyle, 2003).

➤ Some folk remedies may be misdiagnosed as abuse. Three folk practices of Southeast Asians leave marks on the body that providers may interpret as signs of violence or abuse. Cao gio is rubbing the skin with a coin to produce dark blood or ecchymotic strips; it is done to treat colds and flu-like symptoms. Bat gio is skin pinching on the temples to treat headaches or on the neck for sore throat; if petechiae or ecchymoses appear, the treatment is a success. Poua is burning the skin with the tip of dried weed-like grass; it is believed the burning will cause the noxious element that causes the pain to be released (Andrews & Boyle, 2003).

FOCUS ASSESSMENT CRITERIA

Subjective/Objective Data

Assess for subjective (S) and objective (O) cues:

Determine present knowledge of (S)

➤ Illness
  ➤ Severity
  ➤ Susceptibility to complications
  ➤ Prognosis
  ➤ Ability to cure it or control progression

➤ Treatment/diagnosis studies
➤ Preventive measures

Does anything interfere with adherence to the prescribed health behavior? (S)

Learning needs (perceived by client, family) (S)

History of disease

➤ Onset
➤ Effects on lifestyle (relationships, work, leisure, finances)
➤ Symptoms

Stage of adaptation to disease

➤ Disbelief
➤ Anger
➤ Denial
➤ Awareness
➤ Depression
➤ Acceptance

Learning ability (client, family)

➤ Level of education
➤ Language spoken
➤ Ability to read
➤ Language understood

Cultural factors

➤ Health care beliefs and practices
➤ Values
➤ Traditions
➤ Lifestyle

Ability to perform prescribed procedures (O)

➤ Competency
➤ Accuracy

Level of cognitive and psychomotor development (O)

➤ Age
➤ Ability to read and write

Presence of sensory deficits (O)

➤ Vision
➤ Taste (altered or lost)
➤ Hearing
➤ Pain
➤ Smell (altered or lost)

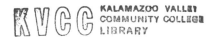

GOAL

The client or primary caregiver will describe disease process, causes and factors contributing to symptoms, and the regimen for disease or symptom control.

Indicators

Relate the intent to practice health behaviors needed or desired for recovery from illness/symptom management and prevention of recurrence or complications.

Describe signs and symptoms that need to be reported.

GENERAL INTERVENTIONS

1. Identify barriers to learning.

➤ Physical condition

Rationale: Pain, fatigue, dyspnea, or other symptoms can interfere with client's motivation and ability to learn.

➤ Sensory status
➤ Intelligence and learning ability:
  ➤ Education
  ➤ Learning disabilities
  ➤ Language difficulties

Rationale: Impaired hearing, vision, cognition, or memory, a learning disability, or a language barrier can interfere with communication and learning. A client with any such problem needs alternative teaching techniques.

➤ Anxiety level: mild, moderate, severe, or panic

Rationale: Extreme anxiety impairs a client's learning and coping abilities.

➤ Specific stressors, nature of concerns

Rationale: Every client experiences some emotional reaction to illness. The nature and degree of this reaction depends on how the client perceives his or her situation and its anticipated effects—physical, psychological, financial, social, occupational, and spiritual. Negative emotional reactions can interfere with motivation and ability to learn.

2. Determine the client's knowledge of his or her condition, prognosis, and treatment measures. Reinforce and supplement the physician's explanation as necessary.

Rationale: Assessing the client's level of knowledge will assist in the development of an individualized learning program. Providing accurate information can decrease the client's anxiety associated with the unknown and unfamiliar.

3. Identify factors that influence learning.

Rationale: The client's ability to learn will be affected by a number of variables that need to be considered. Denial of illness, lack of financial resources, and depression may affect the client's ability and motivation to learn. Cognitive factors associated with this might influence the client's ability to learn new information.

4. Provide the client and family with information about how to utilize the health care system (billing and payment, making appointments, follow-up care, resources available, etc.).

Rationale: Information on how to "work the system" will help the client and family to feel more comfortable and more in control of client's health care. This will positively influence compliance with the health care regimen.

5. Explain and discuss with client and family/caregiver (when possible) the following:

➤ Disease process
➤ Treatment regimen (medications, diet, procedures, exercises, equipment use)
➤ Rationale for regimen
➤ Side effects of regimen
➤ Lifestyle changes needed
➤ Follow-up care needed
➤ Signs or symptoms of complications
➤ Resources, support available
➤ Home environment alterations needed

Rationale: Depending on client's physical and cognitive limitations, it may be necessary to provide the family/caregiver with the necessary information for managing the treatment regimen. To assist the client with postdischarge care, the client needs information about the disease process, treatment regimen, symptoms of complications, as well as resources available for assistance.

6. Promote a positive attitude and active participation of the client and family.

➤ Solicit expression of feelings, concerns, and questions from client and family.
➤ Encourage client and family to seek information and make informed decision.
➤ Explain responsibilities of client/family and how these can be assumed.

Rationale: Active participation in the treatment regimen helps the client and family feel more in control of the illness, which enhances the effective management of the therapeutic regimen.

7. Ensure that the client with visual and/or hearing impairments has glasses and a hearing aid available and uses them during teaching sessions. Provide written teaching materials in the client's first language when possible.

Rationale: Vision and hearing aids, adequate lighting, written materials in client's primary language, and so forth will help to compensate for barriers to learning. Decreasing external stimuli will assist the client to correctly perceive what is being said.

8. Explain that changes in lifestyle and needed learning will take time to integrate.

➤ Provide printed material (in client's primary language when possible).
➤ Explain whom to contact with questions.
➤ Identify referrals or community services needed for follow-up.

Rationale: Explaining that changes are expected to take time to integrate will provide reassurance for the client that he or she does not have to make changes all at once. Support and reassurance will assist the client with compliance. Providing information about available resources also helps the clients to feel supported in his or her efforts.

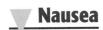 Nausea

Definition

Nausea: The state in which a person experiences an unpleasant wave-like sensation in the back of the throat, epigastrium, or throughout the abdomen that may or may not lead to vomiting.

Defining Characteristics

MAJOR (MUST BE PRESENT)

A vague, unpleasant, subjective sensation of being "sick to stomach" (S)

MINOR (MAY BE PRESENT)

Can be accompanied by watery salivation, pallor, sweating, tachycardia (O)
May precede vomiting (O)

Related Factors

BIOPATHOPHYSIOLOGIC

Related to tissue trauma and reflex muscle spasms secondary to

Acute gastroenteritis
Peptic ulcer disease
Irritable bowel syndrome
Pancreatitis
Infections (e.g., food poisoning)
Drug overdose
Renal calculi
Uterine cramps associated with menses
Motion sickness
Stress

TREATMENT-RELATED

Related to effects of chemotherapy, theophylline, digitalis, antibiotics, antivirals
Related to effects of anesthesia

Key Concepts

GENERIC CONSIDERATIONS

➤ Nausea results from stimulation of the medullary-vomiting center in the brain (Porth, 2002).
➤ Nausea and vomiting, when determined to have emotional origins, may result from developmental adjustment and adaptation. A child learns that vomiting is unacceptable and thus learns to control it. He or she receives approval for not vomiting. Should childhood situations or conflicts resurface, the adult may experience nausea and vomiting.
➤ Nausea is the third most common side effect of chemotherapy after alopecia and fatigue (Foltz et al., 1996).
➤ Inadequate management of previous nausea causes anticipatory nausea before chemotherapy (Eckert, 2001).

FOCUS ASSESSMENT CRITERIA

Assess for subjective data

Onset/duration

➤ Time of day, pattern

Frequency
Vomitus (amount, time of day)

Associated with:

➤ Medications
➤ Activity
➤ Specific foods
➤ Position
➤ Pain

Relief measures

GOAL

The client will report decreased nausea.

Indicators

Name foods or beverages that do not increase nausea.
Describe factors that increase nausea.

GENERAL INTERVENTIONS

1. Explain the cause of the nausea and the duration, if known.
2. Teach how to use antiemetic medications before and after chemotherapy.
3. Promote comfort during nausea and vomiting.

➤ Protect people at risk for aspiration (immobile clients, children).
➤ Address the cleanliness of the person and environment.
➤ Provide an opportunity for oral care after each episode.
➤ Apply a cool damp cloth to the person's forehead, neck, and wrists.

4. Reduce or eliminate noxious stimuli.

Pain

➤ Plan care to avoid unpleasant or painful procedures before meals.
➤ Medicate clients for pain 30 minutes before meals according to physician's orders.
➤ Provide a pleasant relaxed atmosphere for eating (no bedpans in sight; do not rush); try a "surprise" (e.g., flowers with meal).
➤ Arrange the plan of care to decrease or eliminate nauseating odors or procedures near mealtimes.

Fatigue

➤ Teach or assist client to rest before meals.
➤ Teach client to spend minimal energy preparing food (cook large quantities and freeze several meals at a time; request assistance from others).

Odor of food

➤ Teach client to avoid cooking odors—frying food, brewing coffee—if possible (take a walk, select foods that can be eaten cold).

▼ Noncompliance

Definition

Noncompliance: State in which an individual or group desires to comply but factors are present that deter adherence to health-related advice given by health professionals.

Defining Characteristics

MAJOR (MUST BE PRESENT, ONE OR MORE)

Verbalization of noncompliance or nonparticipation or confusion about therapy
And/or
Direct observation of behavior indicating noncompliance

MINOR (MAY BE PRESENT)

Missed appointments
Partially used or unused medications
Persistence of symptoms
Progression of disease process
Undesired outcomes (postoperative morbidity, pregnancy, obesity, addiction, regression during rehabilitation)

Related Factors

PATHOPHYSIOLOGIC

Related to impaired ability to perform tasks because of disability secondary to

Poor memory
Motor and sensory deficits

Related to increasing disease-related symptoms despite adherence to advised regimen

TREATMENT-RELATED

Related to

Side effects of therapy
Past unsuccessful experience with advised regimen
Impersonal aspects of referrals
Nontherapeutic environment
Financial cost of therapy
Complex, unsupervised, prolonged therapy

SITUATIONAL (PERSONAL, ENVIRONMENTAL)

Related to barriers to access secondary to

Mobility problems
Transportation problems
Financial issues
Inclement weather
Lack of child care

Related to concurrent illness of family member
Related to nonsupportive family, peers, community
Related to barriers to care secondary to homelessness
Related to change in employment status
Related to change in health insurance coverage
Related to barriers to comprehension secondary to

Cognitive deficits
Anxiety
Visual effects
Fatigue
Hearing deficits
Decreased attention span
Poor memory
Motivation

Carp's Cue ▶ *Compliance depends on various factors, including motivation, perception of vulnerability, and beliefs about controlling or preventing illness; environment; quality of health instruction; and ability to access resources (cost, accessibility). The diagnosis Noncompliance describes a person desiring to comply but prevented from doing so by certain factors (e.g., lack of understanding, inadequate finances, overly complex instructions). The nurse must attempt to reduce or eliminate these factors to ensure successful interventions.*

The process of informed consent protects a person's right to self-determination. Informed consent has three conditions: the person must be capable of giving consent, must be capable of understanding the advantages and disadvantages of consent, and must not be coerced (Cassells & Redman, 1989). When a person refuses to comply with advice or instructions, it is important for the nurse to assess for and validate the presence of all required elements for informed consent. The nurse is cautioned against using Noncompliance to describe a person who has made an informed autonomous decision not to comply. As Cassells and Redman (1989) state, "human dignity is respected by granting individuals the freedom to make choices in accordance with their own values." When a person must change habits or lifestyle or perform certain activities to manage a health problem, Risk for Ineffective Therapeutic Regimen Management is very useful.

Be careful not to use Noncompliance as Noncompliance related to not following weight loss diet and 10-pound weight gain. Not following the weight loss diet and 10-pound weight gain have not caused or contributed to Noncompliance. They are the signs and symptoms. The diagnosis should be noncompliance related to unknown etiology as evidenced by not following weight loss diet and a 10-pound weight gain.

Key Concepts

GENERIC CONSIDERATIONS

> Compliance is a positive behavior that clients exhibit when moving toward mutually defined therapeutic goals (DeGreest et al., 1998).
> Compliance should be viewed on a continuum rather than as separate states of compliance or noncompliance (Blevins & Lubkin, 1999).
> Partnerships between health care provider and client involve choices and compromises. Some clients desire a passive role, whereas others want complete autonomy.
> Compliance involves a behavioral change, which the following can influence positively (Blevins & Lubkin, 1999):
>> Initial and continuing trust in health care professionals
>> Reinforcement from significant others
>> Perception of own susceptibility to the disease
>> Perception that the disease is serious
>> Evidence that compliance helps control symptoms or the disease
>> Tolerable side effects
>> Less interference with daily activities of client or significant others
>> More benefit than harm provided by therapy
>> Positive sense of self
> The following factors hinder compliance (Blevins & Lubkin, 1999):
>> Inadequate explanation
>> Disagreement between the provider and client
>> Long duration of therapy

> ➤ High complexity or expense of regimen
> ➤ Great number and severity of side effects
> ➤ Noncompliance that follows a period of compliant behavior is termed relapse. It usually happens when nonsupportive environmental influences overcome the person's desire to perform the newly adopted behavior. Causes of relapse can be any of the related factors already listed.

GERIATRIC CONSIDERATIONS

Factors influencing noncompliance in older adults are functional deficits, complicated regimens, costs, inconvenience, and side effects that decrease functional status (e.g., strength, alertness).

FOCUS ASSESSMENT CRITERIA

Subjective/Objective Data

Assess for subjective (S) and objective (O) cues:

Unacceptable side effects of therapy (S)

> ➤ Unpleasant taste
> ➤ Pain
> ➤ Difficulty swallowing
> ➤ Too expensive
> ➤ Time-consuming
> ➤ Inconvenient

Does family member report any of the above problems? (S)
What does the client want from the nurse or physician? (S)
What is the person's general first motivation? (S)

> ➤ Does client seek help as needed?
> ➤ Does client intend to make advised lifestyle alterations?
> ➤ Does client accept diagnosis?

What is the client's perception of his or her present state of health? (S)

> ➤ Does client consider self to be generally well?
> ➤ Does he or she fear a specific illness?
> ➤ Does client believe his or her illness?

How does client view the advised treatment regimen? (e.g., does it make personal sense?) (S)
Situations that interfere with prescribed behavior

> ➤ Family demands
> ➤ Travel (hotels, restaurants)

➤ Stress
➤ Lack of transportation
➤ Occupations
➤ Denial

Evidence of noncompliance (O)

➤ Persistence of symptoms
➤ Problems with medications (pill count, serum drug levels)
➤ Progression of disease
➤ Missed appointments

Obstacles to self-care (O)

➤ Inability to read
➤ Musculoskeletal deficits
➤ Immaturity
➤ Cognitive deficits
➤ Memory lags
➤ Pain

GOAL

The person will report a desire to change or initiate change.

Indicators

Describe reasons for suggested regimen.
Identify barriers to adhering to regimen.

GENERAL INTERVENTIONS

1. Determine person's understanding of presence of or risk for health problem (prognosis, disability).

➤ Vulnerability to problem
➤ Prevention or treatment measures available
➤ Effectiveness of preventive measures
➤ Effectiveness of treatment measures

Rationale: Lack of understanding of the health problem, complications, and the client's own vulnerability contribute to noncompliance (Blevins & Lubkin, 1999).

2. Explore client's feelings regarding

➤ Past attempts at compliance
➤ Present concerns regarding prevention or treatment modalities
➤ Which recommendations are feasible
➤ Level of guidance desired from professional
➤ Support from significant others

Refer to Ineffective Therapeutic Regimen Management for additional interventions.

Rationale: Increasing the person's beliefs that the health behavior change is possible contributes to long-term compliance (DeGreest et al., 1998). Perceived success as a result of one's own efforts enhances self-confidence, which helps to increase adherence (DeGreest et al., 1998).

3. Encourage positive thinking about new health-related behaviors.

Collaborate with client to set goals.

➤ Short-term goals are most useful.
➤ Be flexible.
➤ Be realistic, considering each person's uniqueness.
➤ Avoid imposing your goals for client.

Consider using a contract, a written statement of expected behaviors.

➤ Initially, use short-term contracts with family member, coworker, friend, or nurse.
➤ For the long term, self-contracts work well; the client finds his or her own rewards and reinforces his or her own positive behavior changes.

Self-monitoring is useful to determine positive and negative influences on compliance.

➤ Daily records
➤ Charts
➤ Diary of progress or symptoms, clinical values (e.g., blood pressure), or dietary intake

Rationale: Establishing a consensual regimen and goals validates that the client is the decision maker and the health care professional is the advisor (Blevins & Lubkin, 1999). Contracting involves a commitment to make changes and to be accountable for choices (Blevins & Lubkin, 1999).

4. Review present medication therapy (prescribed and over-the-counter).

➤ Discuss present therapy (names, dosages, time taken, side effects). Don't ask, "Are you taking your medications?" Ask the following:
  ➤ "What medications did you take today? Yesterday?"
  ➤ "What time of day is it difficult for you to take your medications?"
  ➤ "Are there times when you decide not to take one of the doses?"

➤ Determine person's understanding of the need for medication.
  ➤ Emphasize life-long therapy when indicated (e.g., hypertension, diabetes mellitus).
  ➤ Explain the complications of unmanaged disease.
➤ Identify possible adverse interactions among drugs (consult pharmacist).
➤ Commit to working with the person to reduce or eliminate side effects (e.g., change agents or dose).
➤ Help the person identify a reminder to take the medication (e.g., brushing teeth at night, daily favorite TV show, watch timer).
➤ Ask person to call primary provider with problems rather than stopping the medication.
➤ Emphasize that unavoidable side effects are still better than the consequences of no therapy (e.g., stroke, blindness, renal failure).

Rationale: Lack of understanding regarding reasons for drug therapy and options available contributes to noncompliance (Blevins & Lubkin, 1999).

5. Help to reduce side effects.

➤ For gastric irritation, administer drug with milk or food; yogurt may be advisable (unless contraindicated).
➤ For drowsiness, administer medication at bedtime or late in afternoon; consult primary provider for dose reduction.
➤ For leg cramps (hypokalemia), increase foods high in potassium (e.g., oranges, raisins, tomatoes, bananas).
➤ For other side effects, consult pertinent preferences.
➤ Use long-acting intramuscular preparations whenever possible; this includes some antibiotics and antipsychotic medications.
➤ Suggest use of combination pills if available (e.g., Maxzide [hydrochlorothiazide and triamterene] and Triavil [perphenazine and amitriptyline]).
➤ When appropriate, be sure client is taking the fewest pills possible (check dosages to provide the largest dose available in the fewest pills).
➤ To decrease frequency of oral medications, suggest longer-acting drug preparations, including the transdermal patch (e.g., nitroglycerin).
➤ Encourage prescription of generic drugs for people with financial concerns. Determine whether client needs assistance (e.g., pharmaceutical patient assistance program).
➤ When treatments require more than one set of hands, evaluate home help situation.
➤ When expensive equipment is involved for treatments at home, make appropriate referrals to social workers and local agencies.

Rationale: Open discussions about side effects can encourage the person to report problems before discontinuing treatment (Blevins & Lubkin, 1999).

6. Initiate health teaching and referrals, as indicated.

➤ Teach importance of adhering to prescribed regimen.

➤ Provide written drug information tailored to client's needs. Include drug names, dosages, number of tablets to take and when, purpose of drugs, potential side effects and adverse reactions, and directions for relief of side effects.

➤ Offer praise for honesty about compliance and for sharing reasons. For example:

   ➤ "I am glad you told me that you stopped taking Motrin because it made your stomach hurt. Now I understand why your hands still ache. Let's talk about ways we can get you some comfort."

   ➤ "It's good that you told me about your stopping the blood pressure pills. That explains your headaches and higher pressure today. Let's discuss how those pills made you feel."

➤ At discharge from hospital or outpatient setting, provide written names and phone numbers of professionals to call with questions or concerns about prescribed drug regimen.

Rationale: Compliance increases when expectations, responsibilities, and consequences are discussed (Wong, 2003). In children, attempts to engage them in some aspect of self-care can increase independence, initiative, and self-confidence. Contracting is an effective method with older children when they are involved in defining the rules of the agreement (Wong, 2003).

Imbalanced Nutrition: Less Than Body Requirements

Definition

Imbalanced Nutrition: Less Than Body Requirements: State in which a person who is not NPO experiences or is at risk of experiencing reduced weight related to inadequate intake or metabolism of nutrients for metabolic needs

Defining Characteristics

MAJOR (MUST BE PRESENT, ONE OR MORE)

Person who is not NPO reports or has food intake less than recommended daily allowance with or without weight loss
And/or
Actual or potential metabolic needs in excess of intake with weight loss

MINOR (MAY BE PRESENT)

Weight 10% to 20% + below ideal height and frame

Triceps, skinfold, mid-arm circumference, and mid-arm muscle circumference less than 60% standard measurement

Muscle weakness and tenderness

Mental irritability or confusion

Decreased serum albumin

Decreased serum transferring or iron-binding capacity

Related Factors

PATHOPHYSIOLOGIC

Related to increased caloric requirements and difficulty in ingesting sufficient calories secondary to

Burns (postacute phase)

Trauma

Cancer

Chemical dependence

Infection

Related to dysphagia (difficulty swallowing) secondary to

CVA

Parkinson's disease

Muscular dystrophy

Cerebral palsy

Amyotrophic lateral sclerosis

Neuromuscular disorders

Related to decreased absorption of nutrients secondary to

Crohn's disease

Lactose intolerance

Cystic fibrosis

Related to self-induced vomiting, physical exercise in excess of caloric intake, or refusal to eat secondary to anorexia nervosa

Related to reluctance to eat for fear of poisoning secondary to paranoid behavior

Related to anorexia, excessive physical agitation secondary to bipolar disorder

Related to anorexia and diarrhea secondary to protozoal infection

Related to anorexia, impaired protein and fat metabolism, and impaired storage of vitamins secondary to cirrhosis

TREATMENT-RELATED

Related to protein and vitamin requirements for wound healing and decreased intake secondary to

Surgery
Radiation therapy
Wired jaw
Surgical reconstruction of mouth
Medications (chemotherapy)

Related to inadequate absorption as a medication side effect of (specify)

Colchicine
Para-aminosalicylic acid
Neomycin
Antacid
Pyrimethamine

Related to decreased oral intake, mouth discomfort, nausea, and vomiting secondary to

Radiation therapy
Tonsillectomy
Chemotherapy

SITUATIONAL (PERSONAL, ENVIRONMENTAL)

Related to decreased desire to eat secondary to

Anorexia
Nausea and vomiting
Social isolation
Stress
Depression
Fatigue

Related to inability to procure food (physical limitations, financial or transportation problems)
Related to inability to chew (damaged or missing teeth, ill-fitting dentures)
Related to diarrhea secondary to (specify)

Carp's Cue ▶ *Nurses are primarily the diagnosticians and prescribers for improving nutritional status. Although Imbalanced Nutrition is not a difficult diagnosis to validate, interventions for it can challenge the nurse. Many factors influence food habits and nutritional status, personal, family, cultural, financial, functional ability, nutritional knowledge, disease and injury, and treatment regimens. Imbalanced Nutrition: Less Than Body Requirements describes people who can ingest food but eat an inadequate or imbalanced quantity or quality. For instance, the diet may have*

insufficient protein or excessive fat. Quantity may be insufficient because of increased metabolic requirements (e.g., cancer, pregnancy) or interference with nutrient use (e.g., impaired storage of vitamins in cirrhosis). The nursing focus for Imbalanced Nutrition is assisting the person or family to improve nutritional intake. Nurses should not use the collaborative problems PC: Electrolyte Imbalance or PC: Negative Nitrogen Balance to describe those situations unless the person cannot eat.

Key Concepts

GENERIC CONSIDERATIONS

> ➤ For proper metabolic functioning, the body requires adequate carbohydrates, protein, fat, vitamins, minerals, electrolytes, and trace elements. Figure II.1 depicts the food pyramid developed by the US Department of Agriculture. It recommends daily servings of five food groups. The sixth group—fats, oils, and sweets—should be eaten sparingly and should not exceed 30% of total calorie intake.
> ➤ Overall, 54.9% of adult Americans are overweight (15% over ideal weight for height); 18% to 25% of adolescents are overweight. The range for children is 25% to 30% (Dudek, 2001).
> ➤ Obesity is a risk factor for hypertension; type 2 diabetes mellitus; coronary artery disease; cancer of the breast, endometrium, cervix, ovary, colon, rectum, prostate, gallbladder, and biliary tract; and joint and foot disorders (Dudek, 2001).
> ➤ Studies report that US women consume insufficient iron, calcium, and vitamins A and C (Lo, 1995).
> ➤ Americans eat half of the fiber requirement and 20% more fat than needed (Dudek, 2001).
> ➤ The National Research Council (1989) compiled the dietary recommendations outlined in Table II.9.
> ➤ Factors influencing nutrient requirements include age, activity, gender, health status (presence of disease, injuries), and nutrient metabolism (storage, absorption, use, excretion).
> ➤ Drugs can reduce nutrient intake by altering the following (White & Ashworth, 2000):
>> ➤ Appetite (e.g., metformin, digoxin, paroxetine)
>> ➤ Absorption (e.g., neomycin, cimetidine)
>> ➤ Metabolism (e.g., metformin, isoniazid, phenytoin)
> ➤ Figure II.2 is a Basal Metabolic Index (BMI) chart to determine the optimal weight for height.
> ➤ The person with cancer experiences disease- and treatment-related nutritional problems:
>> ➤ Disease-related
>>> ➤ Malabsorption
>>> ➤ Anemia

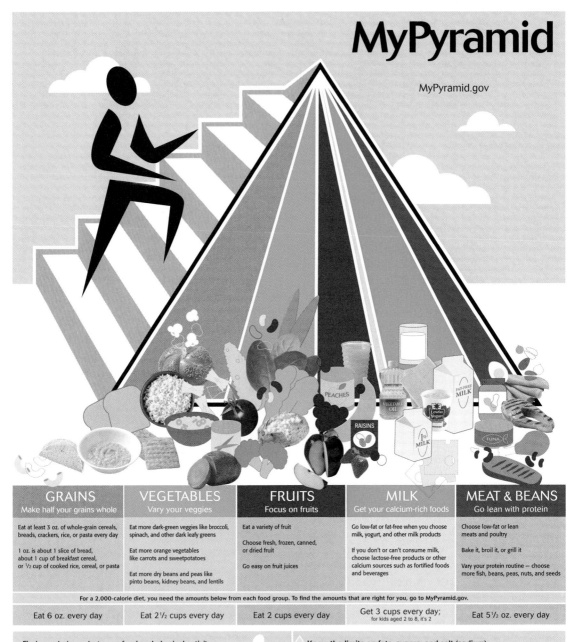

FIGURE II–1. The Food Pyramid. See MyPyramid.gov. Step to a healthier you.

Table II–9. DIETARY RECOMMENDATIONS OF THE NATIONAL RESEARCH COUNCIL REPORT

Reduce total fat intake to 30% or less of calories, saturated fatty acid intake to less than 10% of kilocalories, and cholesterol to less than 300 mg daily.*

Drink 8–10 glasses of water or noncaffeinated beverages.

Increase intake of starches and other complex carbohydrates.

Maintain protein intake at moderate levels.† Increase dry beans, fish.

Increase fiber intake to 25–35 g daily.

Eat 2–4 servings of fruit daily.

Eat 3–5 servings of vegetables daily.

Limit total daily intake of salt (sodium chloride) to 6 g or less.‡

Maintain adequate calcium and iron intake.

Avoid taking dietary supplements in excess of the recommended daily allowance (RDA) in any one day.

Balance food intake and physical activity to maintain appropriate body weight.

For those who drink alcoholic beverages, limit consumption to the equivalent of less than 1 oz of pure alcohol in a single day.§

*The intake of fat and cholesterol can be reduced by substituting fish, poultry without skin, lean meats, and low-fat or nonfat dairy products for fatty meats and whole-milk dairy products; by choosing more vegetables, fruits, cereals, and legumes; and by limiting oils, fats, egg yolks, and fried and other fatty foods.
†Meet at least the RDA for protein; do not exceed twice the RDA.
‡Limit the use of salt in cooking, and avoid adding it to food at the table. Salty, highly processed salty, salt-preserved, and salt-pickled foods should be consumed sparingly.
§The Committee does not recommend alcohol consumption. One ounce of pure alcohol is the equivalent of two cans of beer, two small glasses of wine, or two average cocktails.
National Research Council, Committee on Diet and Health of Food and Nutrition Board. (1989). Diet and health: Implications for reducing chronic disease risk. *Nutrition Reviews, 47*, 142–149; *Food guide pyramid: A guide to daily food choices.* Leaflet No. 572. Washington, DC: US Department of Agriculture; Dudek, S.G. (2001). *Nutrition essentials for nursing practice.* (4th ed.) Philadelphia: Lippincott Williams and Wilkins.

- Diarrhea
- Protein deficits
- Constipation
- Fatigue
➤ Treatment-related
  - Stomatitis
  - Anorexia
  - Diarrhea
  - Fatigue
  - Nausea and vomiting

GERIATRIC CONSIDERATIONS

➤ In general, older adults need the same kind of balanced diet as any other group, but fewer calories. Diets of older clients, however, tend

Body Mass Index

The body mass index (BMI) is used to determine who is overweight.

$$BMI = \frac{703 \times \text{weight in pounds}}{(\text{height in inches})^2} \quad OR \quad \frac{\text{weight in kilograms}}{(\text{height in meters})^2}$$

BMI score is at the intersection of height and weight. A body mass index score of 25 or more is considered overweight and 30 or more is considered obese.

| 25 | Overweight Limit | | Overweight |

Weight	100	105	110	115	120	125	130	135	140	145	150	155	160	165	170	175	180	185	190	195	200	205
Height																						
5'0"	20	21	21	22	23	24	**25**	26	27	28	29	30	31	32	33	34	35	36	37	38	39	40
5'1"	19	20	21	22	23	24	**25**	26	26	27	28	29	30	31	32	33	34	35	36	37	38	39
5'2"	18	19	20	21	22	23	24	**25**	26	27	27	28	29	30	31	32	33	34	35	36	37	37
5'3"	18	19	19	20	21	22	23	24	**25**	26	27	27	28	29	30	31	32	33	34	35	35	36
5'4"	17	18	19	20	21	21	22	23	24	**25**	26	27	27	28	29	30	31	32	33	33	34	35
5'5"	17	17	18	19	20	21	22	22	23	24	**25**	26	27	27	28	29	30	31	32	32	33	34
5'6"	16	17	18	19	19	20	21	22	23	23	24	**25**	26	27	27	28	29	30	31	31	32	33
5'7"	16	16	17	18	19	20	20	21	22	23	23	24	**25**	26	27	27	28	29	30	31	31	32
5'8"	15	16	17	17	18	19	20	21	21	22	23	24	24	**25**	26	27	27	28	29	30	30	31
5'9"	15	16	16	17	18	18	19	20	21	21	22	23	24	24	**25**	26	27	27	28	29	30	30
5'10"	14	15	16	17	17	18	19	19	20	21	22	22	23	24	24	**25**	26	27	27	28	29	29
5'11"	14	15	15	16	17	17	18	19	20	20	21	22	22	23	24	24	**25**	26	26	27	28	29
6'0"	14	14	15	16	16	17	18	18	19	20	20	21	22	22	23	24	24	**25**	26	26	27	28
6'1"	13	14	15	15	16	16	17	18	18	19	20	20	21	22	22	23	24	24	**25**	26	26	27
6'2"	13	13	14	15	15	16	17	17	18	19	19	20	21	21	22	22	23	24	24	**25**	26	26
6'3"	12	13	14	14	15	16	16	17	17	18	19	19	20	21	21	22	22	23	24	24	**25**	26
6'4"	12	13	13	14	15	15	16	16	17	18	18	19	19	20	21	21	22	23	23	24	24	**25**

FIGURE II–2. Body mass index. Source: Shape Up America. National Institutes of Health.

to be insufficient in iron, calcium, and vitamins. The combination of long-established eating patterns, income, transportation, housing, social interaction, and the effects of chronic or acute disease influence nutritional intake and health (Miller, 2004).

➤ The decreased energy needs of many older adults require a change in nutrient intake:

	25 to 50 years of age	**50 years or older**
Carbohydrates	60%	55%
Protein	10%	20%
Fat	30%	25%
Kcal/day		
Women	2,200	1,900
Men	2,900	2,300

➤ People taking diuretics must be observed closely for adequate hydration (intake and output) and electrolyte balance, especially sodium and potassium. Potassium-rich foods should be included regularly in the diet as oranges and bananas.

➤ Iron-deficiency anemia usually occurs over time and may be related to chronic diseases and insufficient dietary iron. Increasing the intake of foods rich in vitamin C, folic acid, and dietary iron can improve the conditions necessary for optimal absorption of iron. Iron supplementation is often necessary.

FOCUS ASSESSMENT CRITERIA

Assess for subjective data

Ability to eat, swallow
Complains of taste changes, decreased appetite, nausea
Diet recall for 24 hours

➤ Is this the usual intake pattern?
➤ Is intake of five basic food groups sufficient?
➤ Is fluid intake sufficient?

Objective Data

General

➤ Appearance
➤ Hair
➤ Height
➤ Mouth
➤ Muscle mass
➤ Skin
➤ Weight, BMI
➤ Teeth
➤ Fat distribution
➤ Nails
➤ BMI
➤ Edema

Anthropometric measurements

➤ Mid-arm circumference
➤ Triceps skinfold
➤ Mid-arm muscle circumference

Laboratory studies

➤ Decreased serum prealbumin
➤ Decreased serum transferring

Assess for related factors

Subjective

Appetite (usual, changes)
Dietary patterns

➤ Food/fluid dislikes, preferences, taboos
➤ Religious dietary practices

Activity level

➤ Occupation, exercise (type, frequency)

Food procurement/preparation (by whom)

➤ Functional ability
➤ Kitchen facilities
➤ Income adequate for food needs
➤ Transportation

Knowledge of nutrition

➤ Basic five food groups
➤ Recommended intake of carbohydrates, fats, salts
➤ Relationship of activity and metabolism

Physiologic risk factors

➤ Neurologic impairment
➤ Chronic illness
➤ Malabsorption
➤ Inflammatory bowel disease

Psychosocial conditions

➤ Alcohol abuse
➤ Isolation
➤ Drug use
➤ Depression
➤ Household status
➤ Institutionalization

Medications (prescribed, over-the-counter)
Reports of

➤ Allergies
➤ Indigestion
➤ Anorexia
➤ Diarrhea
➤ Dysphagia
➤ Vomiting
➤ Constipation

➤ Nausea
➤ Chewing problems
➤ Fatigue
➤ Pain

Objective

Ability to chew, swallow, feed self

➤ For more information on Focus Assessment Criteria, visit http://connection.lww.com

GOAL

The client will ingest daily nutritional requirements in accordance with activity level and metabolic needs.

Imbalanced Nutrition: More Than Body Requirements

Definition

Imbalanced Nutrition: More Than Body Requirements: State in which a person experiences or is at risk of experiencing weight gain related to an intake in excess of metabolic requirements

Defining Characteristics

MAJOR (MUST BE PRESENT, ONE OR MORE)

Overweight (weight 10% over ideal for height and frame or BMI 25.0–29.0), or
Obese (weight 20% or more over ideal for height and frame or BMI over 30)
Triceps skinfold greater than 15 mm in men and 25 mm in women

MINOR (MAY BE PRESENT)

Reported undesirable eating patterns
Intake in excess of metabolic requirements
Sedentary activity patterns

Related Factors

PATHOPHYSIOLOGIC

Related to altered satiety patterns secondary to (specify)
Related to decreased sense of taste and smell

TREATMENT-RELATED

Related to altered satiety secondary to

Medications (corticosteroids, antihistamines, estrogens)
Radiation (decreased sense of taste and smell)

SITUATIONAL (PERSONAL, ENVIRONMENTAL)

Related to risk to gain more than 25 to 30 pounds when pregnant
Related to lack of basic nutrition knowledge

MATURATIONAL
Adult/Older Adult

Related to decreased activity patterns, decreased metabolic needs

 Carp's Cue ▶ *Using this diagnosis to describe people who are overweight or obese places the focus of interventions on nutrition. Obesity is a complex condition with sociocultural, psychological, and metabolic implications. When the focus is primarily on limiting food intake, as with many weight-loss programs, the chance of permanent weight loss is slim. To be successful, a weight-loss program must focus on behavior modification and lifestyle changes. The nursing diagnosis Imbalanced Nutrition: More Than Body Requirements does not describe this focus. Rather, Ineffective Health Maintenance related to intake of excess of metabolic requirements better reflects the need to increase metabolic requirements through exercise and decreased intake. For some people who desire weight loss, Ineffective Coping related to increased eating in response to stressors could be useful in addition to Ineffective Health Maintenance. The nurse should be cautioned against applying a nursing diagnosis for an overweight or obese person who does not want to participate in a weight-loss program. Motivation for weight loss must come from within. Imbalanced Nutrition: More Than Body Requirements does have clinical usefulness in people at risk for or who have experienced weight gain because of pregnancy, taste or smell changes, or medications (e.g., corticosteroids).*

▼ Imbalanced Nutrition: Potential for More Than Body Requirements

Definition

Imbalanced Nutrition: Potential for More Than Body Requirements: State in which a person is at risk of experiencing an intake of nutrients that exceeds metabolic needs.

Defining Characteristics

Reported or observed obesity in one or both parents
Rapid transition across growth percentiles in infants and children
Reported use of solid food as major food source before 5 months of age
Observed use of food as a reward or comfort measure
Reported or observed higher baseline weight at beginning of each pregnancy
Dysfunctional eating patterns

Carp's Cue *This nursing diagnosis is similar to Risk for Imbalanced Nutrition: More Than Body Requirements. It describes a person who has a family history of weight gain (e.g., previous pregnancy). Until clinical research differentiates this diagnosis from other currently accepted diagnoses, use Ineffective Health Maintenance (Actual or Risk for) or Risk for Imbalanced Nutrition: More Than Body Requirements to direct teaching to assist clients and families to identify unhealthy dietary patterns.*

▼ Acute Pain

Definition

Acute Pain: The state in which a person experiences and reports the presence of severe discomfort or an uncomfortable sensation, lasting from 1 second to less than 6 months.

Defining Characteristics

MAJOR (MUST BE PRESENT)

Communication (verbal or coded) of pain (S)

MINOR (MAY BE PRESENT)

Guarding, protective behavior (O)

Self-focusing (S)

Narrowed focus (altered time perception, withdrawal from social contact, impaired thought processes) (O)

Associated behavior (moaning, crying, pacing, restlessness) (O)

Facial mask of pain (lackluster-eyed, "beaten look," fixed or scattered movement, grimace) (O)

Autonomic responses not seen in chronic stable pain (diaphoresis [sweating], changes in blood pressure and pulse, papillary dilation, increased or decreased respiratory rate) (O)

Related Factors

See Impaired Comfort.

Nursing management of pain presents specific challenges. Is acute pain a response that nurses treat as a nursing diagnosis or collaborative problem? Is acute pain the etiology of another response that better describes the condition that nurses treat? Does some cluster of nursing diagnoses represent a pain syndrome or chronic pain syndrome (e.g., Fear, Risk for Ineffective Family Coping, Impaired Physical Mobility, Social Isolation, Ineffective Sexuality Patterns, Risk for Colonic Constipation, Fatigue)? McCafferty and Beebe (1989) cite 18 nursing diagnoses that can apply to people experiencing pain. Viewing pain as a syndrome diagnosis can provide nurses with a comprehensive nursing diagnosis for people in pain to whom many related nursing diagnoses could apply.

Key Concepts

GENERIC CONSIDERATIONS

➤ Pain has been described as an "experience that overwhelms the individual and consumes every aspect of life" (Ferrell, 1995, p. 609).

➤ All pain is real, regardless of its cause. Pure psychogenic pain is probably rare, as is pure organic pain. Most bodily pain is a combination of mental events (psychogenic) and physical stimuli (organic).

➤ Pain has two components: sensory, which is neurophysiologic, and perceptual or experiential, which has cognitive and emotional origins. The interaction of these two components determines the amount of suffering (Schechter, 1989a).

➤ Pain tolerance means the duration and intensity of pain that a person is willing to endure. It differs among people and may vary in one person in different situations. For example, tolerance to pain at night is usually lower than during the day.

> Social and environmental factors that influence pain tolerance are as follows:
>> Knowledge of pain and its cause
>> Ability to control pain
>> Energy level (fatigue)
>> Stress level
>> Response of others (family, friends)
> Studies have shown that diagnosed physiologic pain does respond to placebos, so a positive response to placebo cannot be used to diagnose pain as psychogenic (Perry & Heidrich, 1981).
> Pain can be classified as acute or chronic, according to cause and duration, not intensity.
>> *Acute pain* has a duration of 1 second to less than 6 months. The cause is usually organic disease or injury. With healing, the pain subsides and eventually disappears.
>> *Chronic pain* usually lasts for 6 months or longer. It can be described as limited, intermittent, or persistent.
>> *Limited pain* results from a known physical lesion, and an end of the pain will come (e.g., burns).
>> *Intermittent pain* provides the person with pain-free periods. The cause may or may not be known (e.g., headaches).
>> *Persistent pain* usually occurs daily. The cause may or may not be known and is usually not a threat to life (e.g., low back pain).
> The visible signs of pain (physical and behavioral) are determined by the person's pain tolerance, culture, and the duration of the pain, not the pain intensity.
> The person may respond to acute pain physiologically by diaphoresis (sweating) and increased blood pressure and heart and respiratory rates and behaviorally by crying, moaning, or showing anger.
> The person with chronic pain usually has adapted to it, both physiologically and behaviorally. Thus, he or she may not show visible signs of the pain.
> Nurses' fear of precipitating addiction often makes them reluctant to administer narcotics. Porter and Jick (1980) identified that 4 of 11,000 addicts reported they received Demerol in the hospital.
> Drug tolerance is a physiologic phenomenon in which, after repeated doses, the prescribed dose begins to lose its effectiveness.
> Drug dependence is a physiologic state that results from repeated administration of a drug.
> Withdrawal occurs if a drug is discontinued abruptly. Tapering down the drug dosage manages the withdrawal symptoms.

GERIATRIC CONSIDERATIONS

> Pain is omnipresent in older adults and may be accepted by them and professionals as a normal and unavoidable accompaniment to

aging. Unfortunately, many chronic diseases that are common in older adults, such as osteoarthritis and rheumatoid arthritis, may not receive adequate pain management.

➤ Older adults may not demonstrate objective signs and symptoms of pain because of years of adaptation and increased pain tolerance. They may eventually accept the pain, thereby lowering expectations for comfort and mobility. Pain-coping mechanisms cultivated throughout life are important to identify and reinforce in pain management. Effective pain management can greatly improve overall physical functioning and emotional well-being (Clinton & Eland, 1991).

➤ The effects of narcotic analgesics are prolonged in older adults because of decreased metabolism and clearance of the drug. Also, side effects seem to be more frequent and pronounced, especially anticholinergic effects, extrapyramidal effects, and sedation. For older adults, it is advised that drugs be started at a lower dosage. Because older adults often take multiple drugs, drug interactions should be monitored (Malseed, 1995).

FOCUS ASSESSMENT CRITERIA

See Impaired Comfort.

GOAL

The person will experience a satisfactory relief measure as evidenced by (specify).

GENERAL INTERVENTIONS

1. Assess for factors that decrease pain tolerance.

➤ Disbelief from others
➤ Fear (e.g., of addiction or loss of control)
➤ Monotony
➤ Lack of knowledge
➤ Fatigue

2. Address disbelief from others

➤ Relate your acceptance of the client's response to pain.
  ➤ Acknowledge the pain.
  ➤ Listen attentively to client's discussion of pain.
➤ Convey that you are assessing pain because you want to understand it better (not determine whether it really exists).

➤ Assess the family for any misconceptions about pain or its treatment.
  ➤ Explain the concept of pain as an individual experience.
➤ Discuss why a person may experience increased or decreased pain (e.g., fatigue [increased], distractions [decreased]).
➤ Encourage family members to share their concerns privately (e.g., fear that the person will use pain for secondary gains if he or she receives too much attention).
➤ Assess whether family members doubt the pain; discuss the effects of doubting on the person's pain and on the relationship.
➤ Encourage the family to give attention also when the client does not exhibit pain.

Rationale: Trying to convince health care providers that he or she is experiencing pain will cause the client anxiety, which compounds the pain. Both are energy depleting.

3. Reduce lack of knowledge.

➤ Explain the cause of pain, if known.
➤ Relate the severity of the pain and how long it will last, if known.
➤ Explain diagnostic procedures and tests in detail by relating the discomforts and sensations that the client will feel; approximate the duration (e.g., "During the intravenous pyelogram, you might feel a momentary hot flash through your entire body").
➤ Allow person to see and handle equipment if possible.

Rationale: People who are prepared for painful procedures by explanations of the actual sensations experience less stress than those who receive vague explanations.

4. Reduce fear.

➤ Provide accurate information to reduce fear of addiction.
  ➤ Explore reasons of the fear.
➤ Explain the difference between drug tolerance and drug addiction (see Key Concepts).
➤ Assist in reducing fear of losing control.
  ➤ Provide privacy for the client's pain experience.
  ➤ Attempt to limit the number of health care providers who provide care.
  ➤ Allow client to share intensity of pain; express how well he or she tolerated it.
➤ Provide information to reduce fear that the medication will gradually lose its effectiveness.
  ➤ Discuss drug tolerance.
➤ Discuss interventions for drug tolerance with the physician (e.g., changing the medication, increasing the dose, decreasing the interval).
  ➤ Discuss the effect of relaxation techniques on medication effects.

Rationale: Information given before a potentially stressful event reduces fear of the unknown and assists the person to adapt (Hymovich & Hagopian, 1992).

5. Decrease fatigue.

➤ Determine the cause of fatigue (sedatives, analgesics, sleep deprivation).
➤ Explain that pain contributes to stress, which increases fatigue.
➤ Assess present sleep pattern and the influence of pain on sleep.
➤ Provide opportunities to rest during the day and with periods of uninterrupted sleep at night (must rest when pain is reduced).
➤ Consult with physician for an increased dose of pain medications at bedtime.

Refer to Disturbed Sleep Patterns for specific interventions to enhance sleep.

Rationale: Inadequate sleep decreases the ability to tolerate pain and depletes the energy needed to participate in social activities (Eland, 1988).

6. Reduce monotony.

➤ Discuss with client and family the therapeutic uses of distraction, along with other methods of pain relief.
➤ Emphasize that the degree to which a person can be distracted from the pain is not at all related to the existence or intensity of the pain.
➤ Explain that distraction usually increases pain tolerance and decreased pain intensity; however, after the distraction ceases, the person may have an increased awareness of pain and fatigue.
➤ Vary the environment if possible.
   ➤ If the client is on bed rest:
      ➤ Encourage personnel to wear seasonal pins and bright-colored apparel.
      ➤ Encourage family to decorate the room with flowers, plants, and pictures.
      ➤ Provide music.
      ➤ Consult with a recreational therapist for appropriate tasks.
   ➤ If the client is at home:
      ➤ Encourage person to plan an activity for each day, preferably outside the home.
      ➤ Discuss the possibility of learning a new skill (e.g., a craft, a musical instrument).
      ➤ Teach a method of distraction during acute pain that is not a burden (e.g., count items in a picture, count anything in the room, such as patterns on wallpaper, count silently to self); breathe rhythmically; listen to music and increase the volume as the pain increases.

Rationale: Adults and children who are experiencing pain feel their bodies and their lives are out of control. Attempts must be made to provide some choice or control during their day (Lubkin, 1995).

7. Collaborate with client about possible methods to reduce pain intensity.
   ➤ Consider the following before selecting a specific pain-relief method:
      ➤ Client's willingness (motivation) and ability to participate
      ➤ Preference
      ➤ Support of significant others for method
      ➤ Contraindications (allergy, health problem)
      ➤ Method's cost, complexity, precautions, and convenience
   ➤ Explain the various noninvasive pain-relief methods to the client and family and why they are effective.
   ➤ Discuss the use of heat applications, their therapeutic effects, indications, and related precautions.
      ➤ Hot water bottle
      ➤ Warm tub
      ➤ Hot summer sun
      ➤ Moist heat pack
      ➤ Electric heating pad
      ➤ Thin plastic wrap over heat (e.g., knee, elbow)
   ➤ Discuss the use of cold applications, their therapeutic effects, indications, and related precautions.
      ➤ Cold towels (wrung out)
      ➤ Ice bag
      ➤ Ice massage
      ➤ Cold water immersion for small body parts
      ➤ Cold gel pack
   ➤ Explain the therapeutic uses of topical preparations, such as menthol, capsaicin, massage, and vibration.
   ➤ Teach client to avoid negative thoughts about ability to cope with pain (Gaston-Johnson et al., 2000).
   ➤ Provide distraction (e.g., guided imagery, music).

Rationale: Studies have shown that the human brain secretes endorphins, which have opiate-like properties that relieve pain. The release of endorphins may be responsible for the positive effects of placebos and noninvasive pain-relief measures (McCafferty & Beebe, 1989). Nonpharmacologic interventions provide a major treatment approach for pain, specifically chronic pain (McGuire, Sheidler & Polomano, 2000). They provide clients with an increased sense of control, promote active involvement, reduce stress and anxiety, elevate mood, and raise the pain threshold (McGuire, Sheidler & Polomano, 2000). Cognitive pain interventions try to modify thought processes to relieve pain. Examples are distraction, (e.g., counting, word games, conversation, breathing exercises), imagery, and educational programs about pain management (McGuire, Sheidler & Polomano, 2000). Behavioral methods attempt to modify physiologic reactions to pain. Examples are relaxation, meditation, music therapy, hypnosis, and biofeedback (McGuire, Sheidler & Polomano, 2000). Relaxation and guided imagery effectively manage pain by increasing sense of control, reducing feelings of helplessness and hopelessness, providing a calming diversion, and disrupting the pain–anxiety–tension cycle (Sloman, 1995).

8. Provide optimal pain relief with prescribed analgesics.

➤ Determine preferred route of administration: oral, intramuscular (IM), intravenous (IV), rectal (see Key Concepts).
➤ Assess vital signs, especially respiratory rate, before administration.
➤ Consult with pharmacist for possible adverse interactions with other medications (e.g., muscle relaxants, tranquilizers).
➤ Use a preventative approach.
   ➤ Medicate before an activity (e.g., ambulation) to increase participation, but evaluate the hazard of sedation.
   ➤ Instruct client to request PRN pain medication before the pain is severe.
   ➤ Collaborate with physician or nurse practitioner to order medications on a 24-hour basis rather than PRN.

Rationale: The preventative approach may reduce the total 24-hour dose compared with the PRN approach; it provides a constant blood level of the drug, it reduces craving for the drug, and it reduces the anxiety of having to ask and wait for PRN relief (Agency of Health Care Policy and Research [AHCPR], 1992).

9. Assess client's response to pain-relief medication.

➤ After administration, return in 30 minutes to assess effectiveness.
➤ Ask client to rate severity of pain before the medication and amount of relief received.
➤ Ask person to indicate when pain began to increase.
➤ Consult with physician if a dosage or interval change is needed; the dose may be increased by 50% until effective (AHCPR, 1992).

Rationale: Adults and children who are experiencing pain feel their bodies and their lives are out of control. Attempts must be made to provide some choice or control during their day (Lubkin, 1995).

10. Reduce or eliminate common side effects of narcotics.

Sedation

➤ Assess whether the cause is the narcotic, fatigue, sleep deprivation, or other drugs (sedatives, antiemetics).
➤ Inform person that drowsiness usually occurs the first 2 to 3 days and then subsides.

➤ If drowsiness is excessive, consult with physician to slightly reduce the dose.

Constipation

➤ Explain the effects of narcotics on peristalsis.
➤ For long-term drug use, consult with a physician on the use of a stool softener.
➤ Increase fiber. Add prune juice to diet.

Nausea and vomiting

➤ Instruct the person that nausea usually subsides after a few doses.
➤ Refrain from withholding narcotic doses because of nausea; rather, secure an order for antiemetic.
➤ If nausea persists, consult with a physician for a change of narcotic that produces less nausea (e.g., morphine).

Dry mouth

➤ Explain that narcotics decrease saliva production.
➤ Instruct person to rinse mouth often, suck on sugarless sour candies, eat pineapple chunks or watermelon (if permissible), and drink liquids often.
➤ Explain the necessity of good oral hygiene and dental care.

11. Assist family to respond optimally to client's pain experience.

➤ Assess family's knowledge of pain and response to it.
➤ Give accurate information to correct misconceptions (e.g., addiction, doubt of pain).
➤ Provide each family member with opportunities to discuss fears, anger, and frustrations privately; acknowledge the difficulty of the situation.
➤ Incorporate family members in the pain-relief modality, if possible (e.g., stroking, massage) (Grealish, 2000).
➤ Praise their participation and concern.

Rationale: Addiction is a psychological syndrome characterized by compulsive drug-seeking behavior generally associated with a desire for drug administration to produce euphoria or other effects, not pain relief. Addiction is believed to be rare, and there is no evidence that adequate administration of opioids for pain reduces addiction. Pain is an intense experience for the client and family members. Interventions focus on helping families understand pain's effects on roles and relationships (Lubkin, 1995).

12. Assist with the aftermath of pain.

➤ Inform the person when the cause of pain has been removed or decreased (e.g., spinal tap).
➤ Encourage person to discuss the pain experience.

➤ Praise client for his or her endurance and convey that he or she handled the pain well, regardless of actual behavior.

Rationale: Providing an opportunity to discuss the pain experience will clarify misconceptions and increase a sense of control.

13. Initiate health teaching, as indicated.

➤ Discuss with client and family noninvasive pain-relief measures (relaxation, distraction, massage).
➤ Teach the techniques of choice to the person and family.
➤ Explain the expected course of the pain (resolution) if known (e.g., fractured arm, surgical incision).

Rationale: Management of pain will continue at home.

▼ Chronic Pain

Definition

Chronic Pain: The state in which a person experiences pain that is persistent or intermittent and lasts for more than 6 months.

Defining Characteristics

MAJOR (MUST BE PRESENT)

The person reports that pain has existed for more than 6 months (may be the only assessment data present) (S)

MINOR (MAY BE PRESENT)

Discomfort (S)
Anger, frustration, depression because of situation (S)
Facial mask of pain (O)
Anorexia, weight loss (O)
Insomnia (O)
Guarded movement (O)
Muscle spasms (O)
Redness, swelling, heat (O)

Related Factors

See Impaired Comfort.

Chronic pain is a complex nursing diagnosis. Chronic pain affects all aspects of one's life: physical, social, cognitive, emotional, sexual, spiritual, and work. As a beginning student, this diagnosis in its entirety is beyond your abilities. The focus of this book on this diagnosis will be limited. Consult with your instructor regarding the need for an experienced nurse to address the more complex effects of chronic pain (e.g., depression).

Key Concepts

Refer to Acute Pain.

FOCUS ASSESSMENT CRITERIA

See Impaired Comfort.

GOAL

The person will relate improvement of pain and increased daily activities.

Indicators

Relate that others validate that their pain exists.
Practice selected noninvasive pain-relief measures.

GENERAL INTERVENTIONS

1. Assess person's pain experience.

➤ Determine the intensity of pain at its worst and best.
➤ Ask person to rate pain using a scale of 0 to 10 (0 = no pain; 10 = worst pain) or 0 to 5.
　➤ Rate it at its best.
　➤ Rate it after a pain-relief measure.
　➤ Rate it at its worst.
　➤ Rate that he/she can tolerate.
➤ Explore with person how he or she manages the pain at home.
➤ Add these self-care pain relief measures to care plan.

Rationale: The person is an expert on his or her pain. The personal pain experience can be managed by the use of cognitive and physical techniques (Holmes, 1998).

   2. Assess for factors that decrease pain tolerance.

➤ See Acute Pain.

   3. Reduce or eliminate factors that increase pain.

➤ See Acute Pain.

   4. Allow person to share the effects of chronic pain on his or her life (Ferrell, 1995).

➤ Physical well-being (fatigue, strength, appetite, sleep, function, constipation, nausea)
➤ Psychological well-being (anxiety, depression, coping, control, concentration, sense of usefulness, fear, enjoyment)
➤ Spiritual well-being (religiosity, uncertainty, positive changes, sense of purpose, hopefulness, suffering, meaning of pain, transcendence)
➤ Social well-being (family support, family distress, sexuality, affection, employment, isolation, financial burden, appearance, roles, relationships)

   5. Assist client and family to reduce the effects of depression on lifestyle.

➤ Explain the relationship between chronic pain and depression.
➤ Encourage verbalization concerning difficult situations.
➤ Listen carefully.

   6. Collaborate with client to initiate appropriate noninvasive pain-relief measures.

➤ See Acute Pain.

   7. Provide pain relief with prescribed analgesics.

➤ Determine preferred route of administration: oral, IV, IM, rectal (refer to Key Concepts).
➤ Assess client's response to the medication. For those admitted to acute care settings:
   ➤ After administration, return in 30 minutes to assess effectiveness.
➤ Ask person to rate severity of pain before the medication and amount of relief received.
➤ Ask client to indicate when the pain began to increase.
➤ Consult with the physician if a dosage or interval change is needed.
➤ For outpatients:
   ➤ Ask person to keep a record of when he or she takes medication and kind of relief received.
   ➤ Instruct person to consult physician with questions concerning medication dosage.

➤ Encourage the use of oral medications as soon as possible.
  ➤ Consult with physician for a schedule to change from IM to oral.
  ➤ Explain to client and family that oral medications can be as effective as IM.
➤ Explain how the transition will occur:
  ➤ Begin oral medication at a larger dose than necessary (loading dose).
  ➤ Continue PRN IM medication dose.
  ➤ Gradually reduce IM medication dose.
  ➤ Use the person's account of pain to regulate oral doses.
➤ Consult with physician about possibly adding aspirin or acetaminophen to medication regimen.

Rationale: The scheduled approach may reduce the total 24-hour drug dose as compared with the PRN approach and may reduce the client's anxiety associated with having to ask for and wait for PRN medications. The PRN approach is effective for breakthrough pain or to manage additional pain from treatments and procedures.

8. Reduce or eliminate common side effects of narcotics.

➤ See Acute Pain.

9. Assist family to respond optimally to the client's pain experience.

➤ See Acute Pain.
  ➤ Encourage family to seek assistance if needed for specific problems, such as coping with chronic pain: family counselor, financial and service agencies (e.g., American Cancer Society).

Rationale: The person with chronic pain may respond with withdrawal, depression, anger, frustration, and dependency, all of which can affect the family in the same way.

10. Promote optimal mobility.

➤ Discuss the value of exercise to strengthen and stretch muscles, decrease stress, and promote sleep.
➤ Plan daily activities when pain is at its lowest level.

Rationale: A regular amount of exercise will increase strength, decrease pain, and fatigue.

11. Initiate health teaching and referrals as indicated.

➤ Discuss with client and family various treatment modalities available:
  ➤ Family therapy
  ➤ Behavior modification
  ➤ Hypnosis
  ➤ Exercise program

➤ Group therapy
➤ Biofeedback
➤ Aqua therapy
➤ Acupuncture

Rationale: Individual therapies can increase sense of control. Group activities can increase socialization and coping abilities.

▼ Risk for Peripheral Neurovascular Dysfunction

Definition

Risk for Peripheral Neurovascular Dysfunction: State in which a person is at risk of experiencing a disruption in circulation, sensation, or motion of an extremity.

Risk Factors

Presence of risk factor (see Related Factors).

Related Factors

PATHOPHYSIOLOGIC

Related to increased volume of (specify extremity) secondary to

Bleeding (e.g., trauma, fractures)
Arterial obstruction
Coagulation disorder
Venous obstruction/pooling

Related to increased capillary filtration secondary to

Allergic response (e.g., insect bites)
Severe burns (thermal, electrical)
Frostbite
Trauma
Venomous bites (e.g., snake)
Hypothermia
Nephrotic syndrome

Related to restrictive envelope secondary to

Circumferential burns of extremities
Excessive pressure

TREATMENT-RELATED

Related to increased volume secondary to

Infiltration of intravenous infusion
Nonpatent wound drainage system
Excessive movement
Dislocated prosthesis (knee, hip)

Related to increased capillary filtration secondary to

Total knee replacement
Total hip replacement

Related to restrictive envelope secondary to

Tourniquet
Circumferential dressings
Cast
Premature or tight closure of fascial defects
Antishock trousers
Ace wraps
Brace
Restraints
Blood pressure cuff
Excessive traction
Air splints

This diagnosis represents a situation that nurses can prevent by identifying who is at risk and implementing measures to reduce or eliminate causative or contributing factors. Risk for Peripheral Neurovascular Dysfunction can change to compartmental syndrome. PC: Compartmental Syndrome is inadequate tissue perfusion in a muscle, usually an arm or leg, caused by edema, which obstructs venous and arterial flow and compresses nerves. The nursing focus for compartmental syndrome is diagnosing its presence and notifying the physician. The medical interventions required to treat the problem are surgical, such as evacuation of hematoma, repair of damaged vessels, or fasciotomy. Refer to PC: Compartmental Syndrome, if indicated. Another misuse of this diagnosis is Risk for Peripheral Neurovascular Dysfunction related to thrombus in left leg. This situation does not represent a high-risk situation that a nurse can prevent; rather, it is a situation that requires nurse- and physician-prescribed interventions. The collaborative problem PC: Thrombus left leg would accurately describe this situation.

Key Concepts

GENERIC CONSIDERATIONS

➤ The most frequent cause of medical litigation in North America is failure to diagnose neurovascular compromise, which advances to compartmental syndrome (Bourne & Rorabeck, 1989).

➤ After trauma or surgery or with certain therapeutic measures, obstruction of blood flow can result from
  ➤ Edema
  ➤ Embolus (air, fat, blood)
  ➤ Clot formation
  ➤ Blood vessel trauma
  ➤ Pressure on the vessels (cast, tourniquet, restraints, constrictive nature of burned tissue)
➤ Neurovascular compromise occurs when tissue pressure increases in a space-limiting envelope or site (Pellino et al., 1998).
➤ Factors that can limit a space are anatomic, such as skin or muscle fascia, pathophysiologic, such as circumferential burns of extremities, or treatment-related, such as casts (Fahey & Milzarek, 1999).
➤ Factors that can increase tissue pressure or envelope content are bleeding, edema formation, or anything that decreases arterial pressure or increases arterial pressure (Pellino et al., 1998).
➤ Vascular insufficiency and nerve compression from edema can reduce blood supply to an extremity and result in peripheral nerve damage. Permanent damage can result within 4 to 12 hours (Fahey & Milzarek, 1999).
➤ Compartments are areas of muscle, nerve, and blood vessels encased in elastic boundaries of skin, muscle, fascia, and bone. The body has 46 compartments, with 38 found in the arms or legs (Kracun & Wooten, 1998).
➤ The effects of venous compression and the resulting signs and symptoms are outlined in Figure II.3.
➤ Lower leg pain that is worse after running may indicate chronic compartmental syndrome. The achy pounding leg pain occurs after muscles warm up (usually 5 to 10 minutes) and can persist for several minutes to hours.

FOCUS ASSESSMENT CRITERIA

Assess for related factors

Subjective Data

History of

➤ Compromised peripheral circulation
➤ Peripheral thrombosis

Tobacco use

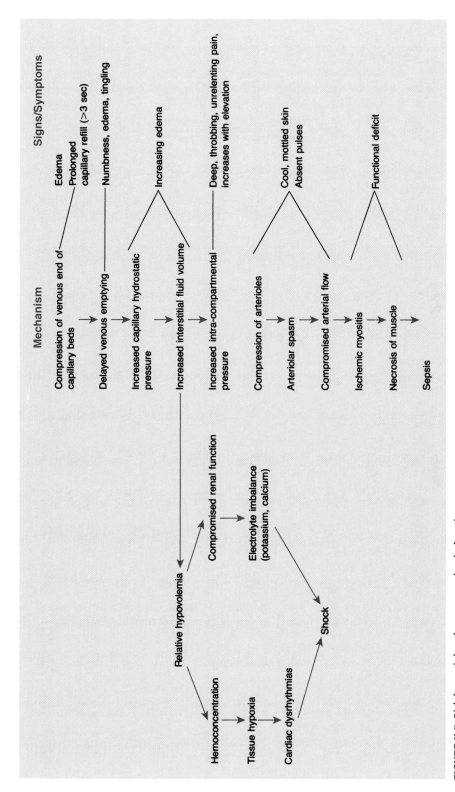

FIGURE II.3 Risk for peripheral neurovascular dysfunction.

Objective Data

Edema; postoperative
Pressure on vessels

➤ Cast

Bleeding within compartment
Venipuncture
Restraints
Trauma

GOAL

The person will demonstrate intact peripheral sensation or movement.

Indicators

Palpable peripheral pulses
Warm extremities
Capillary refill less than 3 seconds

GENERAL INTERVENTIONS

1. Assess and evaluate neurovascular status at least every hour for first 24 hours; compare with unaffected limb, if possible.

➤ Skin
  ➤ Temperature (cool, warm)
  ➤ Color (pale, dependent, rubor, flushed, cyanotic)
➤ Bilateral pulses (radial, posterior tibial, dorsalis pedis)
  ➤ Rate, rhythm
➤ Volume
  ➤ 0 = Absent, nonpalpable
  ➤ Thready, weak, fades in and out
  ➤ Present, but diminished
  ➤ Normal, easily palpable
  ➤ Aneurysmal
➤ Edema (location, pitting); measure circumference at widest diameter of leg or arm
➤ Capillary refill (normal, less than 3 seconds)
➤ Document findings

Rationale: Trauma causes tissue edema and blood loss that reduces tissue perfusion. Inadequate circulation and edema damage peripheral nerves, resulting in decreased sensation, movement, and circulation (Porth, 2002).

2. Instruct client to report unusual, new, or different sensations, such as tingling, numbness, and decreased ability to move toes or fingers.

Rationale: Neurovascular compromise often begins as minor sensations; early detection can enable prompt intervention to prevent serious complications (Pellino et al., 1998).

3. Reduce edema or its effects on function.

➤ Remove jewelry from affected limb.
➤ Elevate limbs unless contraindicated.
➤ Advise client to move fingers or toes of affected limb two to four times an hour.
➤ Monitor drainage (characteristics, amount) from wounds or incision.
➤ Maintain patency of the wound drainage system.
➤ Apply ice bags around injured site if not contraindicated. Place cloth between ice bag and skin.

Rationale: Swelling that cannot be controlled causes increased tissue pressure and occlusion of the blood supply to nerve and muscle tissue, resulting in anoxia. This complication is compartmental syndrome.

4. Notify the physician if the following occur:

➤ Change in sensation
➤ Change in movement ability
➤ Pale, mottled, or cyanotic skin
➤ Capillary refill greater than 3 seconds
➤ Diminished or absent pulse
➤ Increasing pain or pain not controlled by medication
➤ Pain with passive stretching of muscle
➤ Pain increased with elevation

5. If above signs or symptoms occur, discontinue elevation and ice application.

➤ Promote circulation in affected limb.
➤ Ensure optimal hydration to maximize circulation.
➤ Monitor traction apparatus and splints for pressure on vessels or nerves. Remove at least every hour and perform ROM.
➤ Encourage active ranges of motion of unaffected body parts and ambulation, if permissible.

Rationale: These measures will decrease tissue pressure and restore local blood flow.

➤ Document changes and nursing response.

6. Initiate health teaching, as indicated.

➤ Teach client and family to watch for and report the following symptoms:
  ➤ Severe pain
  ➤ Numbness or tingling
  ➤ Swelling
  ➤ Skin discoloration
  ➤ Paralysis or reduced movement
  ➤ Cool white toes or fingertips
  ➤ Foul odor, warm spots, soft areas, or cracks in the cast
➤ Emphasize the importance of follow-up evaluations.

Rationale: A sudden change in temperature, drop in pressure, or no pulse indicates graft thrombosis. Changes in sensation or motor function can indicate compartmental syndrome (Kracun & Wooten, 1998).

▽ Impaired Physical Mobility

▽ Impaired Bed Mobility

▽ Impaired Walking

▽ Impaired Wheelchair Mobility

▽ Impaired Wheelchair Transfer Ability

Definition

Impaired Physical Mobility: State in which a person experiences or is at risk of experiencing limitation of physical movement but is not immobile.

Defining Characteristics (Levinc, Kreinovitch, Bahrenburg & Mitchell, 1989)

MAJOR (ONE OR MORE MUST BE PRESENT)

Compromised ability to move purposefully within the environment (e.g., bed, mobility, transfers, ambulation)
ROM limitations

MINOR (MAY BE PRESENT)

Imposed restriction of movement
Reluctance to move

Related Factors

PATHOPHYSIOLOGIC

Related to decreased strength and endurance secondary to

Autoimmune alterations (e.g., multiple sclerosis, arthritis)
Nervous system diseases (e.g., Parkinson's disease, myasthenia gravis)
Muscular dystrophy
Partial paralysis (spinal cord injury, stroke)
CNS tumor

➤ Increased intracranial pressure
➤ Sensory deficits
➤ Musculoskeletal impairment
➤ Fractures
➤ Connective tissue disease (systemic lupus erythematosus)

Related to edema

TREATMENT-RELATED

Related to external devices (casts or splints, braces, IV tubing)
Related to insufficient strength and endurance for ambulation with (specify)

Prosthesis
Crutches
Walker

SITUATIONAL (PERSONAL, ENVIRONMENTAL)

Related to

Fatigue
Motivation
Pain

MATURATIONAL

Children

Related to abnormal gait secondary to

Congenital skeletal deficiencies
Legg-Calvé-Perthes disease
Osteomyelitis

Older Adult

Related to decreased motor agility
Related to muscle weakness

Impaired Physical Mobility describes a person with limited use of arm(s) or leg(s) or limited muscle strength. Nurses should not use this diagnosis to describe complete immobility; in this case, Disuse Syndrome is more applicable. Limitation of physical movement also can be the etiology of other nursing diagnoses, such as Self-Care Deficit and Risk for Injury. Nursing interventions for Impaired Physical Mobility focus on strengthening and restoring function and preventive deterioration. If the limited mobility affects self-care, use a self-care deficit diagnosis also.

Key Concepts

GENERIC CONSIDERATIONS

➤ According to Miller (2004), mobility is one of the most significant aspects of physiologic functioning, because it greatly influences the maintenance of independence.

➤ Activity, mobility, and flexibility are integral to a person's lifestyle. Compromised mobility seriously affects self-concepts and lifestyle.

➤ The four ROM categories are passive, active assistive, and active, and active resistive (Adams & Clough, 1998):

  ➤ Passive ROM is movement of the client's muscles by another person with the client's help.

  ➤ Active assistive ROM is active contraction of a muscle with assistance by an external force such as a therapist, mechanical, appliance, or the uninvolved extremity.

  ➤ Active ROM is active contraction of a muscle against the force of gravity, such as straight leg lift.

  ➤ Active resistive ROM is active contraction of a muscle against resistant, such as weights.

➤ Isometric exercises are when muscles contract or tense without joint movement. They are contraindicated in people with cardiac conditions because they increase left ventricular function. When performed, muscles should be tensed for 5 to 15 seconds (Pellino et al., 1998).

➤ Ambulation is a complex three-dimensional activity involving the legs, pelvis, trunk, and upper extremities. Gait is a complex movement involving the musculoskeletal, neurologic, and cardiovascular systems. Cognitive factors such as mentation and orientation are critical for safe ambulation (Addams & Clough, 1998).

GERIATRIC CONSIDERATIONS

➤ About 10% of un-institutionalized older adults report some limitation in mobility; of institutionalized older adults, more than 90% are dependent in at least one ADL (Miller, 2004). Mobility problems are often the reason for nursing home admission or extensive in-home care. Assessment of mobility determines the extent of functional impairment as a result of disease or disability.

➤ Effects of immobility are particularly dangerous in older adults. Muscle weakness, atrophy, and decreased endurance occur quickly, and biochemical and physiologic effects such as nitrogen loss and hypercalciuria are important to consider (Porth, 2002). Permanent functional loss is more likely with prolonged immobility, and older adults also are vulnerable to new morbidity such as pneumonia, pressure sores, falls and fracture, osteoporosis, incontinence, confusion, and depression. Every effort toward prevention and mobilization should be made (Miller, 2004).

➤ Age-related changes in joint and connective tissue impair flexion and extension movements, decrease flexibility, and reduce cushioning protection for joints (Miller, 2004).

FOCUS ASSESSMENT CRITERIA

Subjective Data

Assess for subjective (S) and objective (O) cues:

History of symptoms (complaints of) (S)

➤ Pain
➤ Muscle weakness
➤ Fatigue
   ➢ Attributed to?
   ➢ Amount of time out of bed
   ➢ Induced by?
   ➢ Amount of time sleeping or resting

History of systemic disorders (O)

➤ Neurologic
   ➢ Head trauma
   ➢ Birth defect
   ➢ Multiple sclerosis
   ➢ Increased intracranial pressure
   ➢ CVA
   ➢ Guillain-Barré syndrome
   ➢ Polio

- ➤ Tumor
- ➤ Myasthenia gravis
- ➤ Spinal cord injury
- ➤ Cardiovascular
  - ➤ Myocardial infarction
  - ➤ Congenital heart anomaly
  - ➤ Congestive heart failure
- ➤ Musculoskeletal
  - ➤ Osteoporosis
  - ➤ Arthritis
  - ➤ Fractures
- ➤ Respiratory
  - ➤ Chronic obstructive
  - ➤ Pneumonia
  - ➤ Dyspnea on exertion
  - ➤ Pulmonary disease (COPD)
  - ➤ Orthopnea
- ➤ Debilitating diseases
  - ➤ Cancer
  - ➤ Renal disease
  - ➤ Endocrine disease

History of recent trauma or surgery (O)
Current drug therapy (O)
Dominant hand (O)
Motor function (O)

Right arm	Strong	Weak	Absent	Spastic
Left arm	Strong	Weak	Absent	Spastic
Right leg	Strong	Weak	Absent	Spastic
Left leg	Strong	Weak	Absent	Spastic

Mobility (O)

Ability to turn self	Yes	No	Assistance needed (specify)
Ability to sit	Yes	No	Assistance needed (specify)
Ability to stand	Yes	No	Assistance needed (specify)
Ability to get up	Yes	No	Assistance needed (specify)
Ability to transfer	Yes	No	Assistance needed (specify)
Ability to ambulate	Yes	No	Assistance needed (specify)

Weight-bearing (assess both right and left sides)

- ➤ Full
- ➤ As tolerated
- ➤ Partial
- ➤ Non–weight-bearing

Gait (O)

- ➤ Stable
- ➤ Unstable

Assistive devices (O)

➤ Crutches
➤ Wheelchair
➤ Cane
➤ Prosthesis
➤ Braces
➤ Walker
➤ Other

Restrictive devices (O)

➤ Cast or splint
➤ Foley
➤ Traction
➤ IV line
➤ Braces
➤ Monitor
➤ Ventilator
➤ Dialysis
➤ Drain

ROM (neck, shoulders, elbows, arms, spine, hips, legs) (O)

➤ Full
➤ Limited (specify)
➤ None

Endurance (see Activity Intolerance for additional information)

Assess (O)

➤ Resting pulse, blood pressure, respirations
➤ Blood pressure, respirations, and pulse immediately after activity
➤ Pulse every 2 minutes until pulse returns to within 10 beats of resting pulse

After activity, assess for indicators of hypoxia (showing intensity, frequency, or duration of activity must be decreased or discontinued) as follows:

Blood pressure (O)

➤ Failure of systolic rate to increase
➤ Increase in diastolic of 155 mm Hg

Respirations (O)

➤ Excessive rate increases
➤ Decrease in rate
➤ Irregular rhythm
➤ Dyspnea

Cerebral and other changes (O)

➤ Confusion
➤ Incoordination
➤ Change in equilibrium
➤ Weakness
➤ Pallor
➤ Cyanosis

Peripheral circulation (O)

➤ Capillary refill time (normal, less than 3 seconds)
➤ Skin color, temperature, and turgor
➤ Peripheral pulses (rate, quality)
  ➤ Brachial
  ➤ Posterior tibial
  ➤ Radial
  ➤ Popliteal
  ➤ Femoral
  ➤ Pedal

Motivation (as perceived by nurse and/or stated by person) (O)

➤ Excellent
➤ Satisfactory
➤ Poor

GOAL

The person will report increased strength and endurance of limbs.

Indicators

Demonstrate the use of adaptive devices to increase mobility.
Use safety measures to minimize potential for injury.
Describe rationale for interventions.
Demonstrate measures to increase mobility.

GENERAL INTERVENTIONS

1. Assess causative factors.

➤ Trauma (e.g., cartilage tears, fractures, amputations)
➤ Surgical procedure (e.g., joint replacement, reduction of fractures, vascular surgery)
➤ Debilitating disease (e.g., diabetes, cancer, rheumatoid arthritis, multiple sclerosis, stroke)

2. Promote motivation and adherence (Addams & Clough, 1998).

➤ Explain the problem and the objective of each exercise.
➤ Ensure that initial exercises are easy and require submaximal strength and coordination.
➤ Progress only if the client is successful at the present exercise.
➤ Provide written instructions for prescribed exercises after demonstrating and observing return demonstration.
➤ Document and discuss improvement specifically (e.g., can lift leg 2 inches higher).

Rationale: Promoting the client's feelings of control and self-determination may improve compliance with the exercise program.

3. Increase limb mobility. Determine type of ROM appropriate for person (passive, active assistive, active, active resistive).

➤ Perform passive or active assistive ROM exercises (frequency determined by client's condition):
  ➢ Teach client to perform active ROM on affected limbs at least four times a day, if possible.
  ➢ Perform passive ROM on affected limbs. Do the exercises slowly to allow the muscles time to relax, and support the extremity above and below the joint to prevent strain on joints and tissues.
  ➢ During ROM, the client's legs and arms should move gently to within his or her pain tolerance; perform ROM slowly to allow the muscles time to relax.
  ➢ For passive ROM, the supine position is most effective. The client who performs ROM himself or herself can use a supine or sitting position.
  ➢ Do ROM daily with bed bath, three or four times daily if there are specific problem areas. Try to incorporate into ADLs.
➤ Support extremity with pillows to prevent or reduce swelling.
➤ Medicate for pain as needed, especially before activity (see Impaired Comfort).
➤ Apply heat or cold to reduce pain, inflammation, and hematoma.
➤ Apply cold to reduce swelling after injury (usually first 48 hours).
➤ Encourage client to perform exercise regimens for specific joints as prescribed by physician or physical therapist (e.g., isometric, resistive).

Rationale: Active ROM increases muscle mass, tone, and strength and improves cardiac and respiratory functioning. Passive ROM improves joint mobility and circulation.

4. Position in alignment to prevent complications.

➤ Use a foot board.
➤ Avoid prolonged sitting or lying in the same position.
➤ Change position of the shoulder joints every 2 to 4 hours.

➤ Use a small pillow or no pillow when in Fowler's position.
➤ Support the hand and wrist in natural alignment.
➤ If the client is supine or prone, place a rolled towel or small pillow under the lumbar curvature or under the end of the rib cage.
➤ Place a trochanter roll or sandbags alongside the hips and upper thighs.
➤ If the client is in the lateral position, place pillow(s) to support the leg from groin to foot and a pillow to raise the shoulder and elbow slightly; if needed, support the lower foot in dorsal flexion with a sandbag.
➤ For upper extremities:
  ➤ Arms abducted from the body with pillows
  ➤ Elbows in slight flexion
  ➤ Wrist in a neutral position, with fingers slightly flexed, and thumb abducted and slightly flexed
  ➤ Position of shoulder joints changes during the day (e.g., adduction, abduction, range of circular motion)

Rationale: Prolonged immobility and impaired neurosensory function can cause permanent contractures.

5. Maintain good body alignment when mechanical devices are used.

➤ Traction devices
  ➤ Assess for correct position of traction and alignment of bones.
  ➤ Observe for correct amount and position of weights.
  ➤ Allow weights to hang freely, with no blankets or sheets on ropes.
  ➤ Assess for changes in circulation; check pulse quality, skin temperature, color of extremities, and capillary refill (should be less than 3 seconds).
  ➤ Assess for changes in circulation (numbness, tingling, pain).
  ➤ Assess for changes in mobility (ability to flex/extend unaffected joints).
  ➤ Assess for signs of skin irritation (redness, ulceration, blanching).
  ➤ Assess skeletal traction pin sites for loosening, inflammation, ulceration, and drainage; clean pin insertion sites (procedure may vary with type of pin and physician's order).
  ➤ Encourage isometrics and prescribed exercise program.
➤ Casts
  ➤ Assess for proper fit of cast (should not be to loose or too tight).
  ➤ Assess circulation to the encased area every 2 hours (numbness, tingling, pain).
  ➤ Assess motion of uninvolved joist (ability to flex and extend).
  ➤ Assess for skin irritation (redness, ulceration, or complaints of pain under the cast).
  ➤ Keep cast clean and dry; do not allow sharp objects to be inserted under cast; petal rough edges with adhesive tape; place soft cotton under edges that seem to be causing pressure points.

- ➤ Allow cast to air dry while resting on pillows to prevent dents.
- ➤ Observe cast for areas of softening or indentation.
- ➤ Exercise joints above and below cast if allowed (e.g., wiggle fingers and toes every 2 hours).
- ➤ Assist with prescribed exercise regimens and isometrics of muscles enclosed in casts.
- ➤ Keep extremities elevated after cast application to reduce swelling.
- ➤ Braces
  - ➤ Assess for correct positioning of braces.
  - ➤ Observe for signals of skin irritation (redness, ulceration, blanching, itching, pain).
  - ➤ Assist with exercises prescribed for specific joints.
  - ➤ Have the client demonstrate correct application of the brace.
- ➤ Prosthetic devices
  - ➤ Observe for signs of skin irritation of the stump before applying prosthetic device (stump should be clean and dry; Ace bandage should be rewrapped and securely in place).
  - ➤ Have the client demonstrate correct application of the prosthesis.
  - ➤ Assess for gait alterations or improper walking technique.
  - ➤ Proceed with health teaching, if indicated.
- ➤ Ace bandages
  - ➤ Assess for correct position of Ace bandage.
  - ➤ Apply Ace bandage with even pressure, wrapping from distal to proximal portions and making sure that the bandage is not too tight or too loose.
  - ➤ Observe for bunching of the bandage.
  - ➤ Observe for signs of irritation of skin (redness, ulceration, excessive tightness).
  - ➤ Rewrap Ace bandages twice daily or as needed, unless contraindicated (e.g., if the bandage is a postoperative compression dressing, it should be left in place).
  - ➤ When wrapping lower extremity, leave the heel exposed, using figure-8 technique.
- ➤ Slings
  - ➤ Assess for correct application; sling should be loose around neck and should support elbow and wrist above level of the heart.
  - ➤ Remove slings for ROM.

Note: Some mechanical devices may be removed for exercises, depending on nature of injury or type and purpose of device. Consult with the physician to ascertain when the person may remove the device.

Rationale: Ambulatory aids must be used correctly and safely to ensure effectiveness and prevent injury. Prolonged immobility and impaired neurosensory function can cause permanent contractures. Pressure from mechanical devices can cause damage to skin and tissue.

6. Provide progressive mobilization.

➤ Assist slowly to sitting position.
  ➢ Allow client to dangle legs over the side of the bed for a few minutes before standing.
  ➢ Limit time to 15 minutes, three times a day, the first few times out of bed.
➤ Increase time out of bed, as tolerated, by 15-minute increments.
➤ Progress to ambulation with or without assistive devices.
➤ If client cannot walk, assist him or her out of bed to a wheelchair or chair.
➤ Encourage ambulation for short frequent walks (at least three times daily), with assistance if unsteady.
➤ Increase lengths of walks progressively each day.

Rationale: A regular exercise program including ROM, isometrics, and selected aerobic activities can help maintain the integrity of joint function (Addams & Clough, 1998). Prolonged bed rest or decreased blood volume can cause a sudden drop in blood pressure; increased activity reduces fatigue and increases endurance (Porth, 2002).

7. Encourage use of affected arm when possible.

➤ Encourage the person to use affected arm for self-care activities (e.g., feeding self, dressing, brushing hair).
➤ For post-CVA neglect of upper limb, see Unilateral Neglect.
➤ Instruct client to use unaffected arm to exercise the affected arm.
➤ Use appropriate adaptive equipment to enhance the use of arms.
  ➢ Universal cuff for feeding in clients with poor control in both arms, hands
  ➢ Large-handled or padded silverware to assist clients with poor fine motor skills
  ➢ Dishware with high edges to prevent food from slipping
  ➢ Suction-cup aids to prevent sliding of plate
➤ Use a warm bath to alleviate early-morning stiffness and improve mobility.
➤ Encourage client to practice handwriting skills, if able.
➤ Allow time to practice using affected limb.

Rationale: Exercise enhances independence. Incorporating ROM exercises into a person's daily routine encourages regular performances.

8. Ensure that physical therapy program has been scheduled before discharge.

Rationale: Physical therapy will need to be continued until the person has reached their potential to continue exercises on own.

▼ Impaired Bed Mobility

Definition

Impaired Bed Mobility: State in which a person experiences, or is at risk of experiencing, limitation of movement in bed.

Defining Characteristics

Impaired ability to turn side to side
Impaired ability to move from supine to sitting to supine
Impaired ability to "scoot" or reposition self in bed
Impaired ability to move from supine to prone or prone to supine
Impaired ability to move from supine to long sitting or long sitting to
    supine

Carp's Cue ▶ Impaired Bed Mobility may be a clinically useful diagnosis when a person is a candidate for rehabilitation to improve strength, ROM, and movement. The nurse can consult with a physical therapist for a specific plan. This diagnosis is inappropriate for an unconscious or terminally ill person.

Related Factors

Refer to Impaired Physical Mobility

Key Concepts

Refer to Impaired Physical Mobility

FOCUS ASSESSMENT CRITERIA

Refer to Impaired Physical Mobility

GOAL

Refer to Impaired Physical Mobility

GENERAL INTERVENTIONS

Refer to Impaired Physical Mobility

▼ Impaired Walking

Definition

Impaired Walking: State in which a person experiences, or at risk of experiencing, limitation in walking.

Defining Characteristics

Impaired ability to climb stairs.
Impaired ability to walk required distances
Impaired ability to walk on an incline
Impaired ability to walk on uneven surfaces
Impaired ability to navigate curbs

Related Factors

Refer to Impaired Physical Mobility

Key Concepts

Refer to Impaired Physical Mobility

FOCUS ASSESSMENT CRITERIA

Refer to Impaired Physical Mobility

GOAL

The person will increase walking distances.

Indicators

Demonstrate safe mobility
Use mobility aids correctly

GENERAL INTERVENTIONS

Refer to Impaired Physical Mobility

▼ Impaired Wheelchair Mobility

Definition

Impaired Wheelchair Mobility: State in which a person experiences or is at risk for experiencing difficulty with wheelchair and safety.

Defining Characteristics

Impaired ability to operate manual or power wheelchair on an even or uneven surface
Impaired ability to operate manual or powered wheelchair on an incline
Impaired ability to operate wheelchair on curbs

Related Factors

Refer to Impaired Physical Mobility

Key Concepts

Refer to Impaired Physical Mobility

FOCUS ASSESSMENT CRITERIA

Refer to Impaired Physical Mobility

Impaired Wheelchair Mobility and Impaired Wheelchair Transfer Ability is a nursing diagnosis that requires most nurses to consult with a physical therapist. After the consultation or therapy, the nurse can then reinforce the techniques prescribed by physical therapy. The plan of care would specify the techniques.

GOAL

The person will report satisfactory safe wheelchair mobility.

Indicators

Demonstrate safe use of wheelchair
Demonstrate safe transfer to wheelchair

GENERAL INTERVENTIONS

➤ Determine factors interfering with proper wheelchair use (i.e., knowledge, strength, mentation).
➤ Consult with physical therapist for specific techniques.
➤ Teach transfer techniques (weight-bearing and non–weight-bearing) as prescribed by physical therapy.
➤ Have person demonstrate technique; evaluate effectiveness and safety.

Rationale: Interventions for this diagnosis are to evaluate causes of problem and to reinforce the prescriptions of physical therapy each shift.

▼ Impaired Wheelchair Transfer Ability

Definition

Impaired Wheelchair Transfer Ability: State in which a person experiences or is at risk for experiencing difficulty with transfer to and from the wheelchair.

Defining Characteristics

Impaired ability to transfer from bed to chair and chair to bed
Impaired ability to transfer on or off a toilet or commode
Impaired ability to transfer in or out of tub or shower

Impaired ability to transfer between uneven levels
Impaired ability to transfer from chair to floor or floor to chair
Impaired ability to transfer from chair to car or car to chair
Impaired ability to transfer from floor to chair or chair to floor
Impaired ability to transfer standing to floor or floor to standing

Related Factors

Refer to Impaired Physical Mobility

FOCUS ASSESSMENT CRITERIA

Refer to Impaired Physical Mobility

GOAL

The person will demonstrate transfer to and from the wheelchair.

Indicators

Identify when assistance is needed.
Demonstrate ability to transfer in varied situations (e.g., toilet, bed, car, chair, uneven levels).

GENERAL INTERVENTIONS

1. Consult with a physical therapist to determine how much assistance the client needs.

   ➤ None
   ➤ Verbal cuing
   ➤ Support by clinician's hand
   ➤ Physical assistance
   ➤ Mechanical device (e.g., lifts)

Rationale: Refer to Impaired Physical Mobility

2. Advise that ability may fluctuate; encourage client to request assistance.

Rationale: This is to prevent injury

▼ **Ineffective Protection**

▼ **Impaired Tissue Integrity**

▼ **Impaired Skin Integrity, Risk For**

▼ **Impaired Skin Integrity**

▼ **Impaired Oral Mucous Membrane**

▼ **Impaired Oral Mucous Membrane, Risk for**

Definition

Ineffective Protection: State in which a person experiences a decrease in the ability to guard against internal or external threats, such as illness or injury.

Defining Characteristics

MAJOR (MUST BE PRESENT, ONE OR MORE)

Deficient immunity
Impaired healing
Altered clotting
Maladaptive stress response
Neurosensory alterations

MINOR (MAY BE PRESENT)

Chills
Insomnia
Perspiration
Fatigue
Dyspnea
Anorexia
Cough
Weakness
Itching

Immobility
Restlessness
Disorientation
Pressure sores

This broad diagnosis describes a person with compromised ability to defend against microorganisms, bleeding, or both because of immunosuppression, myelosuppression, abnormal clotting factors, or all these. Use of this diagnosis entails several potential problems.

The nurse is cautioned against substituting Ineffective Protection for an immune system compromise, AIDS, disseminated intravascular coagulation, diabetes mellitus, or other disorders. Rather, the nurse should focus on diagnoses describing the person's functional abilities that are or may be compromised by altered protection, such as Fatigue, Risk for Infection, and Risk for Social Isolation. The nurse also should address the physiologic complications of altered protection that require nursing and medical interventions for management, identifying appropriate collaborative problems.

It is problematic if the nurse uses Ineffective Protection in each of these three cases: Mr. A, who has leukemia, leukopenia, and no evidence of infection; Mr. B, who is experiencing sickle cell crisis; and Mr. C, who has AIDS. The problem is that this diagnosis does not describe the specific focus of nursing but describes situations in which more specific responses can be diagnosed. For Mr. A, the nursing diagnosis of Risk for Infection related to compromised immune system would apply. For Mr. B., the collaborative problem PC: Sickle Cell Crisis best describes his situation, which the nurse monitors and manages using physician- and nurse-prescribed interventions. The nursing diagnosis Risk for Infection and the collaborative problem PC: Opportunistic Infections would apply to Mr. C.

As these examples show, in most cases, the nursing diagnosis Risk for Infection and selected collaborative problems prove more clinically useful than Ineffective Protection.

Impaired Tissue Integrity has limited clinical use. One use is Risk for Impaired Tissue Integrity related to prolonged contact lens use and improper care of lens.

Impaired Tissue or Skin Integrity should not be used as a new label or name for surgical incisions, tracheostomies, or burns. Instead, ask yourself how has the burn, incision, or tracheostomy affected the person's ability to function and what problems can they cause that the nurse can prevent. Examples are nursing diagnoses such as Risk for Infection, Impaired Communication, Acute Pain, and collaborative problems of PC: Bleeding, PC: Electrolyte Imbalances.

▼ Impaired Tissue Integrity

Definition

Impaired Tissue Integrity: State in which a person experiences or is at risk for damage to the integumentary, corneal, or mucous membranous tissues of the body.

Defining Characteristics

MAJOR (MUST BE PRESENT)

Disruptions of corneal, integumentary, or mucous membranous tissue or invasion of body structure (incision, dermal ulcer, corneal ulcer, oral lesion)

MINOR (MAY BE PRESENT)

Lesions (primary, secondary)
Dry mucous membrane
Edema
Leukoplakia
Erythema
Coated tongue

Related Factors

PATHOPHYSIOLOGIC

Related to inflammation of dermal–epidermal junctions secondary to

Autoimmune alterations

➤ Lupus erythematosus
➤ Scleroderma

Metabolic and endocrine alterations

➤ Diabetes mellitus
➤ Jaundice
➤ Hepatitis
➤ Cancer
➤ Cirrhosis
➤ Thyroid dysfunction
➤ Renal failure

Bacterial

➤ Impetigo
➤ Folliculitis
➤ Cellulitis

Viral

➤ Herpes zoster (shingles)
➤ Herpes simplex
➤ Gingivitis

AIDS
Fungal

➤ Ringworm (dermatophytosis)
➤ Athlete's foot
➤ Vaginitis

Related to decreased blood and nutrients to tissues secondary to

Diabetes mellitus

➤ Peripheral vascular alterations
➤ Anemia
➤ Cardiopulmonary disorders
➤ Venous stasis
➤ Arteriosclerosis

Nutritional alterations

➤ Obesity
➤ Emaciation
➤ Edema
➤ Dehydration
➤ Malnutrition

TREATMENT-RELATED

Related to decreased blood and nutrients to tissues secondary to

Therapeutic extremes in body temperature
NPO status
Surgery
Prolonged use of contact lenses

Related to imposed immobility secondary to sedation
Related to mechanical trauma

Therapeutic fixation devices

➤ Wired jaw
➤ Casts
➤ Traction

Orthopedic devices/braces

Related to effects of radiation on epithelial and basal cells

Related to effects of mechanical irritants or pressure secondary to

Inflatable or foam donuts
Tourniquets
Footboards
Restraints
Dressings, tape, solutions
External urinary catheters
Nasogastric (NG) tubes
Endotracheal tubes
Oral prostheses/braces
Contact lenses

SITUATIONAL (PERSONAL, ENVIRONMENTAL)

Related to chemical trauma secondary to

Excretions
Secretions
Noxious agents/substances

Related to environmental irritants secondary to

Radiation—sunburn
Humidity
Bites (insect, animal)
Poisonous plants
Temperature
Parasites
Inhalants

Related to the effects of pressure of immobility secondary to

Pain
Fatigue
Cognitive, sensory, or motor deficits
Motivation
Related to inadequate personal habits (hygiene/dental/dietary/sleep)
Related to impaired mobility secondary to (specify)
Related to thin body frame

MATURATIONAL

Related to dry thin skin and decreased dermal vascularity secondary to aging

Impaired Tissue Integrity is the broad diagnosis under which the more specific diagnoses of Impaired Skin Integrity and Impaired Oral Mucous Membranes fall. Because tissue is composed of epithelium, connective tissue, muscle, and nervous tissue, Impaired Tissue Integrity correctly describes some pressure ulcers that are deeper than the dermis. Impaired Skin Integrity should be used to describe disruptions of epidermal and dermal tissue only.

When a pressure ulcer is stage IV, necrotic, or infected, it may be more appropriate to label the diagnosis a collaborative problem, such as PC: Stage IV Pressure Ulcer. This would represent a situation that a nurse manages with physician- and nurse-prescribed interventions. When a stage II or III pressure ulcer needs a dressing that requires a physician's order in an acute care setting, the nurse should continue to label the situation a nursing diagnosis, because it would be appropriate and legal for a nurse to treat the ulcer independently in other settings (e.g., in the community).

If a client is immobile and multiple systems are threatened (respiratory, circulatory, musculoskeletal as well as integumentary), the nurse can use Disuse Syndrome to describe the entire situation. If a client is at risk for damage to corneal tissue, the nurse can use a diagnosis such as Risk for Impaired Corneal Tissue Integrity related to corneal drying and lower lacrimal production secondary to unconscious state.

Key Concepts

GENERIC CONSIDERATIONS

➤ "At any given time, more than 1 million Americans are estimated to have pressure ulcers" (Maklebust, 1999, p. 861). Pressure ulcer incidence ranges from 2.7% to 29.5% in acute care settings, as high as 41% in critical care populations, and from 2.4% to 23% in skilled nursing facilities and nursing homes (Maklebust, 1999).

➤ Tissues are groupings of specialized cells that unite to perform specific functions. The human body is composed of four basic types of tissue: epithelial, connective (including skeletal tissue and blood), muscle, and nervous.

➤ The external covering of the body is composed of epithelial tissue, called the integument. Wherever the body exposes large openings to the outside (e.g., the mouth), its outer covering changes from integument to an inner lining called the mucous membrane. Each layer of the integument has its counterpart in a complete mucous membrane. The integument includes both the skin and the subcutaneous tissue.

➤ The skin is a complex organ consisting of two layers: the outer epidermis and the deeper dermis. The epidermis is approximately 0.04 mm thick, and the dermis is about 0.5 cm thick (Porth, 2002).

➤ The epidermis functions as a barrier to protect inner tissues (from injury, chemicals, organisms); as a receptor for a range of sensations (touch, pain, heat, cold); as a regulator of body temperature through radiation (giving off heat), conduction (transfer of heat), and convection (movement of warm air molecules away from the body); as a regulator of water balance by preventing water and electrolyte loss; and as a receptor for vitamin D from the sun (Maklebust & Sieggreen, 1996).

➤ The skin's responses to antigens are capillary dilation (erythema), arteriole dilation (flare), and increase capillary permeability (wheal), which all contribute to localized edema, spasms, and pruritus.

➤ Causes of tissue destruction can be mechanical, immunologic, bacterial, chemical, or thermal. Mechanical destruction includes physical trauma and incision. Immunologic destruction occurs as an allergic response. Bacterial destruction results from an overgrowth of organisms. Chemical destruction results when a caustic substance contacts unprotected tissue. Thermal destruction occurs when tissue is exposed to temperature extremes that are incompatible with cell life (Maklebust & Sieggreen, 1996).

Wound Healing

➤ Wound healing is a complex sequence of events initiated by injury to the tissues. The components are coagulation of bleeding, inflammation, epithelialization, fibroplasia and collagen metabolism, collagen maturation, scar remodeling, and wound contraction (Wysocki, 1999).

➤ A wound must be considered in relation to the entire person. Major factors that affect wound healing are nutrition, vitamins, minerals, anemia, blood volume and tissue oxygenation, steroids and antiinflammatory drugs, diabetes mellitus, chemotherapy, and radiation.

➤ Wound healing requires the following intrinsic factors (Boynton et al., 1999):

   ➢ Increased protein—carbohydrate intake sufficient to prevent negative nitrogen balance, hypoalbuminemia, and weight loss

   ➢ Increased daily intake of vitamins and minerals

      ➣ Vitamin A, 10,000 to 50,000 IU

      ➣ Vitamin D, 0.5 to 1.0 mg/1,000 diet calories

      ➣ Vitamin B_2, 0.25 mg/1,000 diet calories

      ➣ Vitamin B_6, 2 mg

      ➣ Niacin, 15 to 20 mg

      ➣ Vitamin B_{12}, 400 mg

      ➣ Vitamin C, 75 to 300 mg

      ➣ Vitamin D, 400 mg

> Vitamin E, 10 to 15 IU
> Traces of zinc, magnesium, calcium, copper, manganese
> Adequate oxygen supply and the blood volume and ability to transport it

GERIATRIC CONSIDERATIONS

➤ Some older adults exhibit shiny, loose, thin, transparent skin, primarily on the backs of the hands and the forearms. Subcutaneous fat decreases with aging, reducing the cushioning of bony prominences and putting older adults at increased risk for pressure ulcers.

➤ Aging causes diminished immunocompetence and decreased angiogenesis, which delays wound healing (Boynton et al. 1999).

➤ Age-related decreases in sebum secretion and the number of sebaceous glands cause drier coarser skin that is more prone to fissures and cracks.

➤ In older adults, cells are larger and proliferate more slowly, fibroblasts decrease in number, and dermal vascularity decreases. All these factors contribute to slower wound healing.

➤ With aging, the thermal threshold for sweating increases and the sweat output decreases.

➤ Aging nails become dull, brittle, and thickened due to decreased blood supply to the nailbed. Splitting of the nails can occur, increasing the risk of infection. Thickening of the toenails causes the distal portion of the nail to lift from the nailbed; debris collection creates a risk of fungal infection.

TRANSCULTURAL CONSIDERATIONS

➤ The darker the person's skin, the more difficult it is to assess for changes in color. A baseline must be established in daylight or with at least a 60-watt bulb. Baseline skin color should be assessed in areas with the least amount of pigmentation (e.g., palms of hands, soles of feet, underside of forearms, abdomen, and buttocks; Weber & Kelley, 2003).

➤ All skin colors have an underlying red tone. Pallor in black-skinned people is seen as an ashen or gray tone. Pallor in brown-skinned people appears as a yellowish-brown color. Pallor can be assessed in mucous membranes, lips, nailbeds, and conjunctiva of the lower eyelids (Andrews & Boyle, 2003).

➤ Assessment of capillary refill time can be done on the second or third finger, lips, or earlobes (Andrews & Boyle, 2003).

➤ To assess for rashes and skin inflammations in dark-skinned people, the nurse should rely on palpation for warmth and induration, not observation (Giger & Davidhizar, 2004).

FOCUS ASSESSMENT CRITERIA

Assess for Related Factors.

Subjective Data

History of symptoms

➤ Onset
➤ Precipitated by what?
➤ Relieved by what?
➤ Frequency

History of exposure (if allergy is suspected)

➤ Carrier of contagious disease
➤ Chemicals, paints, cleaning agents, plants, animals
➤ Heat or cold
➤ Medical, surgical, and dental history; use of tobacco, alcohol

Current drug therapy

➤ What drugs?
➤ How often?
➤ When was last dose taken?
➤ Effects on symptoms

Factors contributing to the development or extension of tissue destruction (assess for)

Skin deficits

➤ Dryness
➤ Thinness
➤ Edema
➤ Excessive perspiration
➤ Obesity
➤ Aging skin

Mucous membrane deficits

➤ Mouth pain
➤ Oral lesions or ulcers
➤ Bleeding gums
➤ Oral plaque
➤ Coated tongue
➤ Dryness

Corneal deficits

➤ Absence of blink reflex
➤ Diminished tearing

➤ Corneal ulcers
➤ Contact lens wear
➤ Ptosis
➤ Sensory deficits
➤ Excessive tearing

Impaired oxygen transport

➤ Edema
➤ Anemia

Peripheral vascular disorders

➤ Arteriosclerosis
➤ Venous stasis
➤ Cardiopulmonary disorders

Chemical/mechanical irritants

➤ Radiation
➤ Contact lenses
➤ Casts, splints, braces
➤ Oral prostheses
➤ Incontinence (feces, urine)

Nutritional deficiencies

➤ Protein
➤ Vitamin
➤ Mineral and trace elements
➤ Dehydration

Systemic disorders

Refer to Related Factors (Pathophysiologic).

Sensory deficits

➤ Decreased level of consciousness
➤ Neuropathy
➤ Visual or taste alterations
➤ Brain or cord injury
➤ Confusion

Immobility

Assess for defining characteristics.

Objective Data

Skin

➤ Color
➤ Texture

➤ Turgor
➤ Vascularity
➤ Moisture
➤ Temperature

Lesions

➤ Type
➤ Shape
➤ Location
➤ Size
➤ Distribution
➤ Drainage
➤ Color

Circulation

➤ Do capillaries refill within 3 seconds after blanching?
➤ Does erythema subside within 30 mm after pressure is removed?

Edema

➤ Note degree and location.
➤ Palpate over bony prominences for sponginess (indicates edema).

Oral mucous membrane

Refer to Focus Assessment Criteria for Impaired Oral Mucous Membrane.

▼ Risk for Impaired Skin Integrity

Definition

Risk for Impaired Skin Integrity: State in which a person is at risk for damage to the epidermal and dermal tissue.

Risk Factors

See Impaired Tissue Integrity.

 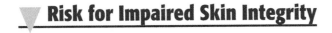 *See Impaired Tissue Integrity*

Key Concepts

See Impaired Tissue Integrity

FOCUS ASSESSMENT CRITERIA

See Impaired Tissue Integrity

GOAL

The person will demonstrate skin integrity free of pressure ulcers (if able).

Indicators

Participate in risk assessment.
Express willingness to participate in prevention of pressure ulcers.
Describe etiology and prevention measures.
Explain rationale for interventions.

GENERAL INTERVENTIONS

1. Use the agency's assessment scale to identify individual risk.

Factors in addition to activity and mobility deficits (e.g., the Braden Scale, Worton Score [AHCPR, 1992])

➤ Assess for skin deficits
  ➤ Dryness
  ➤ Edema
  ➤ Obesity
  ➤ Thinness
  ➤ Excessive Perspiration
➤ Assess for impaired oxygen transport
  ➤ Edema
  ➤ Anemia
  ➤ Peripheral vascular disorders
  ➤ Arteriosclerosis
  ➤ Cardiopulmonary disorders
➤ Assess for chemical/mechanical/thermal irritants
  ➤ Radiation
  ➤ Incontinence (feces, urine)
  ➤ Casts, splints, braces
  ➤ Spasms
➤ Assess for nutritional deficits
  ➤ Protein
  ➤ Vitamin

> ➤ Mineral and trace element
> ➤ Dehydration
- ➤ Assess for systemic disorders
  - ➤ Infection
  - ➤ Diabetes mellitus
  - ➤ Cancer
  - ➤ Hepatic or renal disorders
- ➤ Assess for sensory deficits
  - ➤ Neuropathy
  - ➤ Confusion
  - ➤ Head injury
  - ➤ Cord injury
- ➤ Assess for immobility

Rationale: To prevent pressure ulcers, individuals at risk must be identified so that risk factors can be reduced through interventions.

2. Attempt to modify contributing factors to lessen the possibility of a pressure ulcer developing.

- ➤ Incontinence of urine or feces
- ➤ Determine etiology of incontinence.
- ➤ Maintain sufficient fluid intake for adequate hydration (approximately 2,500 ml daily, unless contraindicated); check oral mucous membranes for moisture and check urine specific gravity. Establish a schedule for emptying bladder (begin with every 2 hours).
- ➤ If person is confused, determine what his or her incontinence pattern is and intervene before incontinence occurs.
- ➤ Explain problem to client; secure his or her cooperation for the plan.
- ➤ When incontinent, wash perineum with a liquid soap that does not alter skin pH.
- ➤ Apply a protective barrier to the perineal region (incontinence film barrier spray, or wipes).
- ➤ Check person frequently for incontinence when indicated.

For additional interventions, refer to Impaired Urinary Elimination.

Rationale: Maceration is a mechanism by which the tissue is softened by prolonged wetting or soaking. If the skin becomes waterlogged, the cells are weakened and the epidermis is easily eroded.

3. Reduce immobility.

- ➤ Encourage ROM exercises and weight-bearing mobility, when possible, to increase blood flow to all areas.
- ➤ Promote optimal circulation when in bed.
  - ➤ Use repositioning schedule that relieves vulnerable area most often (e.g., if vulnerable area is the back, turning schedule would

be left side to back, back to right side, right side to left side, and left side to back); post "turn clock" at bedside.

➤ Turn or instruct client to turn or shift weight every 30 minutes to 2 hours, depending on other causative factors and the ability of the skin to recover from pressure.

➤ Increase frequency of the turning schedule if any reddened areas that appear do not disappear within 1 hour after turning.

➤ Place person in normal or neutral position with body weight evenly distributed (Fig. 11.5). Use 30-degree laterally inclined position when possible.

➤ Keep bed as flat as possible to reduce shearing forces; limit semi-Fowler's position to only 30 minutes at a time.

➤ Use foam blocks or pillows to provide a bridging effect to support the body above and below the high-risk or ulcerated area so affected area does not touch bed surface. Do not use foam donuts or inflatable rings because these increase the area of pressure

➤ Alternate or reduce the pressure on the skin with an appropriate support surface.

➤ Suspend heels off bed surface.

➤ Use enough personnel to lift person up in bed or chair rather than pull or slide skin surfaces.

➤ Have person wear long-sleeved top and socks to reduce friction on elbows and heels.

➤ To reduce shearing forces, support feet with footboard to prevent sliding.

➤ Promote optimal circulation when person is sitting.

➤ Limit sitting time for person at high risk for ulcer development.

➤ Instruct person to lift self using chair arms every 10 minutes, if possible, or assist person in rising up off the chair at least every hour, depending on risk factors present.

➤ Do not elevate legs unless calves are supported, to reduce the pressure over the ischial tuberosities. Pad chair with pressure-relieving cushion.

➤ Inspect areas at risk of developing ulcers with each position change:

➤ Ears
➤ Elbows
➤ Occiput
➤ Trochanter
➤ Heels
➤ Ischia
➤ Sacrum
➤ Scapula
➤ Scrotum

➤ Observe for erythema and blanching and palpate for warmth and tissue sponginess with each position change.

➤ Do not rub reddened areas. To avoid damaging the capillaries, do not perform massage.

Malnourished state

➤ Consult a dietitian.
➤ Increase protein and carbohydrate intake to maintain a positive nitrogen balance; weigh the person daily and determine serum albumin level weekly to monitor status.
➤ Ascertain that daily intake of vitamins and minerals is maintained through diet or supplements (see Key Concepts for recommended amounts).

See Imbalanced Nutrition: Less Than Body Requirements for additional interventions.

Rationale: Adequate nutrition (protein, vitamins, minerals) is vital for healing wounds, preventing infection, preserving immune function, and minimizing loss of strength (Maklebust & Sieggreen, 1996). Pressure is a compressing downward force on a given area. If pressure against soft tissue is greater than intracapillary blood pressure (approximately 32 mm Hg), the capillaries can be occluded, and the tissue can be damaged as a result of hypoxia. Shear is a parallel force in which one layer of tissue moves in one direction and another layer moves in the opposite direction. If the skin sticks to the bed linen and the weight of the sitting body makes the skeleton slide down inside the skin, the subepidermal capillaries may become angulated and pinched, resulting in decreased perfusion of the tissue. Friction is the physiologic wearing away of tissue. If the skin is rubbed against the bed linens, the epidermis can be denuded by abrasion.

▼ Impaired Skin Integrity

Definition

Impaired Skin Integrity: State in which a person is at risk for damage to the epidermal and dermal tissue.

Defining Characteristics

MAJOR (MUST BE PRESENT)

Disruptions of epidural and dermal tissue.

MINOR (MAY BE PRESENT)

Divided skin
Lesions (primary, secondary)
Erythema

Related Factors

See Impaired Tissue Integrity

GOAL

The person will demonstrate progressive healing of dermal ulcer.

Indicators

Identify causative factors for pressure ulcers.
Identify rationale for prevention and treatment.
Participate in the prescribed treatment plan to promote wound healing.

GENERAL INTERVENTIONS

1. Identify the stage of pressure ulcer development.

➤ Stage I: Nonblanchable erythema of intact skin
➤ Stage II: Ulceration of epidermis and/or dermis
➤ Stage III: Ulceration involving subcutaneous fat
➤ Stage IV: Extensive ulceration penetrating muscle, bone, or supporting structure

Rationale: The stage of pressure ulcer will determine treatment, nursing, and medicine.

2. Reduce or eliminate factors that contribute to the extension of pressure ulcers; refer to Risk for Impaired Skin Integrity Related to Immobility.
3. Prevent deterioration of the ulcer.

➤ Wash reddened area gently with mild soap, rinse area thoroughly to remove soap, and pat dry.
➤ Avoid massage of bony prominence to stimulate circulation. Protect the healthy skin surface with one or a combination of the following:
  ➤ Apply a thin coat of liquid copolymer skin sealant.
  ➤ Cover area with moisture-permeable film dressing.

➤ Cover area with a hydrocolloid wafer barrier and secure with strips of 1-inch tape; leave in place for 2 to 3 days.

Rationale: When wounds are left uncovered, epidermal cells must migrate under the scab and over the fibrous tissue below. When wounds are semioccluded and the surface of the wound remains moist, epidermal cells migrate more rapidly over the surface. Appropriate use of dressings may promote moist wound. Use of semiocclusive film dressings or hydrocolloid barrier wafers mechanically protect and properly humidify wounds that are epidermal or dermal. These dressings bathe the wound in serous exudate and do not adhere to the wound surface when they are removed. A physician's order may be required.

4. Increase dietary intake to promote wound healing.

➤ Initiate calorie count. Consult dietitian.
➤ Increase protein and carbohydrate intake to maintain a positive nitrogen balance.
➤ Weigh daily and determine serum albumin level weekly to monitor status.
➤ Ascertain that client maintains daily intake of vitamins and minerals through diet or supplements (see Key Concepts for recommended amounts).

See Imbalanced Nutrition: Less Than Body Requirements for additional interventions.

Rationale: Poor nutrition leads to decreased resistance to infection and interferes with wound healing.

5. Devise plan for pressure ulcer management using principles of moist wound healing (Maklebust & Sieggreen, 1996).

➤ Assess status of pressure ulcer.
➤ Assess size—measure longest and widest wound surface.
➤ Assess depth:
  ➤ No break in skin
  ➤ Abrasion or shallow crater
  ➤ Deep crater
  ➤ Necrosis
  ➤ Involved tendon, joint capsule
➤ Assess edges.
  ➤ Attached
  ➤ Not attached
  ➤ Fibrotic

Assess undermining:
  ➤ <2 cm
  ➤ 2 to 4 cm

➤ >4 cm
➤ Tunneling
➤ Assess necrotic tissue type (color, consistency, adherence) and amount.
➤ Assess exudate type and amount.
➤ Assess surrounding skin color.
➤ Check for any peripheral edema and induration.
➤ Assess for granulation tissue.
➤ Assess for epithelialization.
➤ Debride necrotic tissue (collaborate with physician).
➤ Flush ulcer base with sterile saline solution. Avoid use of harsh antiseptic solutions.
➤ Protect granulating wound bed from trauma and bacteria. Insulate wound surface.
➤ Cover pressure ulcer with a sterile dressing that maintains a moist environment over the ulcer base (e.g., film dressing, hydrocolloid wafer dressing, moist gauze dressing). Do not occlude ulcers on immunocompromised patients.
➤ Avoid the use of drying agents (heat lamps, Maalox, Milk of Magnesia).
➤ Monitor for clinical signs of wound infection.
➤ Measure pressure ulcer weekly to determine progress of wound healing.

Rationale: Rationales for topical treatment (Maklebust & Sieggreen, 1996; Parish, Witkowski & Crissey, 1997) are as follows:

➤ Remove necrotic tissue, which delays wound healing by prolonging the inflammatory phase.
➤ Cleanse wound bed to decrease bacterial count. Bacterial counts above 10 may produce infection by overwhelming the host.
➤ Absorb excess exudate, which macerates surrounding skin and increases risk of infection in wound bed.
➤ Maintain a moist wound surface, which promotes cellular migration. Dry wound surfaces delay epithelialization secondary to difficult cellular migration.
➤ Insulate the wound surface; this enhances blood flow and increases epidermal migration.
➤ Protect the healing wound from trauma and bacterial invasion. Open wounds are vulnerable to abrasion, contamination, drying, and shear mechanisms.

6. Consult with nurse specialist or physician for treatment of necrotic, infected, or deep pressure ulcers.
7. Initiate health teaching and referrals, as indicated.

➤ Instruct person and family on care of ulcers.
➤ Teach the importance of good skin hygiene and optimal nutrition.
➤ Refer to community nursing agency if additional assistance at home is needed.

▼ Impaired Oral Mucous Membrane

Definition

Impaired Oral Mucous Membrane: State in which a person experiences or is at risk for disruptions in the oral cavity.

Defining Characteristics

MAJOR (MUST BE PRESENT)

>Gingivitis
>Leukoplakia
>Oral Lesions
>Stomatitis
>Fissures
>Oral pain

MINOR (MAY BE PRESENT)

>Coated tongue
>Xerostomia (dry mouth)
>Edema
>Sensitive tongue
>Foul taste
>Oral tumors
>Purulent drainage
>Taste changes

Related Factors

PATHOPHYSIOLOGIC

Related to inflammation secondary to

>Diabetes mellitus
>Periodontal disease
>Oral cancer
>Infection

TREATMENT-RELATED

Related to drying effects of

>NPO more than 24 hours
>Radiation to head or neck
>Prolonged use of steroids or other immunosuppressives

Use of antineoplastic drugs
Related to mechanical irritation secondary to
Endotracheal tube
NG tube

SITUATIONAL (PERSONAL, ENVIRONMENTAL)

Related to chemical irritants secondary to

Acidic foods
Drugs
Noxious agents
Alcohol
Tobacco

Related to mechanical trauma secondary to

Broken or jagged teeth, ill-fitting dentures
Braces

Related to malnutrition
Related to dehydration
Related to mouth breathing
Related to inadequate oral hygiene
Related to lack of knowledge of oral hygiene
Related to decreased salivation

Impaired Oral Mucous Membrane is a useful nursing diagnosis as an actual and risk diagnosis. As a beginning student you can routinely use Risk for Impaired Oral Mucous Membrane.

Key Concepts

GENERIC CONSIDERATIONS

➤ Oral health directly influences many ADLs (eating, fluid intake, breathing) and interpersonal relations (appearance, self-concept, communication).
➤ Many oral diseases begin quietly and are painless until significant involvement has taken place.
➤ Common causes of decreased salivation are dehydration, anemia, radiation treatment to head and neck, vitamin deficiencies, removal of salivary glands, allergies, and side effects of drugs (e.g., antihistamines, anticholinergics, phenothiazine, narcotics, chemotherapy).
➤ Excessive use of hydrogen peroxide for mouth care may predispose client to an oral yeast infection. Rinse afterward with normal saline (Kemp & Brackett, 2001).

➤ Lemon and glycerin swabs should be used only on clean healthy mouths as a source of refreshment for an NPO client.

➤ Alcohol and tobacco are chronic irritants to oral mucosa and may lead to oral carcinoma.

➤ Stomatitis and mucositis denote inflammation and ulceration of the oral cavity. Stomatitis is associated with chemotherapy; mucositis is associated with radiation therapy. Mucositis refers to any oral mucosal inflammation, regardless of cause. It may progress from dry, red, inflamed, cracked areas to open sores of the mucosa and bleeding ulcers anywhere in the mouth, esophagus, vagina, or rectum. Mucous membranes are highly susceptible to toxicity because of their rapidly proliferating cells. Persons exposed to multiple therapies or who have predisposing risk factors such as poor oral hygiene, dental caries, and tobacco or alcohol use are more likely to develop mucositis. Stomatitis usually begins 2 to 5 days after chemotherapy; mucositis usually occurs 1 to 2 weeks after radiation therapy.

➤ Chemotherapy or direct radiation also can cause xerostomia, which is a decrease in the quality and quantity of saliva (Beck, 2001).

GERIATRIC CONSIDERATIONS

➤ Age-related changes in oral mucosa include loss of elasticity, atrophy of epithelial cells, and diminished blood supply to connective tissue (Miller, 2004).

➤ Dry mouth and vitamin deficiencies in older adults increase vulnerability to oral ulcerations and infection (Miller, 2004).

➤ Older adults commonly exhibit increased saliva viscosity and diminished saliva quantity (Miller, 2004).

FOCUS ASSESSMENT CRITERIA

Assess for defining characteristics.

Subjective Data

Complaints of

Mouth pain, irritation, burning, or dryness
Inability to eat, drink, or swallow own saliva
Bad taste or odor in mouth
Xerostomia (dry mouth)
Change in tolerance to temperature of food (cold, hot)
Chewing difficulties
Change in taste

Poorly fitting dentures
Change in tolerance to acidic or highly seasoned food

Objective Data

Lips

➤ Color
➤ Cracks
➤ Blisters
➤ Fissures
➤ Ulcers/lesions

Tongue

➤ Color
➤ Masses
➤ Cracks, dryness
➤ Lesions
➤ Exudates
➤ Hairy extensions

Oral mucosa (gums, floor of mouth, inner cheeks, palate)

➤ Color
➤ Moisture
➤ Bleeding
➤ Plaques
➤ Swelling (along gum lines)
➤ Lesions (red, white patches)

Saliva

➤ Watery
➤ Absent
➤ Thick
➤ Color

Assess for related factors.

Subjective Data

Medical/surgical
Medication use (prescribed, over-the-counter)
Use of tobacco

➤ Type (cigarettes, pipe, cigars, snuff)
➤ Frequency (packs per day, how many years)

Use of alcohol

➤ Type
➤ Amount (daily, weekly)

Oral hygiene

➤ Frequency of dental checkups
➤ Personal hygiene
  ➢ "Describe your oral care procedure."
  ➢ Frequency
  ➢ Type of equipment (brush, floss)
➤ Possible barriers to performing oral care
  ➢ Cannot hold standard brush
  ➢ Cannot close hand
  ➢ Limited arm movement
  ➢ Semicomatose
  ➢ Lack of knowledge

Nutritional Status (Refer to Imbalanced Nutrition for specific assessment criteria.)

➤ Daily intake of basic five food groups
➤ Daily fluid intake
➤ Difficulty in chewing or swallowing
➤ Are certain foods avoided? Why?

Objective

Teeth

➤ Sharp edges
➤ Looseness
➤ Chips

Dentures/prosthetics

➤ Condition
➤ Fit
➤ Sharp edges
➤ Cracks
➤ Loose parts
➤ Chips

GOAL

The person will be free of oral mucosa irritation or exhibit signs of healing with decreased inflammation.

Indicators

Describe factors that cause oral injury.
Demonstrate knowledge of optimal oral hygiene.

GENERAL INTERVENTIONS

1. Assess for causative or contributing factors.

➤ Poor oral hygiene, preexisting dental problems
➤ Malnourishment
➤ History of heavy alcohol intake and tobacco use
➤ Chemotherapeutic drugs with mucous membrane toxicity
➤ Radiation to head or neck
➤ Immunosuppression
➤ Dehydration
➤ Steroid therapy
➤ Antibiotics

Rationale: Factors that contribute to stomatitis are poor oral hygiene, preexisting oral disease, irritants (spicy foods, citrus fruits, coarse foods [hard bread, pizza], ill-fitting dental prostheses, too-cold/too-hot foods, tobacco or alcohol), dehydration, malnutrition, and drug therapy [antibiotics, steroids]). Some factors can be eliminated.

2. Promote healing and reduce progression of stomatitis.

➤ Inspect oral cavity three times daily with tongue blade and light; if stomatitis is severe, inspect mouth every 4 hours.
➤ Ensure that oral hygiene regimen is done every 2 hours while awake and every 6 hours (every 4 hours if severe) during the night.
➤ Use normal saline solution as a mouthwash.
➤ Floss teeth only once in 24 hours.
➤ Omit flossing if bleeding is excessive; use extreme caution with people with platelet counts less than 50,000.

Rationale: Proper oral hygiene eliminates microorganisms and reduces risks of infection.

3. Reduce oral pain and maintain adequate food and fluid intake.

➤ Assess person's ability to chew and swallow.
➤ Administer mild analgesic every 3 to 4 hours as ordered by physician.
➤ Instruct client to
  ➤ Avoid commercial mouthwashes, citrus fruit juices, spicy foods, extremes in food temperature (hot, cold), crusty or rough foods, alcohol, and mouthwashes with alcohol.

- ➤ Eat bland, cool foods (sherbets).
- ➤ Drink cool liquids every 2 hours and PRN.
➤ Consult with dietitian for specific interventions.
➤ Refer to Impaired Nutrition: Less Than Body Requirements related to anorexia for additional interventions.
➤ Consult with physician for an oral pain relief solution.
- ➤ Xylocaine Viscous 2% oral, swish and expectorate every 2 hours and before meals (if throat is sore, the solution can be swallowed; if swallowed, Xylocaine produces local anesthesia and may affect the gag reflex).
- ➤ Mix equal parts of Xylocaine Viscous, 0.5 aqueous Benadryl solution, and Maalox, swish and swallow 1 oz of mixture every 2 to 4 hours PRN.
- ➤ Mix equal parts of 0.5 aqueous Benadryl solution and Kaopectate; swish and swallow every 2 to 4 hours or PRN.

Rationale: Decreased salivary flow and increased viscosity of saliva reduce the removal of debris (food, bacteria) from the mouth (Kemp & Brackett, 1997). Dry oral mucosa causes discomfort and increases the risk of breakdown and infection.

4. Initiate health teaching and referrals, as indicated.

Rationale: The frequency of oral health maintenance varies according to a person's health status and self-care ability. All clients should have their teeth and mouths cleaned at least once after meals and at bedtime. High-risk clients (e.g., NG tubes, cancer, poorly nourished) should have oral assessments daily. Clients in chronic care settings should have oral assessment at least once a week.

 Risk For Impaired Oral Mucous Membrane

Definition

See Impaired Oral Mucous Membrane

Risk Factors

See Related Factors under Impaired Oral Mucous Membrane

GOAL

The person will demonstrate integrity of the oral cavity.

Indicators

Be free of harmful plaque to prevent secondary infection.
Be free of oral discomfort during food and fluid intake.
Demonstrate optimal oral hygiene.

GENERAL INTERVENTIONS

1. Assess for causative or contributing factors.

➤ Lack of knowledge
➤ Lack of motivation
➤ Impaired ability to use hands
➤ Fatigue
➤ Altered consciousness

Rationale: Factors that contribute to oral disease are excessive use of alcohol and tobacco, microorganisms, inadequate nutrition (quantity, quality), inadequate hygiene, and trauma (NO tubes, ill-fitting dentures, sharp-edged teeth, sharp-edged prostheses, improper use of cleaning devices).

2. Discuss the importance of daily oral hygiene and periodic dental examinations.

➤ Explain the relationship of plaque to dental and gum disease.
➤ Evaluate person's ability to perform oral hygiene.
➤ Allow person to perform as much oral care as possible.
➤ Teach correct oral care.
　➤ Have person sit or stand upright over sink (if he or she cannot get to a sink, place an emesis pan under the chin).
　➤ Remove and clean dentures and bridges daily.
　➤ Fill wash bowl half full of water (place washcloth on bottom to keep denture from breaking if dropped).
　➤ Brush dentures with a denture brush or stiff, hard toothbrush inside and outside; rinse in cool water before replacing.
　➤ Remove stains and odors from dentures by soaking them overnight in 8 oz of water and 1 tsp of laundry bleach (avoid bleach on any appliance with metal).
　➤ Remove hard deposits by soaking dentures in white (not brown) vinegar overnight. Commercial liquid denture cleaners still require brushing.

➤ Floss teeth (every 24 hours).
  ➤ With a piece of dental floss approximately 25 inches long, floss each tooth by wrapping the floss around the second and third fingers of each hand.
  ➤ Begin with the back teeth; insert the floss between each tooth gently to avoid injuring the gum. Wrap floss around tooth, making a C, and gently pull floss up and down over the back of each tooth.
  ➤ Repeat this in reverse to floss the front of the tooth.
  ➤ Remove the floss either by pulling straight up or by releasing one end and pulling the floss through (minor bleeding may occur).
  ➤ Rinse.
  ➤ Floss holders can make flossing easier (back teeth cannot be reached with a floss holder).
➤ Brush teeth (after meals and before sleep).
  ➤ Use a soft toothbrush (avoid hard brushes) with a nonabrasive toothpaste or sodium bicarbonate (1 tsp in 8 oz of water; may be contraindicated in people with sodium restrictions).
  ➤ Brush back and forth or in a small circle, starting at the back of the mouth and brushing one or two teeth at a time.
  ➤ Gently brush tongue and inner sides of cheeks.
  ➤ Rinse with water.
  ➤ Inspect mouth for lesions, sores, or excessive bleeding.

Rationale: Plaque, microbial flora found in the mouth, is the primary cause of dental cavities and periodontal disease. Daily removal of plaque through brushing and flossing can help prevent dental decay and disease.

3. Perform oral hygiene on person who is unconscious or at risk for aspiration as often as needed.

➤ Preparation
  ➤ Tell person what you are going to do.
  ➤ Turn person on the side, supporting the back with a pillow (protect bed with an absorbent pad).
  ➤ Place a tongue blade or bite block to keep mouth open.
  ➤ Wear gloves to protect self.
➤ Brushing procedure
  ➤ For people with their own teeth, brush following the procedure outlined above. Instead of toothpaste, use hydrogen peroxide and water (1:4), sodium bicarbonate (1 tsp:8 oz water), or normal saline solution (may be contraindicated in people with sodium restrictions).
  ➤ For people with dentures, remove dentures and clean as above. Leave dentures out for people who are semicomatose and store in water (in denture cup).
  ➤ If gums are inflamed, use moist cotton-tipped applicators or soft foam Toothettes.

> Use a bulb syringe to rinse mouth; aspirate rinse with suction or use an aspirating toothbrush.
> Move tongue blade or bite block for access to other areas; do not put fingers on tops or edges of teeth.
> Brush tongue and inner cheek tissue gently.
> Pat mouth dry and apply lip lubricant.
> Lightly wipe gums and teeth four to six times a day to prevent drying (e.g., swab with mineral oil or saline, but use sparingly to prevent aspiration).

Rationale: Preventive oral hygiene must be provided for those who are unable to perform this self-care activity. Techniques are used to prevent aspiration.

4. Initiate health teaching and referrals, as indicated.

> Identify clients who need toothbrush adaptations to perform own mouth care.
>> For clients with difficulty closing hands tightly (Danielson, 1988), tape a wide elastic band to toothbrush tightly enough so client can hold brush snugly in hand.
>> For clients with limited hand mobility, enlarge toothbrush handle with a sponge hair roller, wrinkled aluminum foil, or a bicycle handlebar grip attached with a small amount of plaster of Paris.
>> For clients with limited arm movement, extend handle of standard toothbrush by attaching handle of an old toothbrush (after cutting off bristle end) to a new toothbrush with strong cord or plastic cement, or by attaching toothbrush to a plastic rod (the toothbrush can be curved by gently heating and then bending it).
> Refer clients with tooth and gum disorders to a dentist.

Rationale: Clients with specific problems need adaptations and referral to specialist.

Geriatric interventions

> Explain high-risk age-related factors (Miller, 2004).
>> Degenerative bone disease
>> Diminished oral blood supply
>> Dry mouth
>> Vitamin deficiencies

Rationale: Age-related changes and nutritional deficiencies increase vulnerability to oral ulcerations and infections (Miller, 2004).

> Explain that some medications cause dry mouth.
>> Laxatives
>> Antibiotics
>> Antidepressants

➤ Anticholinergics
➤ Analgesics
➤ Iron sulfate
➤ Cardiovascular medications

Rationale: Agents that dry the mouth increase irritation and inflammation.

➤ Determine any barriers to dental care.
  ➤ Financial
  ➤ Mobility
  ➤ Dexterity
  ➤ Lack of knowledge

Rationale: Depending on the specific barrier, selected referrals are indicated.

➤ Factors that contribute to oral disease are excessive use of alcohol and tobacco, microorganisms, inadequate nutrition (quantity, quality), inadequate hygiene, and trauma (NO tubes, ill-fitting dentures).
➤ Teach person and family the factors that contribute to stomatitis and its progression.
➤ Teach diet modifications to reduce oral pain and to maintain optimal nutrition.
➤ Have client describe or demonstrate home care regimen.
➤ Factors that contribute to stomatitis are poor oral hygiene, preexisting oral disease, irritants (spicy foods, citrus fruits, coarse foods [hard bread, pizza], ill-fitting dental prostheses, too-cold or too-hot foods, tobacco or alcohol), dehydration, malnutrition, and drug therapy [antibiotics, steroids]; Beck, 2001).
➤ Proper hydration must be maintained to liquefy secretions and prevent drying of oral mucosa.

▼ Risk for Ineffective Respiratory Function

Definition

Risk for Ineffective Respiratory Function: State in which a person is at risk of experiencing a threat to the passage of air through the respiratory tract and/or to the exchange of gases (O_2—CO_2) between the lungs and the vascular system

Risk Factors

Presence of risk factors that can change respiratory function (see Related Factors)

Related Factors

PATHOPHYSIOLOGIC

Related to excessive or thick secretions secondary to

Infection
Inflammation
Allergy
Cardiac or pulmonary disease
Smoking

Related to immobility, stasis of secretions, and ineffective cough secondary to

Diseases of the nervous system (e.g., Guillain-Barré syndrome, multiple
    sclerosis, myasthenia gravis)
CNS depression/head trauma
CVA (stroke)
Quadriplegia

TREATMENT-RELATED

Related to immobility secondary to

Sedating effects of medications (specify)
Anesthesia, general or spinal

Related to suppressed cough reflex secondary to (specify)
Related to effects of tracheostomy (altered secretions)

SITUATIONAL (PERSONAL, ENVIRONMENTAL)

Related to immobility secondary to

Surgery or trauma
Fatigue
Pain
Perception/cognitive impairment
Fear
Anxiety

Related to extremely high or low humidity
For infants, related to placement on stomach for sleep
Exposure to cold, laughing, crying, allergens, smoke

Carp's Cue ▶ Nursing's many responsibilities associated with problems of respiratory function include identifying and reducing or eliminating risk (contributing) factors, anticipating
potential complications, monitoring respiratory status, and managing acute
respiratory dysfunction.

The author has added Risk for Ineffective Respiratory Function to describe a state that may affect the entire respiratory system, not just isolated areas, such as airway clearance or gas exchange. Allergy and immobility are examples of factors that affect the entire system; thus, it is incorrect to say Impaired Gas Exchange related to immobility, because immobility also affects airway clearance and breathing patterns. The nurse can use the diagnoses Ineffective Airway Clearance and Ineffective Breathing Patterns when nurses can definitely alleviate the contributing factors influencing respiratory function (e.g., ineffective cough, immobility, stress).

The nurse is cautioned not to use this diagnosis to describe acute respiratory disorders, which are the primary responsibility of medicine and nursing together (i.e., collaborative problems). Such problems can be labeled PC: Acute Hypoxia or PC: Pulmonary Edema. Consult with your instructor regarding the use of this diagnosis.

Key Concepts

GENERIC CONSIDERATIONS

➤ Ventilation requires synchronous movement of the walls of the chest and abdomen. With inspiration, the diaphragm moves downward, the intercostal muscles contract, the chest wall lifts up and out, the pressure inside the thorax lowers, and air is drawn in. Expiration occurs as air is forced out of the lungs by the elastic recoil of the lungs and the relaxation of the chest and diaphragm. Expiration is diminished in older adults and those with chronic pulmonary disease, increasing the likelihood of CO_2 retention.

➤ Pulmonary function depends on
  ➤ Adequate perfusion (passage of blood through pulmonary vessels)
  ➤ Satisfactory diffusion (movement of oxygen and carbon dioxide across alveolar capillary membrane)
  ➤ Successful ventilation (exchange of air between alveolar spaces and the atmosphere)

➤ Oxygenation depends on the ability of the lungs to deliver oxygen to the blood and on the ability of the heart to pump enough blood to deliver the oxygen to the microcirculation of the cells.

➤ With pulmonary dysfunction, pulmonary function tests are essential to determine the nature and extent of dysfunction caused by obstruction, restriction, or both. Airway resistance causes obstructive defects. A limitation in chest wall expansion causes restrictive defects. Mixed defects are a combination of obstructive and restrictive problems.

➤ Although arterial blood gases and oxygen saturation studies are very helpful in diagnosing problems with oxygenation, vital signs and mental function are key guides to determining the seriousness of the problem (some clients can tolerate oxygen problems better than others can).

➤ The effects of insufficient oxygenation (hypoxia or hypoxemia) on vital signs are as follows:

Vital Sign	Early Hypoxia/ Hypoxemia	Late Hypoxia/ Hypoxemia
Blood pressure	Rising systolic/ falling diastolic	Falling
Pulse	Rising, bounding, dysrhythmic	Falling, shallow, dysrhythmic
Pulse pressure	Widening	Widened/narrowed
Respirations	Rapid	Slowed/rapid

➤ The effects of insufficient oxygenation on mental function are as follows:

Early Hypoxia/Hypoxemia	Late Hypoxia/Hypoxemia
Irritability	Seizures
Headache	Coma or brain tissue swelling
Confusion	
Agitation	

➤ A cough ("the guardian of the lungs") is accomplished by closure of the glottis and the explosive expulsion of air from the lungs by the work of the abdominal and chest muscles. Although most coughing serves a beneficial purpose, the following may be signs of a medical problem requiring medical intervention:
  ➤ Coughs lasting longer than 2 weeks or associated with high fever
  ➤ Coughs consistently triggered by something (may actually be allergic bronchial asthma)
  ➤ Barking cough, especially in a child

➤ The terms tachypnea, hyperpnea, hyperventilation, bradypnea, and hypoventilation are frequently confused.
  ➤ Tachypnea: rapid shallow respiratory rate
  ➤ Hyperpnea: rapid respiratory rate with increased depth
  ➤ Hyperventilation: increased rate or depth of respiration causing an alveolar ventilation that is above the body's normal metabolic requirements
  ➤ Bradypnea: slow respiratory rate
  ➤ Hypoventilation: decreased rate or depth of respiration, causing a minute alveolar ventilation that is less than the body's requirements

➤ Hypoxia and hypoxemia contribute to increased intracranial pressure, brain swelling, brain damage, and shock. Oxygen demand is greater during febrile illness, exercise, pain, and physical and emotional stress.

➤ Suctioning or instillation of saline should not be used routinely; rather, their use should be based on assessment of individual needs.

➤ Use the following as clinical indicators for need for endotracheal suctioning:

≻ Secretions in the endotracheal tube

≻ Frequent or sustained coughing

≻ Adventitious breath sounds on auscultation (rhonchi, or upper airway gurgles)

≻ Increased peak airway pressure

≻ Decreasing pulse oximetry readings (Sv O_2, PaO_2)

≻ Sudden onset of respiratory distress whenever airway patency is questioned

➤ Instill normal saline based on the client's response to suctioning (secretions sticking to tube or catheter, mucous plugging the airway, suction catheter not eliciting an acceptable cough). Instillation of saline benefits clients only when it causes vigorous cough.

➤ Keep in mind that although endotracheal suctioning is associated with several significant complications, insufficiently frequent or inadequate suction also carries substantial risks. Maintain a delicate balance to minimize all complications.

➤ Nicotine is one of the most toxic and addicting of all poisonous substances. Education, preventive health practices, interventions to enhance tobacco cessation, nicotine dependence treatment, and relapse prevention should be standard nursing practice. Nurses must be persistent in helping their clients to stop smoking by encouraging efforts to quit as often as indicated (in many cases, at each client encounter). Refer to Ineffective Health Maintenance related to Insufficient Knowledge of Effects of Tobacco Use.

GERIATRIC CONSIDERATIONS

➤ Age-related changes in the respiratory system have little effect on function in healthy adults unless they interact with risk factors such as smoking, immobility, or compromised immune system. (Miller, 2004).

➤ Adults 65 years of age and older have a yearly death rate from pneumonia or influenza of 9 per 100,000. When smoking, exposure to air pollutants, or occupational exposure to toxic substances is present, the rate increases to 217 per 100,000. If two or more risk factors are present, the rate rises to 979 per 100,000 (Miller, 2004).

FOCUS ASSESSMENT CRITERIA

Assess for defining characteristics.

Objective Data

Mental status
Respiratory status

➤ Airway
  ➤ Spontaneous nasal
  ➤ Nasal endotracheal tube
  ➤ Spontaneous mouth
  ➤ Oral endotracheal tube
  ➤ Oral airway
  ➤ Tracheostomy
  ➤ Nasal airway
➤ Description
  ➤ Spontaneous, labored, or nonlabored
  ➤ Controlled mechanical ventilation (CMV)
  ➤ Spontaneous intermittent mechanical ventilations (SIMV)
  ➤ Rate (per minute)
  ➤ Rhythm
  ➤ Depth
    ➤ Symmetric
  ➤ Type
    ➤ Splinted/guarded
    ➤ Kussmaul
    ➤ Use of accessory muscle
    ➤ Cheyne-Stokes
➤ Cough
  ➤ Effective (brings forth sputum and clears lungs)
  ➤ Ineffective (does not bring forth mucus or clear lungs)
  ➤ Triggered by what? Relieved by what?
  ➤ Needs assistance with coughing
➤ Sputum
  ➤ Color
  ➤ Character
  ➤ Amount
  ➤ Odor
  ➤ Breath sounds (detected by auscultation: compare right upper and lower lobes to left upper and lower lobes; listen to all four quadrants of the chest)

Circulatory status

➤ Pulse
➤ Blood pressure
➤ Skin color

Assess for related factors

Subjective/Objective

Smoking ("pack-years": number of packs per day times number of
   smoking years)
Smoking within the 8 weeks before anesthesia or surgery
Allergy (medication, food, environmental factors—dust, pollen, other)
Trauma, blunt or overt (chest, abdomen, upper airway, head)
Surgery/pain

➤ Incision of chest/neck/head/abdomen
➤ Recent intubation

Asthma/COPD/sinus problems
Environmental factors

➤ Toxic fumes (cleaning agents, smoke)
➤ Extreme heat or cold
➤ Daily inspired air, work and home (humid, dry, level of pollution,
   level of pollens)

Infection/inflammation
For infant, history of

➤ Placement on stomach to sleep
➤ Prematurity
➤ Low birth weight
➤ Cesarean birth
➤ Complicated delivery
➤ Breast-feeding or formula

GOAL

The person will have a respiratory rate within normal limits.

Indicators

Express willingness to be actively involved in managing respiratory
   symptoms and maximizing respiratory function.
Relate appropriate interventions to maximize respiratory status (varies
   depending on health status).
Have satisfactory pulmonary function, as measured by pulmonary function tests.

GENERAL INTERVENTIONS

1. Determine risk factors.

   ➤ Pain, lethargy
   ➤ Medical order of bed rest
   ➤ Neuromuscular impairment
   ➤ Lack of motivation (to ambulate, to cough and deep breathe)
   ➤ Decreased level of consciousness
   ➤ Lack of knowledge
   ➤ Medications (narcotics, muscle relaxants, other CNS depressants)
   ➤ Inadequate humidity

Rationale: Respiratory effort is reduced due to fatigue, pain, and immobility. These effects, particularly in combination with one or more of the listed risk factors, increase a client's risk of postoperative respiratory problems.

2. Reinforce about the importance of turning, coughing, and deep breathing and leg exercises every 1 to 4 hours.

Rationale: Exercises and movement promote lung expansion and mobilization of secretions. Incentive spirometry promotes deep breathing by providing a visual indicator of the effectiveness of the breathing effort. Coughing assists to dislodge mucous plugs. Coughing is contraindicated in people who have had a head injury, intracranial surgery, eye surgery, or plastic surgery because it increases intracranial and intraocular pressure and tension on delicate tissues (plastic surgery).

3. Eliminate or reduce risk factors, if possible.

   ➤ Assess for optimal pain relief with minimal periods of fatigue or respiratory depression. Coordinate medication regimen with planned activities (e.g., give PRN pain medication with least-sedating side effects 1 hour before physical therapy).
   ➤ Ensure adequate air humidity, providing additional humidification unless contraindicated by heart disease.
   ➤ For nasal stuffiness, use saline nose drops; avoid other nose drops because of rebound effect. Encourage ambulation as soon as consistent with medical plan of care.
   ➤ If client cannot walk, establish a regimen for being out of bed in a chair several times a day (e.g., 1 hour after meals and 1 hour before bedtime).
   ➤ Increase activity gradually. Explain that respiratory function will improve and dyspnea will decrease with practice.
   ➤ For neuromuscular impairment:
       ➤ Vary the position of the bed, thereby gradually changing the horizontal and vertical position of the thorax, unless contraindicated.

➤ Assist client to reposition, turning frequently from side to side (hourly if possible). Encourage deep-breathing and controlled-coughing exercises five times every hour. Teach client to use blow bottle or incentive spirometer every hour while awake (with severe neuromuscular impairment, the person may have to be awakened during the night as well).

➤ For those with quadriplegia, teach person and caregivers the "quad cough" (caregiver places hand on client's diaphragm and thrusts upward and inward).

➤ For child, use colored water in blow bottle; have him or her blow up balloons.

➤ Ensure optimal hydration status.

➤ For the person with a decreased level of consciousness:

  ➤ Position from side to side with set schedule (e.g., left side even hours, right side odd hours); do not leave person lying flat on back.

  ➤ Position client on right side after feedings (NG tube feeding, gastrostomy) to prevent regurgitation and aspiration.

  ➤ Keep head of bed elevated 30 degrees unless contraindicated.

See also Risk for Aspiration.

4. Prevent the complications of immobility.

➤ See Disuse Syndrome

▼ Ineffective Airway Clearance

Definition

Ineffective Airway Clearance: State in which a person experiences a threat to respiratory status related to inability to cough effectively.

Defining Characteristics

MAJOR (MUST BE PRESENT, ONE OR MORE)

Ineffective or absent cough
Inability to remove airway secretions

MINOR (MAY BE PRESENT)

Abnormal breath sounds
Abnormal respiratory rate, rhythm, depth

Related Factors

See Risk for Ineffective Respiratory Function.

 Carp's Cue ▶ *Ineffective Airway Clearance specifically addresses the inability to cough effectively. This is a major nursing focus. This diagnosis can be used especially if the person is high risk for pneumonia. For other persons, especially postsurgical clients, use Risk for Ineffective Respiratory Function.*

Key Concepts

See Risk for Ineffective Respiratory Function.

FOCUS ASSESSMENT CRITERIA

See Risk for Ineffective Respiratory Function.

GOAL

The person will not experience aspiration.

Indicators

Demonstrate effective coughing and increased air exchange.
Explain rationale for interventions to promote coughing.

GENERAL INTERVENTIONS

1. Teach client to sit as erect as possible; use pillows for support if needed.

Rationale: Slouching and cramping positions of the thorax and abdomen interfere with air exchange.

2. Teach client the proper method of deep breathing, which dilates the airways and stimulates controlled coughing.

➤ Breathe deeply and slowly every 1 to 2 hours while sitting up as high as possible.

➤ Use diaphragmatic breathing: hold breath for 3 to 5 seconds and then slowly exhale as much as possible through the mouth. (The lower rib cage and abdomen should sink down.)

➤ Take a second breath, hold, and cough forcefully from the chest (not from the back of the mouth or throat) using two short forceful coughs. Splint the chest with hands or pillow. Check any tube connections. If indicated, use the "huffing" breathing technique as taught preoperatively. Use spirometer three to four times per hour.

Rationale: Deep breathing dilates the airways, stimulates surfactant production, and expands the lung's tissue surface; this improves respiratory gas exchange. Coughing loosens secretions and forces them into the bronchus to be expectorated or suctioned. In some clients, "huffing" breathing may be effective and is less painful.

3. Assess lung fields before and after coughing exercises.

Rationale: Comparison assessments help to evaluate the effectiveness of coughing.

4. If breath sounds are moist-sounding, instruct client to rest briefly and then repeat the exercises.

Rationale: Rales indicate trapped secretions.

5. Assess the current analgesic regimen.

➤ Administer pain medication as needed.
  ➤ Assess its effectiveness: Is the client still in pain?
  ➤ If not, is he or she too lethargic?
  ➤ Note times when client seems to obtain the best pain relief with an optimal level of alertness and physical ability. This is the time to initiate breathing and coughing exercises.

Rationale: Pain or fear of pain can inhibit participation in coughing and breathing exercises. Adequate pain relief is essential.

6. Provide emotional support.

➤ Stay with client for the entire coughing session.
➤ Explain the importance of coughing after pain relief is obtained.
➤ Reassure client that the suture lines are secure and that splinting by hand or pillow will minimize pain on movement.

Rationale: Coughing exercises are fatiguing and painful. Emotional support provides encouragement; warm water can aid relaxation.

7. Maintain adequate hydration and humidity of inspired air.

Rationale: These measures help to decrease viscosity of secretions. Tenacious secretions are difficult to mobilize and expectorate.

8. Move client out of bed to chair postoperative. Early ambulation promotes aeration and day 1 and begin ambulation as can help to minimize pulmonary.

Rationale: Early ambulation promotes aeration and can help to minimize pulmonary complications.

9. Provide motivation and plan strategies to avoid overexertion.

➤ Plan and bargain for adequate rest periods (e.g., "Work hard now, then I'll let you rest.").

➤ Vigorously coach and encourage coughing; use positive reinforcement.

➤ Plan coughing sessions for periods when client is alert and obtaining optimal pain relief.

➤ Allow for rest after coughing sessions and before meals.

Rationale: The client's cooperation enhances the exercises' effectiveness.

10. Evaluate the need for tracheobronchial suctioning.

Rationale: Suctioning will be needed if client is unable to cough effectively

▼ Ineffective Breathing Patterns

Definition

Ineffective Breathing Patterns: State in which a person experiences an actual or potential loss of adequate ventilation related to an altered breathing pattern.

Defining Characteristics

MAJOR (MUST BE PRESENT, ONE OR MORE)

Changes in respiratory rate or pattern (from baseline)
Changes in pulse (rate, rhythm, quality)

MINOR (MAY BE PRESENT)

Orthopnea
Dysrhythmic respirations
Tachypnea, hyperpnea, hyperventilation
Splinted/guarded respirations

Related Factors

See Risk for Ineffective Respiratory Function.

 Carp's Cue ▶ *Ineffective Breathing Patterns as a nursing diagnosis addresses hyperventilation or rapid breathing. Shallow breathing should be addressed as a collaborative problem. PC: Respiratory Insufficiency or Hypoxia is a medical emergency.*

Key Concepts

GENERIC CONSIDERATIONS

➤ Hyperventilation is overbreathing with reduced Pco_2 and respiratory alkalosis.

➤ Causes of hyperventilation syndrome are organic (drug effects, CNS lesions), physiologic (response to high altitude, heat, exercise), emotional (anxiety, hysteria, anger, depression), and habitual faulty breathing habits (rapid shallow breathing; Porth, 2002).

➤ Symptoms of hyperventilation syndrome are headache, dyspnea, numbness and tingling, lightheadedness, chest pain, palpitations, and, occasionally, syncope (Porth, 2002).

➤ Panic can manifest with hyperventilation, and people with panic disorders can hyperventilate.

➤ All nurses involved in caring for clients with COPD must be skilled at teaching pursed-lip breathing, a critical survival skill that these clients must learn to maintain function (Truesdell, 2000). Studies show that pursed-lip breathing decreases respiratory rate, increases tidal volume, decreases arterial CO_2, increases arterial oxygen, and improves exercise performance (Truesdell, 2000).

➤ Teach the client to inhale through the nose, not too deeply. Breathe out through the mouth while holding the lips (except for a section in the center) together. Exhalation should be at least twice as long as inhalation and should be a steady stream of air without blowing too hard (Truesdell, 2000).

GOAL

Indicators

Have respiratory rate within normal limits, compared with baseline (8 to 24/mm).

Express relief of (or improvement in) feelings of shortness of breath.

Relate causative factors and ways of preventing or managing them.

GENERAL INTERVENTIONS

1. Assess history of symptoms and causative factors.

➤ Previous episodes—when, where, circumstances
➤ Causes
   ➤ Organic, physiologic
   ➤ Emotional
   ➤ Faulty breathing habits
   ➤ Explain the cause
   ➤ Stay with person

Rationale: These measures attempt to reduce fear.

2. If fear or panic has precipitated the episode:

➤ Remove cause of fear, if possible.
➤ Reassure client that measures are being taken to ensure safety.
➤ Distract person from thinking about the anxious state by having him or her maintain eye contact with you (or perhaps with someone else he or she trusts); say, "Now look at me and breathe slowly with me like this."

Rationale: Calming a person with shortness of breath by telling him or her that actions are being taken to improve the situation (e.g., "I'm here, and I will get you through this") is an essential intervention to reduce panic and decrease symptoms.

3. Consider use of paper bag as means of rebreathing expired air.

Rationale: Rebreathing expired CO_2 will slow respiratory rate.

4. Reassure person he or she can control breathing; tell him or her that you will help.

Rationale: Interventions focus on slowing breathing pattern and educating the person to control response.

▼ Impaired Gas Exchange

Definition

Impaired Gas Exchange: State in which a person experiences an actual or potential decreased passage of gases (oxygen and carbon dioxide) between the alveoli of the lungs and the vascular system

Defining Characteristics

MAJOR (MUST BE PRESENT)

Dyspnea on exertion

MINOR (MAY BE PRESENT)

Tendency to assume three-point position (sitting, one hand on each knee, bending forward)
Pursed-lip breathing with prolonged expiratory phase
Confusion/agitation
Lethargy and fatigue
Increased pulmonary vascular resistance (increased pulmonary artery/right ventricular pressure)
Decreased gastric motility, prolonged gastric emptying
Decreased oxygen content, decreased oxygen saturation, increased P_{CO_2}, as measured by blood gas analysis
Cyanosis

Respiratory problems that nurses treat as nursing diagnoses are Ineffective Airway Clearance, Ineffective Breathing Pattern, Risk for Ineffective Respiratory Function, Dysfunctional Ventilatory Weaning Response, and Activity Intolerance. If these nursing diagnoses are treated, then it follows that gas exchange should improve. If gas exchange does not improve, then the problem is a collaborative problem and should be labeled as such (e.g., PC: Hypoxemia or PC: Respiratory Insufficiency). In this case, the nursing role is monitoring to detect changes in status. If respiratory status worsens, the nurse manages the situation using nurse- and physician-prescribed interventions.

Some nurses are tempted to use Impaired Gas Exchange to describe the problem of COPD. Labeling COPD as Impaired Gas Exchange does not help in determining nursing interventions. What does the nurse do for Impaired Gas Exchange? The nurse helps the person by treating the Ineffective Airway Clearance, Ineffective Breathing Patterns, and Activity Intolerance and by preventing Ineffective Respiratory Function. The nurse also would assess for functional health patterns that decreased oxygenation has or may have affected, such as sleep, emotional status, and nutrition.

▼ Impaired Spontaneous Ventilation

Definition

Impaired Spontaneous Ventilation: State in which a person is unable to maintain adequate breathing to support life. This is measured by deterioration of arterial blood gases, increased work of breathing, and decreasing energy.

Defining Characteristics

MAJOR (MUST BE PRESENT, ONE OR MORE)

Dyspnea
Increased metabolic rate

MINOR

Increased restlessness
Decreased Po_2
Apprehension
Increased use of accessory muscles
Increased Pco_2
Increased heart rate
Decreased tidal volume
Decreased Sao_2
Decreased cooperation

 Carp's Cue ▶ *This diagnosis represents respiratory insufficiency with corresponding metabolic changes that are incompatible with life. This situation requires emergency nursing and medical management, specifically resuscitation and mechanical ventilation. Inability to sustain spontaneous ventilation is not appropriate as a nursing diagnosis—it is hypoxemia, a collaborative problem. The nursing accountability is to monitor status continuously and to manage changes in status with the appropriate interventions, using protocols.*

This diagnosis even as a collaborative problem is not appropriate for a care plan because it is a medical emergency. The agency's protocol for respiratory arrest should be followed.

▽ Self-Care Deficit Syndrome

▽ Feeding Self-Care Deficit

▽ Bathing/Hygiene Self-Care Deficit

▽ Dressing/Grooming Self-Care Deficit

▽ Toileting Self-Care Deficit

▽ Instrumental Self-Care Deficit

Definition

Self-Care Deficit Syndrome: State in which a person experiences an impaired motor function or cognitive function, causing a decreased ability in performing each of the five self-care activities.

Defining Characteristics

MAJOR (ONE DEFICIT MUST BE PRESENT IN EACH ACTIVITY)

Self-feeding deficits

➤ Unable to cut food or open packages
➤ Unable to bring food to mouth

Self-bathing deficits (include washing entire body, combing hair, brushing teeth, attending to skin and nail care, and applying makeup)

➤ Unable or unwilling to wash body or body parts
➤ Unable to obtain a water source
➤ Unable to regulate temperature or water flow
➤ Unable to perceive need for hygienic measures

Self-dressing deficits (including donning regular or special clothing, not nightclothes)

➤ Impaired ability to put on or take off clothing
➤ Unable to fasten clothing
➤ Unable to groom self satisfactorily
➤ Unable to obtain or replace articles of clothing

Self-toileting deficits

➤ Unable or unwilling to get to toilet or commode
➤ Unable or unwilling to carry out proper hygiene
➤ Unable to transfer to and from toilet or commode
➤ Unable to handle clothing to accommodate toileting
➤ Unable to flush toilet or empty commode

Instrumental self-care deficits

➤ Difficulty using telephone
➤ Difficulty laundering, ironing
➤ Difficulty preparing meals
➤ Difficulty shopping
➤ Difficulty accessing transportation
➤ Difficulty managing money
➤ Difficulty with medication administration

Related Factors

PATHOPHYSIOLOGIC

Related to lack of coordination secondary to (specify)
Related to spasticity or flaccidity secondary to (specify)
Related to muscular weakness secondary to (specify)
Related to partial or total paralysis secondary to (specify)
Related to atrophy secondary to (specify)
Related to muscle contractures secondary to (specify)
Related to comatose state
Related to visual disorders secondary to (specify)
Related to nonfunctioning or missing limb(s)
Related to regression to an earlier level of development
Related to excessive ritualistic behaviors
Related to somatoform deficits (specify)

TREATMENT-RELATED

Related to external devices (specify: casts, splints, braces, intravenous [IV] equipment)
Related to postoperative fatigue and pain

SITUATIONAL (PERSONAL, ENVIRONMENTAL)

Related to cognitive deficits
Related to decreased motivation
Related to fatigue

Related to confusion
Related to pain
Related to disabling anxiety

MATURATIONAL

Older Adult

Related to decreased visual and motor ability, muscle weakness

 Self-care encompasses the activities needed to meet daily needs, commonly known as activities of daily living (ADLs), which are learned over time and become lifelong habits. Self-care activities involve not only what is to be done (hygiene, bathing, dressing, toileting, feeding), but also how much, when, where, with whom, and how (Miller, 2004).

In every person, the threat or reality of an impaired ability to provide self-care evokes panic. Many people report that they fear loss of independence more than death. A self-care deficit affects the core of self-concept and self-determination. For this reason, the nursing focus for self-care deficit should be not on providing the care measure, but on identifying adaptive techniques to allow the person the maximum degree of participation and independence possible.

Currently not on the NANDA list, the diagnosis Self-Care Deficit Syndrome has been added here to describe a person with compromised ability in all five self-care activities. For this person, the nurse assesses functioning in each area and identifies the level of participation of which the person is capable. The goal is to maintain current functioning, to increase participation and independence, or both. The syndrome distinction clusters all five self-care deficits together to enable grouping of interventions when indicated, while also permitting specialized interventions for a specific deficit. The danger of applying a Self-Care Deficit Syndrome diagnosis lies in the possibility of prematurely labeling a person as unable to participate at any level, eliminating a rehabilitation focus. It is important that the nurse classify each person's functional level to promote independence. (Refer to the functional level classification scale in Focus Assessment Criteria). Continuous reevaluation also is necessary to identify changes in the person's ability to participate in self-care.

Key Concepts

GENERIC CONSIDERATIONS

➤ The concept of self-care emphasizes each person's right to maintain individual control over his or her own pattern of living (this applies to both the ill person and the well person).

➤ It is acceptable to be dependent on others to provide basic physiologic and psychological needs for a limited time for those who can progress to more independence.

➤ The following key elements promote relearning of self-care tasks:
  ➤ Providing a structured, consistent environment and routine.
  ➤ Repeating instructions and tasks.
  ➤ Teaching and practicing tasks during periods of least fatigue.
  ➤ Maintaining a familiar environment and teacher
  ➤ Using patience, determination, and a positive attitude (by both learner and teacher)
  ➤ Practice, practice, practice.

Endurance

➤ The endurance or ability of the person to maintain a given level of performance is influenced by the ability to use oxygen to produce energy (related to the optimal functioning of the heart and respiratory systems). Thus, clients with alterations in these systems have increased energy demands or decreased ability to produce energy.

➤ Stress is energy-consuming; the more stressors a person has, the more fatigue he or she experiences. Stressors can be personal, environmental, disease-related, and treatment-related. Examples of possible stressors follows:

Personal	Environmental	Disease-related	Treatment-related
Age	Isolation	Pain	Walker
Support system	Noise	Anemia	Medications
Lifestyle	Unfamiliar setting		Diagnostic studies

➤ Signs and symptoms of decreased oxygen in response to activity (e.g., self-care, mobility) are as follows:
  ➤ Sustained increased heart rate 3 to 5 minutes after ceasing the activity or a change in the pulse rhythm
  ➤ Failure of systolic blood pressure reading to increase with activity or a decrease in value
  ➤ Decrease or excessive increase in respiratory rate and dyspnea
  ➤ Weakness, pallor, cerebral hypoxia (confusion, incoordination)

Refer to Key Concepts under Activity Intolerance for additional information.

GERIATRIC CONSIDERATIONS

➤ Age-related changes do not in themselves cause self-care deficits. Older adults do, however, have an increased incidence of chronic diseases that can compromise functional ability (e.g., arthritis, cardiac disorders, visual impairment).

➤ Older adults with dementia have varying degrees of difficulty with self-care activities depending on memory deficits, ability to follow directions, and judgment (Miller, 2004).

➤ Sixty-three percent of older nursing home residents cannot perform basic ADLs because of cognitive impairment (Miller, 2004).

➤ Caregivers frequently promote excess disability and quicker deterioration in older adults because they believe independent behavior is atypical (Miller, 2004)

FOCUS ASSESSMENT CRITERIA

Evaluate each ADL using the following scale:

0 = Is completely independent
1 = Requires use of assistive device
2 = Needs minimal help
3 = Needs assistance and/or some supervision
4 = Needs total supervision
5 = Needs total assistance or unable to assist

Assess for defining characteristics

Subjective, Objective

➤ Self-feeding abilities
  ➤ Swallowing
  ➤ Selecting foods
  ➤ Using utensils and cutting food
  ➤ Seeing
  ➤ Drinking from cup
  ➤ Chewing
  ➤ Opening
➤ Self-bathing abilities
  ➤ Undressing to bathe
  ➤ Reaching water source
  ➤ Differentiating water temperatures
  ➤ Washing body parts
  ➤ Performing oral care
  ➤ Obtaining equipment (water, soap, towels)
➤ Self-dressing/grooming abilities
  ➤ Putting on or taking off clothing
  ➤ Selecting appropriate clothing
  ➤ Retrieving appropriate clothing
  ➤ Fastening clothing
  ➤ Cleaning/trimming nails
  ➤ Washing and styling hair
  ➤ Shaving

- Brushing teeth
- Plugging in cord
- Using deodorant
- Self-toileting abilities
  - Getting to toilet and undressing
  - Performing hygiene (washing hands)
  - Can use tampon/sanitary napkin
  - Redressing
  - Rising from toilet
  - Sitting on toilet
  - Cleaning self/flushing toilet

Instrumental ADLs

- Telephone
  - Ability to dial
  - Ability to talk, hear
  - Ability to answer
- Transportation
  - Ability to drive
  - Access to transportation
- Laundry
  - Availability of washer
  - Ability to wash, iron
  - Ability to put away
- Food procurement and preparation
  - Ability to cook
  - Ability to select foods
  - Ability to shop
- Medications
  - Ability to remember
  - Ability to administer
- Finances
  - Ability to write checks, pay bills
  - Ability to handle cash transactions (simple, complex)

Assess for real factors

Subjective, Objective

- Ability to remember
- Judgment
- Ability to follow directions
- Ability to identify/express needs
- Ability to anticipate needs (food, laundry)
- Social supports
  - Support people
  - Availability of help with transportation, shopping, money management, laundry

➤ Housekeeping, food preparation
➤ Community resources
➤ Motivation
➤ Endurance

GOAL

The person will participate physically and/or verbally in feeding, dressing, toileting, and bathing activities.

Indicators

Identify preferences in self-care activities (e.g., time, products, location). Demonstrate optimal hygiene after assistance with care.

GENERAL INTERVENTIONS

1. Assess for causative or contributing factors.

➤ Visual deficits
➤ Impaired cognition
➤ Decreased motivation
➤ Impaired mobility
➤ Lack of knowledge
➤ Inadequate social support
➤ Excessive ritualistic behavior
➤ Disabling anxiety
➤ Irrational fears
➤ Developmental regression

Rationale: Specific factors have different interventions.

2. Promote optimal participation.

➤ Assess present level of participation
➤ Determine areas for potentially increased participation in each self-care activity.
➤ Explore the person's goals.
➤ Allow ample time to complete activities without help. Promote independence, but assist when person cannot perform an activity.
➤ Demonstrate how to perform an activity that is problematic.

Rationale: Offering choices and including the client in planning care reduces feelings of powerlessness; promotes feelings of freedom, control, and self-worth and increases the person's willingness to comply with therapeutic regimens.

3. Promote self-esteem and self-determination.

➤ Determine preferences for
  ➤ Schedule
  ➤ Products
  ➤ Methods
  ➤ Clothing selection
  ➤ Hair styling
➤ During self-care activities, provide choices and request preferences.
➤ Do not focus on disability.
➤ Offer praise for independent accomplishments.
➤ Do not allow client to use a disability as a manipulative tool; withdraw attention if person continues to focus on limitations.

Rationale: Enhancing a client's self-care abilities can increase his or her sense of control and independence, promoting overall well-being.

4. Evaluate client's ability to participate in each self-care activity (feeding, dressing, bathing, toileting)

➤ Assign a number value to each activity (refer to the coding scale in focus assessment criteria).
➤ Reassess ability frequently and revise code as appropriate.

Rationale: Optimal education promotes self-care. To teach effectively, the nurse must determine what the learner perceives as his or her own needs and goals, determine what the nurse believes are the learner's needs and goals, and then work to establish mutually acceptable goals.

5. Refer to interventions under each diagnosis—feeding, bathing, dressing, toileting, and instrumental self-care deficit as indicated.

▼ Feeding Self-Care Deficit

Definition

Feeding Self-Care Deficit: State in which a person experiences an impaired ability to perform or complete feeding activities for himself or herself.

Defining Characteristics

Unable to cut food or open food packages
Unable to bring food to mouth

Related Factors

See Self-Care Syndrome

Carp's Cue ▶ *See Self-Care Syndrome*

Key Concepts

See Self-Care Syndrome

FOCUS ASSESSMENT CRITERIA

See Self-Care Syndrome

GOAL

The person will demonstrate increased ability to feed self or report that he or she cannot feed self.

Indicators

Demonstrate ability to make use of adaptive devices, if indicated.
Demonstrate increased interest and desire to eat.
Describe rationale and procedure for treatment.
Describe causative factors for feeding deficit.

GENERAL INTERVENTIONS

1. Assess causative factors.

➤ Visual deficits (blindness, field cuts, poor depth perception)
➤ Affected or missing limbs (casts, amputations, paresis, paralysis)
➤ Cognitive deficits (dementia, trauma, CVA).

Rationale: Interventions are indicated depending on the causative factor.

2. Provide opportunities to relearn or adapt to activity.

➤ Common nursing interventions
  ➤ Ascertain from person or family members what foods the person likes or dislikes.

➤ Ensure client eats meals in the same setting with pleasant surroundings that are not too distracting.

➤ Maintain correct food temperatures (hot foods hot, cold foods cold).

➤ Provide pain relief, because pain can affect appetite and ability to feed self.

➤ Provide good oral hygiene before and after meals.

➤ Encourage person to wear dentures and eyeglasses.

➤ Assist client to the most normal eating position suited to his or her physical disability (best if sitting in a chair at a table).

➤ Provide social contact during eating.

See Imbalanced Nutrition: Less Than Body Requirements.

➤ Specific interventions for people with sensory/perceptual deficits

➤ Encourage client to wear prescribed corrective lenses.

➤ Describe location of utensils and food on tray or table.

➤ Describe food items to stimulate appetite.

➤ For perceptual deficits, choose different colored dishes to help distinguish items (e.g., red tray, white plates).

➤ Ascertain usual eating patterns and provide food items according to preference (or arrange food items in clock-like pattern); record on care plan the arrangement used (e.g., meat, 6 o'clock; potatoes, 9 o'clock; vegetables, 12 o'clock).

➤ Encourage eating of "finger foods" (e.g., bread, bacon, fruit, hot dogs) to promote independence. Avoid placing food to blind side of person with field cut, until visually accommodated to surroundings; then encourage him or her to scan entire visual field.

➤ Specific interventions for people with missing limbs

➤ Provide for eating environment that is not embarrassing to client; allow sufficient time for eating.

➤ Provide only the supervision and assistance necessary for relearning or adaptation.

➤ To enhance independence, provide necessary adaptive devices:

➤ Plate guard to avoid pushing food off plate

➤ Suction device under plate or bowl for stabilization

➤ Padded handles on utensils for a more secure grip

➤ Wrist or hand splints with clamp to hold eating utensils

➤ Special drinking cup

➤ Rocker knife for cutting

➤ Assist with set-up if needed: opening containers, napkins, condiment packages; cutting meat; and buttering bread.

➤ Arrange food so person has enough space to perform the task of eating.

➤ Specific interventions for people with cognitive deficits

➤ Provide isolated quiet atmosphere until person can attend to eating and is not easily distracted from the task.

➢ Supervise feeding program until there is no danger of choking or aspiration.

➢ Orient person to location and purpose of feeding equipment.

➢ Avoid external distractions and unnecessary conversation.

➢ Place person in the most normal eating position he or she can physically assume.

➢ Encourage person to attend to the task but be alert for fatigue, frustration, or agitation.

➢ Provide one food at a time in usual sequence of eating until person can eat the entire meal in normal sequence.

➢ Encourage person to be tidy, to eat in small amounts, and to put food in unaffected side of mouth if paresis or paralysis is present.

➢ Check for food in cheeks.

Refer to Impaired Swallowing for additional interventions.

➤ For a person who is not eating because of fears of being poisoned
  ➢ Allow person to open cans of foods.
  ➢ Serve food family-style, so he or she can witness others eating.

Rationale: Eating has physiologic, psychological, social, and cultural implications. Providing control over meals promotes overall well-being.

3. Initiate health teaching and referrals, as indicated.

➤ Ensure that both person and family understand the reason and purpose of all interventions. Proceed with teaching as needed.

➤ Maintain safe eating methods.

➤ Prevent aspiration.

➤ Use appropriate eating utensils (avoid sharp instruments).

➤ Test temperature of hot liquids and wear protective clothing (e.g., paper bib).

➤ Teach use of adaptive devices.

Rationale: Assistance will be needed at home to maintain or improve self-care ability and prevent injuries.

▽ Bathing/Hygiene Self-Care Deficit

Definition

Bathing/Hygiene Self-Care Deficit: State in which a person experiences an impaired ability to complete bathing/hygiene activities for himself or herself.

Defining Characteristics

Self-bathing deficits (including washing entire body, combing hair, brushing teeth, attending to nail care, and applying makeup)

➤ Unable or unwilling to wash body or body parts
➤ Unable to obtain a water source
➤ Unable to regulate temperature or water flow
➤ Inability to perceive need for hygienic measures

Related Factors

See Self-Care Deficit Syndrome.

 Carp's Cue ➤ *See Self-Care Deficit Syndrome.*

Key Concepts

See Self-Care Deficit Syndrome.

FOCUS ASSESSMENT CRITERIA

See Self-Care Deficit Syndrome.

GOAL

The person will perform bathing activity at expected optimal level or report satisfaction with accomplishments despite limitations.

Indicators

Relate feeling of comfort and satisfaction with body cleanliness.
Demonstrate ability to use adaptive devices.
Describe causative factors of bathing deficit.

GENERAL INTERVENTIONS

1. Assess causative factors.

➤ Visual deficits (blindness, field cuts, poor depth perception)
➤ Affected or missing limbs (casts, amputations, paresis, paralysis, arthritis)
➤ Cognitive deficits (aging, trauma, CVA)

Rationale: Interventions are selected depending on causative factors.

2. Provide opportunities to relearn or adapt to activity.

➤ General nursing interventions for inability to bathe
  ➤ Bathing time and routine should be consistent to encourage optimal independence.
  ➤ Encourage person to wear prescribed corrective lenses or hearing aid.
  ➤ Keep bathroom temperature warm; ascertain client's preferred water temperature.
  ➤ Provide for privacy during bathing routine.
  ➤ Keep environment simple and uncluttered.
  ➤ Observe skin condition during bathing.
  ➤ Provide all bathing equipment within easy reach.
  ➤ Provide for safety in the bathroom (nonslip mats, grab bars).
  ➤ When person is physically able, encourage use of either tub or shower stall, depending on which he or she uses at home (the person should practice in the hospital in preparation for going home).
  ➤ Provide for adaptive equipment as needed.
    ➤ Chair or stool in bathtub or shower
    ➤ Long-handled sponge to reach back or lower extremities
    ➤ Grab-bars on bathroom walls where needed to assist in mobility
    ➤ Bath board for transferring to tub chair or stool
    ➤ Safety treads or nonslip mat on floor of bathroom, tub, and shower
    ➤ Washing mitts with pocket for soap
    ➤ Adapted toothbrushes
    ➤ Shaver holders
    ➤ Hand-held shower spray
  ➤ Provide for relief of pain that may affect ability to bathe self.
➤ Specific interventions for bathing for people with visual deficits
  ➤ Place bathing equipment in location most suitable to individual.
  ➤ Avoid placing bathing equipment to blind side if person has a field cut and is not visually accommodated to surroundings.
  ➤ Keep call bell within reach if person is to bathe alone.
  ➤ Give the person with visual impairment the same degree of privacy and dignity as any other person.
  ➤ Announce yourself before entering or leaving the bathing area.

➤ Observe the person's ability to locate all bathing utensils.

➤ Observe the person's ability to perform mouth care, hair combing, and shaving.

➤ Provide place for clean clothing within easy reach.

➤ Specific interventions for bathing for people with affected or missing limbs

  ➤ Bathe early in morning or before bed at night to avoid unnecessary dressing and undressing.

  ➤ Encourage client to use a mirror during bathing to inspect the skin of paralyzed areas.

  ➤ Encourage the person with amputation to inspect remaining foot or stump for good skin integrity.

  ➤ For limb amputations, bathe stump twice a day and be sure it is dry before wrapping it or applying prosthesis.

  ➤ Provide only the supervision or assistance necessary for relearning the use of extremity or adaptation to the handicap.

  ➤ For lack of sensation, encourage use of the affected area in the bathing process (a person tends to forget the existence of body parts in which there is no sensation).

➤ Specific interventions for bathing for people with cognitive deficits

  ➤ Provide a consistent time for bathing as part of a structured program to help decrease confusion.

  ➤ Keep instructions simple and avoid distractions; orient client to purpose of bathing equipment, put toothpaste on toothbrush.

  ➤ If person cannot bathe the entire body, have him or her bathe one part until he or she does it correctly; give positive reinforcement for success.

  ➤ Supervise activity until person can safely perform the task unassisted.

  ➤ Encourage attention to the task, but be alert for fatigue that may increase confusion.

  ➤ Apply firm pressure to the skin when bathing; it is less likely to be misinterpreted than a gentle touch.

  ➤ Use a warm shower or bath to help a confused or agitated person to relax.

Rationale: Specific interventions with adaptive equipment will improve self-care abilities.

3. Initiate health teaching and referrals, as indicated.

➤ Communicate to staff and family members the person's ability and willingness to learn.

➤ Teach use of adaptive devices.

➤ Ascertain bathing facilities at home and assist in determining if there is any need for adaptations; refer to occupational therapy or social service for help in obtaining needed home equipment. Teach client to use tub or shower stall, depending on what is used at home.

➤ If person is paralyzed, instruct client or family to demonstrate complete skin check on key areas for redness (buttocks, bony prominences).
➤ Teach family to maintain a safe bathing environment.

Rationale: Assistance will be needed at home to maintain or improve self-care abilities and prevent injuries.

▼ Dressing/Grooming Self-Care Deficit

Definition

Dressing/Grooming Self-Care Deficit: State in which a person experiences an impaired ability to perform or complete dressing and grooming activities for himself or herself.

Defining Characteristics

Self-dressing deficits (including donning regular or special clothing, not nightclothes)

➤ Impaired ability to put on or take off clothing
➤ Unable to fasten clothing
➤ Unable to groom self satisfactorily
➤ Unable to obtain or replace articles of clothing

Related Factors

See Self-Care Deficit Syndrome.

 Carp's Cue ▶ *See Self-Care Deficit Syndrome.*

Key Concepts

See Self-Care Deficit Syndrome.

FOCUS ASSESSMENT CRITERIA

See Self-Care Deficit Syndrome.

GOAL

The person will demonstrate increased ability to dress self or report the need to have someone else assist him or her to perform the task.

Indicators

Demonstrate ability to use adaptive devices to facilitate independence in dressing.

Demonstrate increased interest in wearing street clothes.

Describe causative factors for dressing deficits.

Relate rationale and procedures for treatments.

GENERAL INTERVENTIONS

1. Assess causative factors.

➤ Visual deficits (blindness, field cuts, poor depth perception)
➤ Affected or missing limbs (casts, amputations, arthritis, paresis, paralysis)
➤ Cognitive deficits (aging, trauma, CVA)

Rationale: Interventions are selected depending upon causative factor.

2. Provide opportunities to relearn or adapt to activity.

➤ General nursing interventions for self-dressing
   ➣ Encourage person to wear prescribed corrective lenses or hearing aid.
   ➣ Promote independence in dressing through continual and unaided practice.
   ➣ Choose loose-fitting clothing with wide sleeves and pant legs and front fasteners.
   ➣ Allow sufficient time for dressing and undressing, because the task may be tiring, painful, or difficult.
   ➣ Plan for person to learn and demonstrate one part of an activity before progressing further.
   ➣ Lay clothes out in the order in which the client will need them to dress.
   ➣ Provide dressing aids as necessary (some commonly used aids include dressing stick, Swedish reacher, zipper pull, buttonhook, long-handled shoehorn, and shoe fasteners adapted with elastic laces, Velcro closures, or flip-back tongues; all garments with fasteners may be adapted with Velcro closures).

➤ Encourage person to wear ordinary or special clothing rather than nightclothes.

➤ Increase participation in dressing by medicating for pain 30 min before it is time to dress or undress, if indicated.

➤ Provide for privacy during dressing routine.

➤ Provide for safety by ensuring easy access to all clothing and by ascertaining person's performance level.

➤ Specific interventions for dressing for people with visual deficits

➤ Allow person to ascertain the most convenient location for clothing and adapt the environment to accomplish the task best (e.g., remove unnecessary barriers).

➤ Announce yourself before entering or leaving the dressing area.

➤ If person has a field cut, avoid placing clothing to the blind side until he or she is visually accommodated to surroundings; then encourage him or her to turn head to scan entire visual field.

➤ Apply adaptive devices (e.g., hand splints) before dressing activity.

➤ Consult or refer to physical or occupational therapy for teaching application of prosthetics to missing limbs.

➤ Specific interventions for dressing for people with cognitive deficits (Miller, 2004)

➤ Keep verbal communication simple.

➤ Ask yes/no questions.

➤ Use one-step requests (e.g., "put your sock on").

➤ Praise after each step.

➤ Be specific and concise.

➤ Call by name.

➤ Use same word for same thing (e.g., "shirt").

➤ Dress bottom half, then top half.

➤ Prepare an uncluttered environment.

➤ Ensure good lighting.

➤ Make bed; minimize visual clutter.

➤ Lay clothes face down.

➤ Place clothes in order that they will be used.

➤ Allow resident a choice from only two pieces.

➤ Place matching clothes together on hangers.

➤ Remove dirty clothes from dressing area.

➤ Provide nonverbal cues.

➤ Hand one clothing item at a time in correct order.

➤ Place shoes beside correct foot.

➤ Use gestures to explain.

➤ Point or touch body part to be used.

➤ If person cannot complete all the steps, always allow him or her to finish the dressing step, if possible—zipper pants, buckle belt.

➤ Decrease assistance gradually.

Rationale: Specific interventions with adaptive equipment will improve self-care abilities.

3. Initiate health teaching and referrals, as indicated.

➤ Assess understanding and knowledge of client and family for above instructions and rationale.
➤ Proceed with teaching as needed.
➤ Communicate to staff and family members the person's ability and willingness to learn.
➤ Teach use of adaptive devices and techniques that are specific to each disability.
➤ Teach client to maintain a safe dressing environment.
➤ Attempt to be noncritical in correcting errors.

Rationale: Assistance will be needed at home to maintain or improve self-care abilities and prevent injuries.

▼ Toileting Self-Care Deficit

Definition

Toileting Self-Care Deficit: State in which a person experiences an impaired ability to perform or complete toileting activities for himself or herself.

Defining Characteristics

Unable or unwilling to get to toilet or commode
Unable or unwilling to carry out proper hygiene
Unable to transfer to and from toilet or commode
Unable to handle clothing to accommodate toileting
Unable to flush toilet or empty commode

Related Factors

See Self-Care Deficit Syndrome.

 See Self-Care Deficit Syndrome.

Key Concepts

See Self-Care Deficit Syndrome.

FOCUS ASSESSMENT CRITERIA

See Self-Care Deficit Syndrome.

GOAL

The person will demonstrate increased ability to toilet self or report that he or she cannot toilet self.

Indicators

Demonstrate ability to use adaptive devices to facilitate toileting.
Describe causative factors for toileting deficit.
Relate rationale and procedures for treatment.

GENERAL INTERVENTIONS

1. Assess causative factors.

➤ Visual deficits (blindness, field cuts, poor depth perception)
➤ Affected or missing limbs (casts, amputations, paresis, paralysis)
➤ Cognitive deficits (aging, trauma, CVA)

Rationale: Interventions are selected depending on causative factors.

2. Provide opportunities to relearn or adapt to activity.

➤ Common nursing interventions for toileting difficulties
  ➤ Encourage client to wear prescribed corrective lenses or hearing aid.
  ➤ Obtain bladder and bowel history from individual or significant other (see Impaired Bowel Elimination or Impaired Urinary Elimination).
  ➤ Ascertain communication system person uses to express the need to toilet.
  ➤ Maintain bladder and bowel record to determine toileting patterns.
  ➤ Provide adequate fluid intake and balanced diet to promote adequate urinary output and normal bowel evacuation.

- ➤ Promote normal elimination by encouraging activity and exercise within the person's capabilities.
- ➤ Avoid development of "bowel fixation" by less frequent discussion and inquiries about bowel movements.
- ➤ Be alert to possibility of falls when toileting person (be prepared to ease him or her to floor without injuring either of you).
- ➤ Achieve independence in toileting by continual and unaided practice.
- ➤ Allow sufficient time for the task of toileting to avoid fatigue (lack of sufficient time to toilet may cause incontinence or constipation).
- ➤ Avoid use of indwelling and condom catheters to expedite bladder continence (if possible).

➤ Specific interventions for toileting for people with visual deficits
  - ➤ Keep call bell easily accessible so person can quickly obtain help to toilet; answer call bell promptly to decrease anxiety.
  - ➤ If bedpan or urinal is necessary for toileting, be sure it is within person's reach.
  - ➤ Avoid placing toileting equipment to the blind side of a person with field cut (when he or she is visually accommodated to surroundings, you may suggest he or she search entire visual field for equipment).
  - ➤ Announce yourself before entering or leaving toileting area.
  - ➤ Observe person's ability to obtain equipment or get to the toilet unassisted.
  - ➤ Provide for a safe and clear pathway to toilet area.

➤ Specific interventions for toileting for people with affected or missing limbs
  - ➤ Provide only the supervision and assistance necessary for relearning or adapting to the prosthesis.
  - ➤ Encourage person to look at affected area or limb and use it during toileting tasks.
  - ➤ Encourage useful transfer techniques taught by occupational or physical therapy (the nurse becomes familiar with planned mode of transfer).
  - ➤ Provide the necessary adaptive devices to enhance independence and safety (commode chairs, spill-proof urinals, fracture bedpans, raised toilet seats, support siderails for toilets).
  - ➤ Provide for a safe and clear pathway to toilet area.

➤ Specific interventions for toileting for people with cognitive deficits
  - ➤ Offer toileting reminders every 2 hours, after meals, and before bedtime.
  - ➤ When person can indicate the need to toilet, begin toileting at 2-hour intervals, after meals, and before bedtime.
  - ➤ Answer call bell immediately to avoid frustration and incontinence.
  - ➤ Encourage wearing ordinary clothes (many confused people are continent while wearing regular clothing).

➤ Avoid the use of bedpans and urinals; if physically possible, provide a normal atmosphere of elimination in bathroom (the toilet used should remain constant to promote familiarity).

➤ Give verbal cues as to what is expected of the person and positive reinforcement for success. Work to achieve daytime continence before expecting nighttime continence (nighttime incontinence may continue after daytime continence has returned).

Rationale: The client's maximum involvement in toileting activities can reduce the embarrassment associated with needing assistance with toileting (Maher et al., 1998).

3. Initiate health teaching and referrals, as indicated.

➤ Assess the understanding and knowledge of the client and significant others of foregoing interventions and rationales.

➤ Communicate to staff and family members the person's ability and willingness to learn.

➤ Maintain a safe toileting environment.

➤ Reinforce knowledge of transferring techniques.

➤ Teach use of adaptive devices.

➤ Ascertain home toileting needs and refer to occupational therapy or social services for help in obtaining necessary equipment.

▼ Instrumental Self-Care Deficit

Definition

Instrumental Self-Care Deficit: State in which a person experiences an impaired ability to perform certain activities or access certain services essential for managing a household.

Defining Characteristics

Observed or reported difficulty in one or more of the following:

Using a telephone
Accessing transportation
Laundering, ironing
Preparing meals
Shopping (food, clothes)
Managing money
Administering medication

Related Factors

See Self-Care Deficit Syndrome.

 Instrumental Self-Care Deficit is not currently on the NANDA list but has been added here for clarity and usefulness. This diagnosis describes problems in performing certain activities or accessing certain services needed to live in the community (e.g., phone use, shopping, money management). This diagnosis is important to consider in discharge planning and during home visits by community nurses. Consult with your instructor regarding its use.

Key Concepts

GENERIC CONSIDERATIONS

- ➤ Brody (1985) found that, to live in the community, a person has to perform or have assistance with six ADLs as well as additional activities.
- ➤ Instrumental ADLs include housekeeping, preparing and procuring food, shopping, laundering, ability to self-medicate safely, ability to manage money, and access to transportation (Miller, 2004).
- ➤ Instrumental ADLs are more complex tasks than ADLs.
- ➤ Maintaining people in the community, rather than in nursing homes, has significant financial benefit. In 1981, 25% of all US health care expenditures for older adults went to nursing homes, but only 5% of older adults were receiving care in these facilities. Medicaid covers about 90% of public spending for nursing home care (Miller, 2004).
- ➤ Maintaining people in the community, rather than in nursing homes, also maintains autonomy, strengthens family life, and affirms the value of older adults in our society.

FOCUS ASSESSMENT CRITERIA

See Self-Care Deficit Syndrome.

GOAL

The person or family will report satisfaction with household management.

Indicators

Demonstrate use of adaptive devices (e.g., phone, cooking aids).

Describe a method to ensure adherence to medication schedule.

Report ability to make calls and answer telephone.

Report regular laundering by self or others.

Report daily intake of at least two nutritious meals.

Identify transportation options to stores, physician, house of worship, and social activities.

Demonstrate management of simple money transactions.

Identify people who will assist with money matters.

GENERAL INTERVENTIONS

1. Assess for causative and contributing factors.

➤ Visual, hearing deficits
➤ Impaired cognition
➤ Impaired mobility
➤ Lack of knowledge
➤ Inadequate social support

Rationale: Interventions are dependent on specific contributing factors.

2. Assist client to identify self-help devices.

➤ Grooming/dressing aids
  ➢ See Impaired Physical Mobility.
➤ Kitchen/eating aids
  ➢ Dishes with one side built up
  ➢ Built-up handles on cutlery (use plastic foam curlers)
  ➢ Bulldog clip to secure a straw in glass
  ➢ Built-up corner of cutlery board to hold and anchor food or pot (e.g., to butter toast, mash potatoes)
  ➢ Mounted jar opener
  ➢ Nonslip material applied under dishes (same strips used to prevent slipping in bathtub)
  ➢ Two-sided suction holder to hold dishes in place
➤ Communication/security
  ➢ Motion-activated lights near walkway/entrance
  ➢ Nightlight for path to bathroom
  ➢ Light next to bed
  ➢ Specially adapted phones (amplified, big buttons)
➤ Promote self-care and safety for person with cognitive deficit.
➤ Evaluate activities that are achievable.

➤ Teach safety techniques.
  ➣ Turn lights on before dark.
  ➣ Use nightlights.
  ➣ Keep environment simple, uncluttered.
  ➣ Use clocks and calendars as cues.
  ➣ Mark on calendar (using picture symbols) reminders for shopping, laundry, cleaning, doctor's appointments, and the like.
➤ For laundry, teach client to
  ➣ Separate dark and light clothes.
  ➣ Use pictures to illustrate steps for washing clothes.
  ➣ Mark cup with line to indicate amount of soap needed.
  ➣ Minimize ironing.
  ➣ Use an iron with automatic shutoff mechanism.
➤ Evaluate client's ability to select, procure, and prepare nutritious food daily.
  ➣ Prepare a permanent shopping list with cues for essential foods, products.
  ➣ Teach client to review list before shopping, check items needed, and, in the store, check off items selected. (Use a pencil that can be erased to reuse list.)
  ➣ Teach client how to shop for single-person meals (refer to Imbalanced Nutrition for specific techniques).
  ➣ If possible, teach client to use a microwave to reduce the risk of heat-related injuries or accidents.
➤ Offer hints to improve adherence to medication schedule.
  ➣ Have someone place medications in a commercial pill holder divided into 7 days.
  ➣ Take out exact amount of pills for the day. Divide them in small cups, each labeled with time of day.
  ➣ If needed, draw a picture of the pills and the quantity on each cup.
  ➣ Teach client to transfer pills from cup to small plastic bag when planning to be away from home.
➤ Tell client whom to call for instructions if he or she misses a dose.
➤ Determine available sources of transportation.
  ➣ Neighbors, relatives
  ➣ Community center
  ➣ Church group
  ➣ Social service agency
➤ Determine available sources of social support.
  ➣ Discuss the possibility of bartering for services (e.g., wash neighbor's clothes in exchange for shopping help).
  ➣ Identify a person who can provide immediate help (e.g., neighbor, friend, hotline).
  ➣ Identify sources for help with laundry, shopping, and money matters.

Rationale: Interventions focus on assisting the person and family to maintain as much functional independence as possible (Miller, 2004).

3. Initiate health teaching and referrals, as indicated.

➤ Discuss the importance of identifying the need for assistance.
➤ Refer client to community agencies for assistance (e.g., Department of Social Services, area agency on aging, senior neighbors, public health nursing).

Rationale: Community resources can assist the person when caregivers are unavailable (Miller, 2004).

▼ Sleep Deprivation

Definition

Sleep Deprivation: State in which a person experiences prolonged periods of time without sustained, natural, periodic states of relative unconsciousness.

Sleep deprivation is usually a temporary state that can be remedied when the person can go to sleep. External factors can cause sleep deprivation like airline travel, continuous noise, or an unexpected prolonged work schedule. The nursing diagnosis Disturbed Sleep Pattern is more useful for a clinical nurse.

Defining Characteristics

Refer to Disturbed Sleep Pattern.

▼ Disturbed Sleep Pattern

Definition

Disturbed Sleep Pattern: State in which a person experiences or is at risk for experiencing a change in the quantity or quality of his or her rest pattern that causes discomfort or interferes with desired lifestyle.

Defining Characteristics

MAJOR (MUST BE PRESENT)

Difficulty falling or remaining asleep

MINOR (MAY BE PRESENT)

Fatigue on awakening or during the day
Agitation
Dozing during the day
Mood alterations

Related Factors

Many factors can contribute to disturbed sleep patterns. Some common factors are listed below.

PATHOPHYSIOLOGIC

Related to frequent awakenings secondary to

Impaired oxygen transport

➤ Angina
➤ Circulatory disorders
➤ Respiratory disorders
➤ Peripheral arteriosclerosis

Impaired elimination; bowel or bladder

➤ Diarrhea
➤ Dysuria
➤ Retention
➤ Incontinence
➤ Constipation
➤ Frequency

Impaired metabolism

➤ Hyperthyroidism
➤ Hepatic disorders
➤ Gastric ulcers

TREATMENT-RELATED

Related to difficulty assuming usual position secondary to (specify)
Related to excessive daytime sleeping secondary to medications

Tranquilizers
Monoamine oxidase inhibitors
Antidepressants
Amphetamines
Soporifics
Hypnotics
Corticosteroids

  Sedatives
  Barbiturates
  Antihypertensives

SITUATIONAL (PERSONAL, ENVIRONMENTAL)

  Related to excessive hyperactivity secondary to

    Bipolar disorder
    Attention deficit disorder
    Panic anxiety

  Related to excessive daytime sleeping
  Related to depression
  Related to inadequate daytime activities
  Related to pain
  Related to anxiety response
  Related to discomforts secondary to pregnancy
  Related to lifestyle disruptions

    Occupational
    Sexual
    Emotional
    Financial
    Social

  Related to environmental changes (specify):

    Hospitalization (noise, disturbing roommate, fear)
    Travel

  Related to fears
  Related to circadian rhythm changes

MATURATIONAL

Adult Women

  Related to hormonal changes (e.g., perimenopausal)

Carp's Cue▶ *The inability to rest and sleep has been described as "one of the causes as well as one of the accompaniments of disease" (Henderson, 1969). Sleep disturbances can result from physiologic, psychological, social, environmental, and maturational changes or problems.*

  The nursing diagnosis Disturbed Sleep Pattern must be differentiated from sleep disorders, which are chronic conditions (e.g., sleep apnea, narcolepsy) usually not treatable by a nurse. Disturbed Sleep Pattern should be used to describe temporary changes in usual sleep patterns and/or those that a nurse can prevent or reduce (e.g., disruptions for treatments, anxiety response). All clients in the hospital are at risk for Disturbed Sleep Pattern. After you learn routine interventions for all these clients, use only High Risk for Disturbed Sleep Pattern when you need to add more interventions than the usual routine. Consult your instructor about the use of this diagnosis.

Key Concepts

GENERIC CONSIDERATIONS

➤ Sleep involves two distinct stages: rapid eye movement (REM) and non–rapid eye movement (NREM). NREM sleep constitutes about 75% of total sleep time; REM sleep accounts for the remaining 25% (Porth, 2002).

➤ The entire sleep cycle is completed in 70 to 100 minutes; this cycle repeats itself four or five times during the course of the sleep period.

➤ Sleep is a restorative and recuperative process that facilitates cellular growth and repair of damaged and aging body tissues. During NREM sleep, metabolic, cardiac, and respiratory rates decrease to basal levels and blood pressure decreases. There is a profound muscle relaxation, bone marrow mitotic activity, and accelerated tissue repair and protein synthesis. During REM sleep, the sympathetic nervous system accelerates, with erratic increases in cardiac output and heart and respiratory rate. Perfusion to gray matter doubles, and cognitive and emotional information is stored, filtered, and organized (Boyd, 2001).

➤ The active phase of the sleep cycle, REM sleep, is characterized by increased irregular vital signs, penile erections, flaccid musculature, and release of adrenal hormones. REM sleep occurs approximately four to five times a night and is essential to a person's sense of well-being. REM sleep is instrumental in facilitating emotional adaptation; a person needs substantially more REM sleep after periods of increased stress or learning (Blissitt, 2001).

➤ Percentage of time in bed at night actually spent asleep, or sleep efficiency, influences perception of the quality of sleep. Studies report that younger people typically report sleep efficiency of 80% to 95%, whereas older people report 67% to 70% (Hayashi & Endo, 1982).

➤ Sleep deprivation results in impaired cognitive functioning (memory, concentration, judgment) and perception, mental fatigue, reduced emotional control, and increased suspicion, irritability, depression, and disorientation. It also lowers the pain threshold and decreases production of catecholamines, corticosteroids, and hormones (Boyd, 2001; Dines-Kalinowski, 2000).

➤ The average amount of sleep needed according to age follows:

Age	Hours of Sleep
Newborn	14 to 18
6 months	12 to 16
6 months to 4 years	12 to 13
5 to 13 years	7 to 8.5
13 to 21 years	7 to 8.75
Adults younger than 60	6 to 9
Adults older than 60	7 to 8

➤ Hammer (1991) identified three subcategories of Disturbed Sleep Pattern: latency or difficulty falling asleep, interrupted, and early-morning awakening.

➤ People with depression report early-morning awakenings and inability to return to sleep. People with anxiety complain of insomnia and multiple awakenings (Boyd, 2001).

➤ Hypnotics contribute to sleep disturbances by (Abrams, 2004):
   ➤ Requiring increasing dosage as a result of tolerance
   ➤ Depressing CNS function
   ➤ Producing paradoxic effects (nightmares, agitation)
   ➤ Interfering with REM and deep sleep stages
   ➤ Causing daytime somnolence due to a very long half-life

GERIATRIC CONSIDERATIONS

➤ Research has found that sleep efficiency declines with advancing age, so more time is needed in bed to achieve restorative sleep. Sleep time decreases with age (e.g., 6 hours by 70 years). Stages 3 and 4 and REM sleep decrease with aging (Hammer, 1991).

➤ Older adults have more difficulty falling asleep, are more easily awakened, and spend more time in the drowsiness stage and less time in the dream stages than do younger people (Miller, 2004).

➤ Miller (2004) reports that approximately 70% of older adults complain of sleep disturbances, usually involving daytime sleepiness, difficulty falling asleep, and frequent arousals.

FOCUS ASSESSMENT CRITERIA

Assess for defining characteristics.

Subjective Data

Sleep patterns (present, past)

➤ Rate sleep on a scale of 1 to 10 (10 = rested, refreshed)
➤ Usual bedtime and arising time
➤ Difficulty in getting to sleep, staying asleep, awakening

Sleep requirements

➤ To establish the amount of sleep a person needs, have him or her go to bed and sleep until waking in the morning (without an alarm clock). The person should do this for a few days. Calculate the average of the total sleeping hours, subtracting 20 to 30 minutes, which is the time most people need to fall asleep.

History of symptoms

➤ Complaints of
  ➢ Sleeplessness
  ➢ Depression
  ➢ Anxiety
  ➢ Fear (nightmares, dark, maturational situations)
  ➢ Irritability

Objective Data

Physical Characteristics

➤ Drawn appearance
➤ Yawning
➤ Dozing during the day
➤ Decreased attention span
➤ Irritability

Assess for related factors.
Refer to Related Factors.

GOAL

The person will report an optimal balance of rest and activity.

Indicators

Describe factors that prevent or inhibit sleep.
Identify techniques to induce sleep.

GENERAL INTERVENTIONS

Because various factors can disrupt sleep patterns, the nurse should consult the index for specific interventions to reduce specific factors (e.g., pain, anxiety, fear). The following suggests general interventions for promoting sleep and specific interventions for selected clinical situations.

1. Identify causative contributing factors.

   ➤ Pain (see Impaired Comfort)
   ➤ Fear
   ➤ Stress or anxiety (see Anxiety)
   ➤ Immobility or decreased activity
   ➤ Pregnancy
   ➤ Urinary frequency or incontinence (see Impaired Urinary Elimination)
   ➤ Unfamiliar or noisy environment
   ➤ Temperature (too hot/too cold)
   ➤ Insufficient daily stimulation or activity

Rationale: Researchers have reported that the chief deterrents to sleep in critical care clients were activity, noise, pain, physical condition, nursing procedures, lights, vapor tents, and hypothermia.

2. Reduce or eliminate environmental distractions and sleep interruptions.

   ➤ Noise
      ➤ Close door to room.
      ➤ Pull curtains.
      ➤ Unplug telephone.
      ➤ Use "white noise" (e.g., fan, quiet music, tape of rain, waves).
      ➤ Eliminate 24-hour lighting.
      ➤ Provide nightlights.
      ➤ Decrease the amount and kind of incoming stimuli (e.g., staff conversations).
      ➤ Cover blinking lights with tape.
      ➤ Reduce the volume of alarms and television.
      ➤ Place with compatible roommate, if possible.
   ➤ Interruptions
      ➤ Organize procedures to minimize disturbances during sleep period (e.g., when person awakens for medication, also administer treatments and obtain vital signs).
      ➤ Avoid unnecessary procedures during sleep period.
      ➤ Limit visitors during optimal rest periods (e.g., after meals).
      ➤ If voiding during the night is disruptive, have person limit night-time fluids and void before retiring.

Rationale: Sleep cycle includes REM, NREM, and wakefulness. A person typically goes through four or five complete cycles each night. Awakening during a cycle may cause him or her to feel poorly rested in the morning. To feel rested, a person usually must complete an entire rest cycle (70 to 100 minutes) four or five times a night (Cohen & Merritt, 1992; Thelan et al., 1998). Environmental noise that cannot be eliminated or reduced can be masked with "white noise" (e.g., fan, soft music, tape-recorded sounds [rain, ocean waves]; Miller, 2004).

3. Increase daytime activities, as indicated.

> Establish with person a schedule for a daytime program of activity (walking, physical therapy).
> > Discourage naps longer than 90 minutes.
> > Encourage naps in the morning.
> Limit amount and length of daytime sleeping if excessive (e.g., more than 1 hour).
> > Encourage others to communicate with person and stimulate wakefulness.

Rationale: Early-morning naps produce more REM sleep than do afternoon naps. Naps longer than 90 minutes decrease the stimulus for longer sleep cycles in which REM sleep is obtained (Thelan et al., 1998). Irregular sleep patterns can disrupt normal circadian rhythms, possibly leading to sleep difficulties.

4. Promote sleep.

> Assess with person, family, or parents the usual bedtime routine— time, hygiene, practices, rituals (reading, toy)—and adhere to it as closely as possible.
> > Encourage or provide evening care.
> > > Bathroom or bedpan
> > > Personal hygiene (mouth care, bath, shower, partial bath)
> > > Clean linen and bedclothes (freshly made bed, sufficient blankets)
> > Use sleep aids.
> > > Warm bath
> > > Desired bedtime snack (avoid highly seasoned and high-roughage foods)
> > > Reading material
> > > Back rub or massage
> > > Warm milk
> > > Soft music or tape-recorded story
> > > Relaxation/breathing exercises
> > Use pillows for support (painful limb, pregnant or obese abdomen, back).
> Ensure that the person has at least four or five periods of at least 90 minutes each of uninterrupted sleep every 24 hours.
> Document the amount of the person's uninterrupted sleep each shift.

Rationale: A familiar bedtime ritual may promote relaxation and sleep (Cohen & Merritt, 1992). Warm milk contains l-tryptophan, which is a sleep inducer (Hammer, 1991).

5. Provide health teaching and referrals, as indicated.

➤ Teach an at-home sleep routine (Miller, 2004).
➤ Maintain a consistent daily schedule for waking, sleeping, and resting (weekdays, weekends).
➤ Arise at the usual time even after not sleeping well; avoid staying in bed even when awake.
  ➤ Use bed only for activities associated with sleeping.
➤ If awakened and cannot return to sleep, get out of bed and read in another room for 30 minutes.
➤ Avoid caffeine-containing foods and beverages (e.g., chocolate, tea, coffee) during the afternoon and evening.
  ➤ Avoid alcohol.
  ➤ Try a bedtime snack of foods high in L-tryptophan (e.g., milk, peanuts).
➤ Teach the importance of regular exercise (walking, running, aerobic dance) for at least 30 minutes three times a week (if not contraindicated) to reduce stress and promote sleep.
➤ Explain that hypnotic medications are not for long-term use because of the risk for development of tolerance and interference with daytime functioning.
➤ Explain to person and significant others the causes of sleep/rest disturbance and possible ways to avoid or minimize these causes.
➤ Refer a person with a chronic sleep problem to a sleep disorders center.

Rationale: Sedative and hypnotic drugs begin to lose their effectiveness after 1 week of use, requiring increasing dosages and leading to the risk of dependence. Caffeine and nicotine are CNS stimulants that lengthen sleep latency and increase nighttime wakening (Miller, 2004). Alcohol induces drowsiness but suppresses REM sleep and increases the number of awakenings (Miller, 2004).

▼ Spiritual Distress

Definition

Spiritual Distress: State in which a person or group experiences a disturbance in the belief or value system that provides strength, hope, and meaning to life.

Defining Characteristics

MAJOR (MUST BE PRESENT)

Experiences a disturbance in belief system

MINOR (MAY BE PRESENT)

Questions meaning of life, death, suffering
Questions credibility of belief system
Demonstrates discouragement or despair
Chooses not to practice usual religious rituals
Has ambivalent feelings (doubts) about beliefs
Expresses that he or she has no reason for living
Feels a sense of spiritual emptiness
Shows emotional detachment from self and others
Expresses concern—anger, resentment, fear—over meaning of life, suffering, death
Requests spiritual assistance for a disturbance in belief system

Related Factors

PATHOPHYSIOLOGIC

Related to challenge to belief system or separation from spiritual ties secondary to

Loss of body part or function
Pain
Terminal illness
Trauma
Debilitating disease
Miscarriage, stillbirth

TREATMENT-RELATED

Related to conflict between (specify prescribed regimen) and beliefs

Abortion
Isolation
Surgery
Amputation
Blood transfusion
Medications
Dietary restrictions
Medical procedures

SITUATIONAL (PERSONAL, ENVIRONMENTAL)

Related to death or illness of significant other
Related to embarrassment at practicing spiritual rituals
Related to barriers to practicing spiritual rituals:

Restrictions of intensive care
Lack of privacy
Unavailability of special foods/diet
Confinement to bed or room

Related to beliefs opposed by family, peers, health care providers
Related to divorce, separation from loved one

Wellness represents a response to a person's potential for personal growth, involving use of all of a person's resources (social, psychological, cultural, environmental, spiritual, and physiologic). Nurses profess to care for the whole client, but several studies report that they commonly avoid addressing the spiritual dimension of clients, families, and communities (DeYoung, 1984; Martin, Burrows & Pomilio, 1978, Kendrick & Robinson, 2000).

To promote positive spirituality with clients and families, the nurse must possess positive spirituality. The nurse can assist people with spiritual concerns or distress by providing resources for spiritual help, by listening nonjudgmentally, and by providing opportunities for meeting spiritual needs (Stoll, 1984). The nurse should be cautioned against establishing practice patterns that routinely result in referring all spiritual needs of clients and families to religious or spiritual leaders.

Spirituality and religiousness are two different concepts. Burkhart and Solari-Twadell define spirituality as the "ability to experience and integrate meaning and self; others, art, music, literature, nature, or a power greater than oneself" (2001, p. 51). Religiousness is "the ability to exercise participation in the beliefs of a particular denomination of faith community and related rituals" (Burkhart & Solari-Twadell, 2001, p. 51). They can coexist and also exist separately.

Key Concepts

GENERIC CONSIDERATIONS

➤ All people have a spiritual dimension, regardless of whether they participate in formal religious practices (Carson, 1999). An individual is a spiritual person even when disoriented, confused, emotionally ill, irrational, or cognitively impaired.

➤ The nurse must consider the client's spiritual nature as part of total care, along with the physical and psychosocial dimensions.

➤ The spiritual may include, but is not limited to, religion; spiritual needs include religion, values, relationships, transcendence, and affective feeling and communication; creativity and self-expression also may be important to spirituality. Other descriptions of spirituality include inner strength, meaning and purpose, and knowing and becoming.

➤ Health care systems often give spiritual concerns low priority in care planning and delivery. This is less true in hospice organizations, where the spiritual component of care is more likely to be recognized and included (Sheldon, 2000).

➤ Religion influences attitudes and behavior related to right and wrong, family, child-rearing, work, money, politics, and many other functional areas.

➤ To deal effectively with a person's spiritual needs, the nurse must recognize his or her own beliefs and values, acknowledge that these values may not be applicable to others, and respect the client's beliefs when helping him or her to meet perceived spiritual needs.

➤ The value of prayers or spiritual rituals to the believer is not affected by whether they can be scientifically "proved" to be beneficial.

➤ Research indicates that many nurses feel inadequately prepared to provide spiritual care and that fewer than 15% include spirituality in nursing care. "Among the reasons that nurses fail to provide spiritual care are the following: (1) They view religious and spiritual needs as a private matter concerning only an individual and his/her Creator; (2) they are uncomfortable about their own religious beliefs or deny having spiritual needs; (3) they lack knowledge about spirituality and the religious beliefs of others; (4) they mistake spiritual needs for psychosocial needs; and (5) they view meeting the spiritual needs of clients as a family or pastoral responsibility, not a nursing responsibility" (Andrews & Boyle, 2003, p. 426).

➤ To assist people in spiritual distress, the nurse must know certain beliefs and practices of various spiritual groups. Table II.10 provides information on the beliefs and practices that relate most directly to health and illness. It is intended as a reference only. Major religions, denominations, and spiritual groups are arranged alphabetically. Denominations with similar practices and restrictions are grouped together. No attempt is made to discuss the broad beliefs and philosophies of the selected groups; see References/Bibliography for texts supplying such in-depth information.

(*text continues on page 456*)

Table II–10. OVERVIEW OF RELIGIOUS BELIEFS

Agnostic

Beliefs
   It is impossible to know if God exists (specific moral values may guide behavior)

Amish

Illness
   Usually taken care of within family
Texts
   Bible; Ausbund (16th-century German hymnal)
Beliefs
   Rejection of all government aid; rejection of modernization
   Legally exempt from immunizations

Armenian

See Eastern Orthodox

Atheist

Beliefs
   God does not exist (specific moral values may guide behavior)

Baha'i

Illness
   Religion and science are both important
   Usual hospital routines and treatments are usually acceptable
Death
   Burial mandatory; interment near place of death
Beliefs
   Purpose of religion is to promote harmony and peace
   Education very important

Baptist, Churches of God, Churches of Christ, and Pentecostal (Assemblies of God, Foursquare Church)

Illness
   Some practice laying on of hands, divine healing through prayer
   May request Communion
   Some prohibit medical therapy
   May consider illness divine punishment or intrusion of Satan
Diet
   No alcohol (mandatory for most); no coffee, tea, tobacco, pork, or strangled animals
      (mandatory for some)
   Some fasting
Birth
   Oppose infant baptism

Table II–10. **OVERVIEW OF RELIGIOUS BELIEFS** (*Continued*)

Text
  Bible
Beliefs
  Some practice glossolalia (speaking in tongues)

Buddhism

Illness
  May wish counseling by priest
  May refuse treatment on holy days (1/1, 1/16, 2/15, 3/21, 4/8, 5/21, 6/15, 8/1, 8/23, 12/8, 12/31)
Diet
  Strict vegetarianism (mandatory for some)
  Use of alcohol, tobacco, and drugs discouraged
Death
  Last-rite chanting by priest
  Death leads to rebirth; may wish to remain alert and lucid
Texts
  Buddha's sermon on the "eightfold path," the Tripitaka, or "three baskets" of wisdom
Beliefs
  Cleanliness is of great importance
  Suffering is universal

Christian Science

Illness
  Caused by errors in thought and mind
  May oppose drugs; IV fluid; blood transfusions; psychotherapy; hypnotism; physical examinations; biopsies; eye, ear, and blood pressure screening; and other medical and nursing interventions
  Accept only legally required immunizations
  May desire support from a Christian Science reader or treatment by a Christian Science nurse or practitioner (a list of these nonmedical practitioners and nurses may be found in the Christian Science Journal)
  Healing is spiritual renewal
Death
  Autopsy permitted only in cases of sudden death
Text
  Bible; *Science and Health With Key to the Scriptures* by Mary Baker Eddy

Church of Christ

See Baptist

Church of God

See Baptist

(*continued*)

Table II–10. OVERVIEW OF RELIGIOUS BELIEFS (*Continued*)

Confucian

Illness
  The body was given by one's parents and should therefore be well cared for
  May be strongly motivated to maintain or regain wellness
Beliefs
  Respect for family and older people very important

Cults (Variety of Groups, Usually With Living Leader)

Illness
  Most practice faith healing
  May reject modern medicine and condemn health personnel as enemies
  Therapeutic compliance and follow-up are usually poor
  Illness may represent wrong thinking or inhabitation by Satan
Beliefs
  Expansion of cult through conversions important
  May depend on cult environment for definition of reality

Eastern Orthodox (Greek Orthodox, Russian Orthodox, Armenian)

Illness
  May desire Holy Communion, laying on of hands, anointing, or sacrament of
    Holy Unction
  Most oppose euthanasia and favor every effort to preserve life
  Russian Orthodox men should be shaved only if necessary for surgery
Diet
  May fast Wednesdays, Fridays, during Lent, before Christmas, or for 6 hours before
    Communion (seriously ill are exempted)
  May avoid meat, dairy products, and olive oil during fast (seriously ill are exempted)
Birth
  Baptism 8–40 days after birth, usually by immersion (mandatory for some)
  May be followed immediately by confirmation
  Greek Orthodox only: If death of infant is imminent, nurse should baptize infant
    by touching the forehead with a small amount of water three times
Death
  Last rites and administration of Holy Communion (mandatory for some)
  May oppose autopsy, embalming, and cremation
Texts
  Bible; prayer book
  Religious Articles
  Icons (pictures of Jesus, Mary, saints) are very important
  Holy water and lighted candles
  Russian Orthodox wears cross necklace that should be removed only if necessary
Other
  Greek Orthodox opposes abortion
  Confession at least yearly (mandatory for some)

Table II–10. OVERVIEW OF RELIGIOUS BELIEFS (*Continued*)

Holy Communion four times yearly: Christmas, Easter, 6/30, and 8/15
  (mandatory for some)
Dates of holy days may differ from Western Christian calendar

Episcopal

Illness
  May believe in spiritual healing; may desire confession and Communion
Diet
  May abstain from meat on Fridays; may fast during Lent or before Communion
Birth
  Infant baptism is mandatory (nurse may baptize infant when death is imminent
    by pouring water on forehead and saying, "I baptize you in the name of the
    Father, the Son, and the Holy Spirit")
Death
  Last rites optional
Texts
  Bible; prayer book

Friends (Quaker)

No minister or priests; direct, individual, inner experience of God is vital
Diet
  Most avoid alcohol and drugs and favor practice of moderation
Death
  Many do not believe in afterlife
Beliefs
  Pacifism important; many are conscientious objectors to war

Greek Orthodox

See Eastern Orthodox

Hinduism

Illness
  May minimize illness and emphasize its temporary nature
  Viewed as result of karma (actions/fate) of previous life
  Caused by body and spirit not being in harmony or by tension in interpersonal
    relationships
  Belief in healing responses triggered by treatment
  Strong belief in alternative healing practices (e.g., herbal treatments, faith healing)
Diet
  Various doctrines, many vegetarian; many abstain from alcohol (mandatory for
    some); beef and pork are forbidden; prefer fresh cooked foods
Death
  Believe in immortality of the soul
  Seen as rebirth; may wish to be alert; chant prayer   (continued)

Table II–10. OVERVIEW OF RELIGIOUS BELIEFS (*Continued*)

Priest may tie sacred thread around neck or wrist, or body—do not remove
Water is poured into mouth, and family washes body
Cremation preferred—must be soon after death
Beliefs
Physical, mental, and spiritual discipline, and purification of body and
soul emphasized
Believe in the world as a manifestation of Brahman, one divine being pervading
all things
Texts

Vedas	Ramayana
Upanishads	Mahabharata
Bhagavad-Gita	Puranas

Worship
Daily prayers, usually in home; quiet meditation
Rituals may include use of water, fire, lights, sounds, natural objects,
special postures, and gestures

Jehovah's Witness

Illness
Oppose blood transfusions and organ transplantation (mandatory)
May oppose other medical treatments and all modern science
Oppose faith healing; oppose abortion
Diet
Refuses foods to which blood has been added; may eat meats that have been drained
Text
Bible

Judaism

Illness
Medical care emphasized
Rabbinical consultation necessary for donation and transplantation of organs
May oppose surgical procedures on the Sabbath (sundown Friday to sundown
Saturday); seriously ill are exempted
May prefer burial of removed organs or body tissues
May oppose shaving
May wear skull cap and socks continuously, believing head and feet should be covered
Diet
Fasting for 24 hours on holy days of Yom Kippur (in September or October) and
Tishah-b'Ab (in August), Matzo replaces leavened bread during Passover week
(in March or April)
May observe strict Kosher dietary laws (mandatory for some) that prohibit pork,
shellfish, and the eating of meat and dairy products at same meal or with same
dishes (milk products, served first, can be followed by meat in a few minutes;
reverse is not Kosher); seriously ill are exempted

Table II–10. OVERVIEW OF RELIGIOUS BELIEFS (*Continued*)

Birth
  Ritual circumcision 8 days after birth (mandatory for some); fetuses are buried
Death
  Ritual burial; society members wash body
  Burial as soon as possible
  May oppose cremation
  May oppose autopsy and donation of body to science
  Most do not believe in afterlife
  Generally oppose prolongation of life after irreversible brain damage
Texts
  Torah (first five books of Old Testament)
  Talmud
  Prayer book
  Religious Articles
  Menorah (seven-branched candlestick)
  Yarmulke (skull cap, may be worn continuously)
  Tallith (prayer shawl worn for morning prayers)
  Tefillin, or phylacteries (leather boxes on straps containing scripture passages)
  Star of David (may be worn around neck)
Beliefs
  Observation of the Sabbath (Friday evening to Saturday evening) may require
    not writing, traveling, using electrical appliances, or receiving treatment

Krishna

Diet
  Vegetarian diet; no garlic or onions
  No drugs, alcohol; herbal tea only
Death
  Cremation mandatory
Texts
  Vedas
  Srimad-Bhagavatam
Beliefs
  Continual practice of mantra (chant)
  Belief in reincarnation

Lutheran, Methodist, Presbyterian

Illness
  May request Communion, anointing and blessing, or visitation by minister or elder
  Generally encourage use of medical science
Birth
  Baptism by sprinkling or immersion of infants, children, or adults
Death
  Optional last rites or scripture reading   (*continued*)

Table II–10. OVERVIEW OF RELIGIOUS BELIEFS (*Continued*)

Texts
  Bible; prayer book

Mennonite

Illness
  Opposes laying on of hands; may oppose shock treatment and drugs
Texts
  Bible; 18 articles of the Dordrecht Confession of Faith
Beliefs
  Shun modernization; no participation in government, pensions, or health plans

Methodist

See Lutheran

Mormon (Church of Jesus Christ of Latter-Day Saints)

Illness
  May come through partaking of harmful substances such as alcohol, tobacco,
    drugs, and so forth
  May be seen as a necessary part of the plan of salvation
  May desire Sacrament of the Lord's Supper to be administered by a Church
    Priesthood holder
  Divine healing through laying on of hands
  Church may provide financial support during illness
Diet
  Prohibits alcohol, tobacco, and hot drinks (tea and coffee); sparing use of meats
Birth
  No infant baptism; infants are born innocent
Death
  Cremation is opposed
Texts
  Bible; Book of Mormon
  Religious Articles
  Special undergarment may be worn by both men and women and should not be
    removed except during serious illness, childbirth, emergencies, and so forth
Beliefs
  Abortion is opposed
  Vicarious baptism for deceased who were not baptized in life

Muslim (Islamic, Moslem) and Black Muslim

Illness
  Opposes faith healing; favors every effort to prolong life
  May be noncompliant because of fatalistic view (illness is God's will)
  Group prayer may be helpful—no priests

Table II–10. OVERVIEW OF RELIGIOUS BELIEFS (*Continued*)

Diet
  Pork prohibited
  May oppose alcohol and traditional black American foods (cornbread, collard greens)
  Fasts sunrise to sunset during Ramadan (9th month of Muslim year—falls different time each year on Western calendar); seriously ill are exempted
Birth
  Circumcision practiced with accompanying ceremony
  Aborted fetus after 30 days is treated as human being
Death
  Confession of sins before death, with family present if possible; may wish to face toward Mecca
  Family follows specific procedure for washing and preparing body, which is then turned to face Mecca
  May oppose autopsy and organ transplantation
  Funeral usually within 24 hours after death
Texts
  Koran (scriptures); Hadith (traditions)
Prayer
  Five times daily—on rising, midday, afternoon, early evening, and before bed— facing Mecca and kneeling on prayer rug
  Ritual washing after prayer
Beliefs
  All activities (including sleep) restricted to what is necessary for health
  Personal cleanliness very important
  All Muslims: gambling and idol worship prohibited

Pentecostal

See Baptist

Presbyterian

See Lutheran

Quakers

See Friends

Roman Catholic

Illness
  Allowed by God because of man's sins, but not considered personal punishment
  May desire confession (penance) and Communion
  Anointing of sick for all seriously ill patients (some patients may equate this with "Last Rites" and assume they are dying)
  Donation and transplantation of organs permitted
  Burial of amputated limbs (mandatory for some)

(continued)

Table II–10. OVERVIEW OF RELIGIOUS BELIEFS (*Continued*)

Diet
  Fasting or abstaining from meat mandatory on Ash Wednesday and Good Friday
    (seriously ill are exempted); optional during Lent and on Fridays
  Fasts from solid food for 1 hour and abstains from alcohol for 3 hours before
    receiving Communion (mandatory; seriously ill are exempted)
Birth
  Baptism of infants and aborted fetuses mandatory (nurse may baptize in case of
    imminent death by sprinkling water on the forehead and saying, "I baptize you
    in the name of the Father, of the Son, and of the Holy Ghost")
Death
  Anointing of sick (mandatory)
  Extraordinary artificial means of sustaining life are unnecessary
Text
  Bible; prayer book
  Religious Articles
  Rosary, crucifix, saints' medals, statues, holy water, lighted candles
Other
  Attendance at mass required (seriously ill are exempted) on Sundays or late Saturday
    and on holy days (1/1, 8/15, 11/1, 12/8, 12/25, and 40 days after Easter)
  Sacrament of Penance at least yearly (mandatory); opposes abortion

Russian Orthodox

See Eastern Orthodox

Seventh-Day Adventist (Advent Christian Church)

Illness
  May desire baptism or Communion
  Some believe in divine healing
  May oppose hypnosis
  May refuse treatment on the Sabbath (sundown Friday to sundown Saturday)
  Healthful diet and lifestyle are stressed
Diet
  No alcohol, coffee, tea, narcotics, or stimulants (mandatory)
  Some abstain from pork, other meat, and shellfish
Birth
  Opposes infant baptism
Text
  Bible, especially Ten Commandments and Old Testament

Shinto

Illness
  May believe in prayer healing
  Great concern for personal cleanliness

Table II–10. OVERVIEW OF RELIGIOUS BELIEFS (*Continued*)

Physical health may be valued because of emphasis on joy and beauty of life

Family extremely important in giving care and providing emotional support

Beliefs

Worships ancestors, ancient heroes, and nature

Traditions emphasized; aesthetically pleasing area for worship important

Sikhism

Diet

Frequently vegetarian; may exclude eggs and fish

Religious Articles

Men may wear uncut hair, a wooden comb, an iron wrist band, a short sword, and short trousers. These symbols should not be disturbed.

Death

Cremation mandatory, usually within 24 hours after death

Text

Guru Granth Sahib

Taoist

Illness

Illness is seen as part of the health–illness dualism

May be resigned to and accepting of illness

May consider medical treatment as interference

Death

Seen as natural part of life; body is kept in house for 49 days

Mourning follows specific ritual patterns

Text

Tao-te-ching by Lao-tzu

Beliefs

Aesthetically pleasing area for meditation important

Unitarian Universalist

Illness

Reason, knowledge, and individual responsibility are emphasized, so may prefer not to see clergy

Birth

Most do not practice infant baptism

Death

Prefer cremation

Zen

Meditation using lotus position (many hours and years are spent in meditation and contemplation): goal is to discover simplicity

Illness

May wish consultation with Zen master

GERIATRIC CONSIDERATIONS

> ➤ Factors that contribute to spiritual distress and put older adults at risk include questions concerning life after death as the person ages, separation from formal religious community, and a value–belief system that is continuously challenged by losses and suffering.

> ➤ Older people tend to participate in formal religious groups more than younger people. Participation increases dramatically with age, and the desire to participate in church activities remains constant throughout their lives. Older people may find religious services difficult to attend and participate in because of physical impairments. Factors such as lack of transportation, inaccessible toileting facilities, poor acoustics and sound systems for hearing-impaired, and small-print hymn books or prayer books can diminish active involvement in formal religious activities.

> ➤ A common coping method for older adults, prayer increases feelings of self-worth and hope by reducing sense of aloneness and abandonment. In addition to private prayer and meditation, television and radio often provide adjunct stimuli for spiritual life.

> ➤ Older adults may rely on spiritual life more than most young people because of other limitations in their lives. The spiritual realm allows for satisfying connectedness with others. An older person can counterbalance some of the negative, isolating aspects of aging by identifying with tradition and institutional values. Private religion can help to motivate and provide purpose to life.

> ➤ Older adults commonly intertwine their religious beliefs with beliefs about health and illness. The nurse must assess these beliefs appropriately to facilitate the person's understanding of his illness in the context of his religion.

TRANSCULTURAL CONSIDERATIONS

> ➤ Religious beliefs, an integral component of culture, may influence a client's explanation of the causes of illness, perception of its severity, and choice of healer. In times of crisis, such as serious illness and impending death, religion may be a source of consolation for the client and family and may influence the course of action believed to be appropriate (Andrews & Boyle, 2003).

> ➤ Belonging to a specific cultural group does not imply that the person subscribes to that culture's dominant religion. In addition, even when a person identifies with a particular religion, he or she may not accept all its beliefs or practices (Andrews & Boyle, 2003).

> ➤ The nurse's role is not "to judge the religious virtues of individuals but rather to understand" those aspects related to religion that are important to the client and family members (Andrews & Boyle, 2003,

p. 143). Table II.10 was compiled with the intent to assist nurses with this understanding.

FOCUS ASSESSMENT CRITERIA

Assess for defining characteristics.

Subjective Data

What is your source of spiritual strength or meaning?
What is your source of peace, comfort, faith, well-being, hope, or worth?
How do you practice your spiritual beliefs?
Are any practices important for your spiritual well-being?
Do you have a spiritual leader?
Has being ill or hurt affected your spiritual beliefs?

Assess for related factors.

How can I help you maintain your spiritual strength (e.g., contact spiritual leader, provide privacy at special times, request reading materials)?

Objective Data

Current practices
Any religious or spiritual articles (clothing, medals, texts)
Visits from spiritual leader
Visits to place of worship or meditation
Requests for spiritual counseling or assistance
Response to interview on spiritual needs

➤ Grief
➤ Doubt
➤ Anger
➤ Anxiety

Participation in spiritual practices
Rejection or neglect of previous practices
Increased interest in spiritual matters

GOAL

The person will maintain usual spiritual practices not detrimental to health.

Indicators

Express his or her feelings related to beliefs.
Describe spiritual belief system positively.

GENERAL INTERVENTIONS

1. Explore whether the client desires to engage in an allowable religious or spiritual practice or ritual. If so, provide opportunity for him or her to do so.

Rationale: For a client who places a high value on prayer or other spiritual practices, these practices can provide meaning and purpose and can be a source of comfort and strength.

2. Express your understanding and acceptance of the importance of the client's religious or spiritual beliefs and practices.

Rationale: Conveying a nonjudgmental attitude may help reduce the client's uneasiness about expressing his or her belief and practices.

3. Provide privacy and quiet for spiritual rituals, as the client desires and as practicable.

Rationale: Privacy and quiet provide an environment that enables reflection and contemplation.

4. If you wish, offer to pray with the client or read from the religious text.

Rationale: The nurse—even one who does not subscribe to the same religious beliefs or values of the client—can still help him or her meet his or her spiritual needs.

5. Offer to contact a religious leader or hospital clergy to arrange for a visit. Explain available services (e.g., hospital chapel, Bible).

Rationale: These measures can help the client maintain spiritual ties and practice important rituals.

6. Explore whether any usual hospital practices conflict with the client's beliefs (e.g., diet, hygiene, treatments). If so, try to accommodate the client's beliefs to the extent that policy and safety allow.

Rationale: Many religions prohibit certain behaviors.

7. If angry, allow client to express feelings.

➤ Express to person that anger toward God is a common reaction to illness/suffering/death.
➤ Help client recognize and discuss feelings of anger.
➤ Allow client to problem solve to find ways to express and relieve anger.
➤ Offer to contact usual spiritual leader.
➤ Offer to contact other spiritual support person (e.g., pastoral care, hospital chaplain) if person cannot share feelings with usual spiritual leader.

Rationale: The client may view anger at God and a religious leader as "forbidden" and may be reluctant to initiate discussions of spiritual conflicts.

8. Engage in spiritual listening (Cameron, 1998).

➤ Avoid lecturing, criticizing, and giving advice.
➤ Avoid using religious dogma as responses.
➤ Use nondirective communication techniques.
➤ Help person to determine what is right for them.

Rationale: The nurse should function as an advocate in recognizing and respecting the client's spiritual needs, which other health professionals may sometimes overlook or ignore.

▼ Impaired Swallowing

Definition

Impaired Swallowing: State in which a person has decreased ability voluntarily to pass fluids and/or solid foods from the mouth to the stomach.

Defining Characteristics (Jeng et al., 2001)

MAJOR (MUST BE PRESENT, ONE OR MORE)

Observed evidence of difficulty in swallowing

and/or

Stasis of food in oral cavity
Coughing
Choking

MINOR (MAY BE PRESENT)

> After food or fluid intake
> Nasal-sounding voice
> Slurred speech
> Apraxia (ideational, constructional, or visual)
> Drooling

Related Factors

PATHOPHYSIOLOGIC

> Related to decreased/absent gag reflex, mastication difficulties, or decreased sensations secondary to

> > Neurologic/neuromuscular disorders

> > - ➤ Cerebral palsy
> > - ➤ Poliomyelitis
> > - ➤ Guillain-Barré syndrome
> > - ➤ Amyotrophic lateral sclerosis
> > - ➤ CVA
> > - ➤ Right or left hemispheric brain damage
> > - ➤ Neoplastic disease affecting the brain
> > - ➤ Cranial nerve damage
> > - ➤ Myasthenia gravis
> > - ➤ Muscular dystrophy
> > - ➤ Parkinson's disease

> > Related to tracheoesophageal tumors, edema

TREATMENT-RELATED

> Related to surgical reconstruction of the mouth, throat, jaw, or nose
> Related to decreased consciousness secondary to anesthesia
> Related to mechanical obstruction secondary to tracheostomy tube
> Related to esophagitis secondary to radiotherapy

SITUATIONAL (PERSONAL, ENVIRONMENTAL)

> Related to altered level of consciousness
> Related to fatigue
> Related to limited awareness
> Related to irritated oropharyngeal cavity
> Related to decreased saliva

MATURATIONAL

Older Adult

Related to reduction in saliva, taste

 Impaired swallowing can cause Imbalanced Nutrition and Risk for Aspiration. Interventions for these two diagnoses can be incorporated in the plan. If this person also is experiencing anorexia, the diagnosis of Imbalanced Nutrition can be used in addition to Impaired Swallowing. If the person is also experiencing nausea, the Nausea diagnosis would be used in addition to Impaired Swallowing.

Key Concepts

GENERIC CONSIDERATIONS

- Swallowing has an intellectual as well as a physical component.
- The swallowing process occurs in three stages with select cranial nerve involvement (Porth, 2002):
  - Stage 1. Oral: Food is placed in oral cavity, the lips close, and swallowing is initiated as a reflex. The tongue maneuvers the food, and the soft palate and uvula close off the nasopharynx.
  - Stage 2. Pharyngeal: The food passes the anterior fossa arches and triggers the swallow reflex. The tongue prevents the food from returning to the oral cavity by elevation and contraction of the soft palate. Pharyngeal peristalsis begins, causing the food to move downward.
  - Stage 3. Esophageal: Pharyngeal peristalsis pushes the food downward. The larynx elevates and the cricopharyngeal muscles relax, allowing the food to move from the pharynx into the esophagus. The larynx wave pushes the food down the esophagus to the stomach.
- Cranial nerves V, VII, IX, X, and XI are involved in swallowing.
- Impairment of cranial nerve function can cause the following swallowing problems (Hickey, 2002):
  - Trigeminal (V): loss of sensation and ability to move mandible
  - Facial (VII): increased salivation
  - Glossopharyngeal (IX): diminished taste sensation, salivation, and gag reflex
  - Vagus (X): decreased peristalsis
  - Hypoglossal (XI): poor tongue control
- A cough reflex is essential for rehabilitation, but a gag reflex is not.
- Do not confuse the ability to chew with the ability to swallow. See also Imbalanced Nutrition: Less Than Body Requirements.

FOCUS ASSESSMENT CRITERIA

Assess for defining characteristics.

Subjective Data

History of problem with swallowing

➤ Onset
➤ History of nasal regurgitation, hoarseness, choking, or coughing

Problem foods or liquids
Nonproblem foods or liquids

Objective Data

Decreased or absent swallowing, coughing, or gag reflex
Poor coordination of tongue
Observed choking or coughing with food or fluid

Assess for related factors.

Subjective Data

Assess for neurologic conditions that can affect eating and swallowing:

CVA
Brain lesions
Oral surgery
Parkinson's disease
Head trauma
Multiple sclerosis
Tracheoesophageal tumors

Objective Data

Assess for the presence of

Facial muscle weakness
Decreased saliva production
Impaired use of tongue
Thick secretions
Chewing difficulties
Impaired cognition

For more information on focus assessment criteria, visit http://connection. lww.com

GOAL

The person will report improved ability to swallow.

Indicators

The person and/or family will

Describe causative factors when known
Describe rationale and procedures for treatment

GENERAL INTERVENTIONS

1. Consult with speech pathologist for evaluation and a specific plan.

Rationale: The speech pathologist has the expertise needed to perform the swallowing evaluation.

2. Establish a visual method to communicate at bedside to staff that client is dysphagic.

Rationale: The risk of aspiration can be reduced if all staff is alerted.

3. Plan meals when client is well rested; ensure that reliable suction equipment is on hand during meals. Discontinue feeding if client is tired.

Rationale: Fatigue can cause the risk of aspiration.

4. If indicated, use modified supraglottic swallow technique:

➤ Position the head of the bed in a semi- or high Fowler's position with the client's neck flexed forward slightly and chin tilted down.

Rationale: This position uses the force of gravity to aid downward motion of food and decreases risk of aspiration.

➤ Use cutout cup (remove and round out ½ of side of foam cup).

Rationale: This prevents neck extension, which will open airway and risk aspiration.

➤ Take bolus of food and hold in strongest side of mouth for 1 to 2 seconds, then immediately flex the neck with chin tucked against the chest.
➤ Without breathing, swallow as many times as needed.
➤ When client's mouth is emptied, raise chin and clear throat.

Rationale: This maneuver triggers the protective mechanisms of epiglottis movement, laryngeal, and vocal cord adduction (closure). Straws hasten transit time and increase the risk of aspiration.

5. Offer high viscous foods first at meal (e.g., mashed bananas, mashed potatoes, gelatin, gravy).

Rationale: Post-CVA clients may have slowed peristalsis. Viscous foods increase peristaltic pump action.

6. Offer thick liquids (e.g., milk shakes, slushes, nectars, or cream soups).

Rationale: Thicker fluids have a slower transit time and allow more time to trigger the swallow reflex.

7. Establish a goal for fluid intake.

Rationale: These clients are at risk for dehydration because of self-imposed fluid restrictions related to fear of choking.

8. If drooling is present, use a quick-stretch stimulation just before each meal and toward the end of the meal.

➤ Digitally apply short, rapid, downward strokes to edges of bottom lip mostly on affected side.
➤ Use a cold washcloth over finger for added stimulation.

Rationale: Poor tongue control with impaired oral sensation allows food into affected side.

9. If a bolus of food is pocketed in the affected side, teach client how to use tongue to transfer food or apply external digital pressure to cheek to help remove the trapped bolus.

Rationale: Poor tongue control with impaired oral sensation allows food into affected side.

10. For a client with cognitive deficits, do the following:

➤ Divide eating tasks into the smallest steps possible.
➤ Describe and point out food.
➤ Provide a verbal command for each step.
➤ Progress slowly. Limit conversation.
➤ Continue verbal assistance at each meal as needed.

➤ Provide several small meals to accommodate short attention span.
➤ Provide a written checklist for other staff.

Rationale: A confused client needs repetitive simple instructions.

11. Reduce the possibility of aspiration.

➤ Before beginning feeding, assess that the client is adequately alert and can control the mouth, has cough/gag reflex, and can swallow own saliva.
➤ Have suction equipment available.
➤ Position client correctly.
➤ Keep client focused on task by giving directions until he or she has finished swallowing each mouthful.
➤ Keep client's mouth fresh and clean. Mix 1 teaspoon baking soda in 1 quart water. Client should rinse and gargle every 2 hours.
➤ Avoid very hot fluids.
➤ Start with small amount and progress slowly as person learns to handle each step.
➤ If the above strategies are unsuccessful, consultation with a physician may be necessary for alternative feeding techniques such as tube feedings or parenteral nutrition.

Rationale: Impaired reflexes and fatigue increase the risk of aspiration. Exercise can strengthen muscles to improve chewing and tongue movement of bolus to back of mouth to stimulate swallowing reflex (Porth, 2002)

▼ Ineffective Tissue Perfusion (Specify: Renal, Cerebral, Cardiopulmonary, GI)

Definition

Ineffective Tissue Perfusion: State in which a person experiences or is at risk of experiencing a decrease in nutrition and respiration at the cellular level because of a decrease in capillary blood supply.

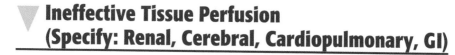

Tissue perfusion depends on many physiologic factors, both within body systems and at the cellular level. A person's response to ineffective tissue perfusion can disrupt some or all functional health patterns and can cause physiologic complications; for example, a person with chronic renal failure is at risk for fluid/electrolyte imbalances, acidosis, nutritional problems, edema, fatigue, pruritus, and disturbed self-concept. Does the diagnosis Ineffective Renal Tissue Perfusion describe these varied responses, or does it simply rename renal failure or renal calculi?

The use of any Ineffective Tissue Perfusion diagnosis other than Peripheral merely provides new labels for medical diagnoses, labels that do not describe the nursing focus or accountability. The following represent incorrect examples of Ineffective Tissue Perfusion diagnoses with associated goals:

> ➤ Ineffective Tissue Perfusion related to hypovolemia secondary to GI bleeding
>   > ➤ Goal: Tissue perfusion improves, as evidenced by stabilized vital signs.
>   > ➤ Correct: PC: GI Bleeding
> ➤ Ineffective Cerebral Tissue Perfusion related to increased intracranial pressure
>   > ➤ Goal: Intracranial pressure is no greater than 15 mm Hg; clinical signs of intracranial pressure are decreased.
>   > ➤ Correct: PC: Increased Intracranial Pressure
> ➤ Ineffective Tissue Perfusion related to vaso-occlusive nature of sickling secondary to sickle cell crisis
>   > ➤ Goal: Client demonstrates improved tissue perfusion, as evidenced by adequate urine output, absence of pain, and strong peripheral pulses.
>   > ➤ Correct: PC: Sickling Crisis

All the above outcomes represent criteria that nurses use to assess the client's status to determine the appropriate nursing and medical interventions indicated. Thus, these situations are better described as collaborative problems.

Ineffective Peripheral Tissue Perfusion can be a clinically useful nursing diagnosis if used to describe chronic arterial or venous insufficiency or potential thrombophlebitis. (In contrast, acute embolism and thrombophlebitis represent collaborative problems.) A nurse focusing on preventing thrombophlebitis in a postoperative client would write the diagnosis Risk for Ineffective Peripheral Tissue Perfusion related to postoperative immobility and dehydration.

▼ Ineffective Peripheral Tissue Perfusion

Definition

Ineffective Peripheral Tissue Perfusion: State in which a person experiences or is at risk of experiencing a decrease in nutrition and respiration at the peripheral cellular level because of a decrease in capillary blood supply.

Defining Characteristics

MAJOR (MUST BE PRESENT, ONE OR MORE)

Presence of one of the following types (see Key Concepts for definitions):

➤ Claudication (arterial)
➤ Rest pain (arterial)
➤ Aching pain (arterial or venous)

Diminished or absent arterial pulses (arterial)
Skin color changes

➤ Pallor (arterial)
➤ Reactive hyperemia (arterial)
➤ Cyanosis (venous)

Skin temperature changes

➤ Cooler (arterial)
➤ Warmer (venous)

Decreased blood pressure (arterial)
Capillary refill longer than 3 seconds (arterial)

MINOR (MAY BE PRESENT)

Edema (venous)
Change in sensory function (arterial)
Change in motor function (arterial)
Trophic tissue changes (arterial)

➤ Hard, thick nails
➤ Loss of hair
➤ Nonhealing wound

Related Factors

PATHOPHYSIOLOGIC

Related to compromised blood flow secondary to

Arteriosclerosis
Varicosities
Buerger's disease
Alcoholism
Diabetes mellitus
Hypotension
Blood dyscrasias

Renal failure
Cancer/tumor

TREATMENT-RELATED

Related to immobilization
Related to presence of invasive lines
Related to pressure sites/constriction (elastic compression bandages, stockings, restraints)
Related to blood vessel trauma or compression

SITUATIONAL (PERSONAL, ENVIRONMENTAL)

Related to pressure of enlarging uterus on pelvic vessels
Related to pressure of enlarged abdomen on pelvic vessels
Related to vasoconstricting effects of tobacco
Related to decreased circulating volume secondary to dehydration
Related to dependent venous pooling
Related to hypothermia
Related to pressure of muscle mass secondary to weight lifting

 Carp's Cue ▶ *See Ineffective Peripheral Tissue Perfusion*

Key Concepts

GENERIC CONSIDERATIONS

➤ Cellular nutrition and respiration depend on adequate blood flow through the microcirculation.
➤ Adequate cellular oxygenation depends on the following processes (Porth, 2002):
  ➤ The ability of the lungs to exchange air adequately (O_2–CO_2)
  ➤ The ability of the pulmonary alveoli to diffuse oxygen and carbon dioxide across the cell membrane to the blood
  ➤ The ability of the red blood cells (hemoglobin) to carry oxygen
  ➤ The ability of the heart to pump with enough force to deliver the blood to the microcirculation
  ➤ The ability of intact blood vessels to deliver blood to the microcirculation
➤ Hypoxemia (decreased oxygen content of the blood) results in cellular hypoxia, which causes cellular swelling and contributes to tissue injury.
➤ Arterial blood flow is enhanced by a dependent position and inhibited by an elevated position (gravity pulls blood downward, away from the heart).

➤ When an alteration in peripheral tissue perfusion exists, the nurse must consider its nature; the two major components of the peripheral vascular system are the arterial and the venous systems. Signs, symptoms, etiology, and nursing interventions are different for problems in each of these two systems and therefore are addressed separately.

➤ Changes in arterial walls increase the incidence of stroke and coronary artery disease (Porth, 2002).

GERIATRIC CONSIDERATIONS

➤ Age-related vascular changes include stiffened blood vessels, which cause increased peripheral resistance, impaired baroreceptor functioning, and diminished ability to increase organ blood flow (Miller, 2004). These age-related changes cause the veins to become more dilated and less elastic. Valves of the large leg veins become less efficient. Age-related reductions in muscle mass and inactivity further reduce peripheral circulation (Miller, 2004).

➤ Physical deconditioning or lack of exercise accentuates the functional consequences of age-related cardiovascular changes. Contributing factors to deconditioning include acute illness, mobility limitations, cardiac disease, depression, and lack of motivation (Miller, 2004).

FOCUS ASSESSMENT CRITERIA

See Tables II.11 and II.12.
Assess for defining characteristics.

Subjective Data

Pain (associated with, time of day)
Pallor, cyanosis, paresthesias
Change in motor function
Temperature change

Objective Data

Skin

➤ Temperature (cool, warm)
➤ Color (pale, dependent rubor, flushed, cyanotic, brown discolorations)
➤ Ulcerations (size, location, description of surrounding tissue)

Table II–11. ARTERIAL INSUFFICIENCY VS. VENOUS INSUFFICIENCY: A COMPARISON OF SUBJECTIVE DATA

Symptom	Arterial Insufficiency	Venous Insufficiency
Pain		
Location	Feet, muscles of legs, toes	Ankles, lower legs
Quality	Burning, shocking, prickling, cramping, sharp, throbbing	Aching, tightness Varies with fluid intake, use of support hose
Quantity	Increase in severity with increased muscle activity or elevation	Decreased muscle activity
Chronology	Brought on predictably by exercise	Greater in evening than in morning
Setting	Use of affected muscle groups	Increases during course of day with prolonged standing or sitting
Aggravating factors	Exercise Extremity elevation	Immobility Extremity dependence
Alleviating factors	Cessation of exercise Extremity dependence	Extremity elevation Compression stockings or Ace wraps
Paresthesia	Numbness, tingling, burning, decreased touch sensation	No change unless arterial system or nerves are affected

Bilateral pulses (radial, femoral popliteal, posterior tibial, dorsalis pedis)

➤ Rate, rhythm weak
➤ Volume normal, easily palpable
➤ Absent, nonpalpable aneurysmal

Paresthesia (numbness, tingling, burning)
Edema (location, pitting)
Capillary refill (normal less than 3 seconds)
Motor ability (normal, compromised)

Risk Factors

Smoking (never quit, years)
Immobility
History of phlebitis
Sedentary lifestyle
Family history of heart disease, vascular disease, stroke, kidney disease, or diabetes mellitus

Table II–12. ARTERIAL INSUFFICIENCY VS. VENOUS INSUFFICIENCY: A COMPARISON OF OBJECTIVE DATA

Sign	Arterial Insufficiency	Venous Insufficiency
Temperature	Cool skin	Warm skin
Color	Pale on elevation, dependent rubor (reactive hyperemia)	Flushed, cyanotic Typical brown discoloration around ankles
Capillary filling	>3 seconds	Nonapplicable
Pulses	Absent or weak	Present unless there is concomitant arterial disease or edema may obscure them
Movement	Decreased motor ability with nerve and muscle ischemia	Motor ability unchanged unless edema is severe enough to restrict joint mobility
Ulceration	Occurs on foot at site of trauma, area of greatest pressure from chronic venous stasis due to valvular incompetence	Occurs around ankle or at tips of toes (most distal to be perfused)
	Ulcers are deep with well-defined margins	Ulcers shallow with irregular edges
	Surrounding tissue is shiny and taut with thin skin	Surrounding tissue edematous with engorged veins

Stress
Medications

➤ Type
➤ Side effects
➤ Dosage

GOAL

The individual will report a decrease in pain.

Indicators

Define peripheral vascular problem in own words.
Identify factors that improve peripheral circulation.
Identify necessary lifestyle changes.
Identify medical regimen, diet, medications, activities that promote vasodilation.

Identify factors that inhibit peripheral circulation.
State when to contact physician or health care professional.

GENERAL INTERVENTIONS

1. Assess causative and contributing factors.

➤ Underlying disease
➤ Inhibited arterial blood flow
➤ Inhibited venous blood flow
➤ Fluid volume excess or deficit
➤ Hypothermia or vasoconstriction
➤ Activities related to symptom/sign onset

Rationale: Different interventions are indicated for different contributing factors.

2. Promote factors that improve arterial blood flow.

➤ Keep extremity in a dependent position.
➤ Keep extremity warm (do not use heating pad or hot water bottle, because the person with a peripheral vascular disease may have a disturbance in sensation and will not be able to determine whether the temperature is hot enough to damage tissue; the use of external heat also may increase the metabolic demands of the tissue beyond its capacity).
➤ Reduce risk for trauma.
➤ Change positions at least every hour.
➤ Avoid leg crossing.
➤ Reduce external pressure points (inspect shoes daily for rough lining).
➤ Avoid sheepskin heel protectors (they increase heel pressure and pressure across dorsum of foot).
➤ Encourage ROM exercises.
➤ Discuss smoking cessation (see Ineffective Health Maintenance Related to Tobacco Use).

Rationale: Arterial blood flow is enhanced by dependent position.

3. Promote factors that prove venous blood flow.

➤ Elevate extremity above the level of the heart (may be contraindicated if severe cardiac or respiratory disease is present).
➤ Avoid standing or sitting with legs dependent for long periods.
➤ Consider the use of elastic compression bandages or below-knee elastic stockings to prevent venous pooling.

➤ Reduce or remove external venous compression that impedes venous flow.
  ➤ Avoid pillows behind the knees or Gatch bed, which is elevated at the knees.
  ➤ Avoid leg crossing.
  ➤ Change positions, move extremities, or wiggle fingers and toes every hour.
  ➤ Avoid garters and tight elastic stockings above the knees.
➤ Measure baseline circumference of calves and thighs if person is at risk for deep venous thrombosis or if it is suspected.

Rationale: Venous blood flow is enhanced by an elevated position and inhibited by a dependent position.

4. Discuss the implications of condition and choices.

➤ Encourage client to share feelings, concerns, and understanding of risk factors, disease process, and effect on life.
➤ Assist client to select lifestyle behaviors that he or she chooses to change.
  ➤ Avoid multiple changes.
  ➤ Consider personal abilities, resources, and overall health.
  ➤ Be realistic and optimistic.

Rationale: The effects of nicotine on the cardiovascular system contribute to coronary artery disease, stroke, hypertension, and peripheral vascular disease (Porth, 2002). Attaining short-term goals can foster motivation to continue to change. Discuss the effects of smoking on circulation and quitting options available.

5. Plan a daily walking program.

➤ Provide reasons for program.
➤ Teach client to avoid fatigue.
➤ Instruct client to avoid increase in exercise until assessed by physician for cardiac problems.
➤ Reassure client that walking does not harm the blood vessels or the muscles; "walking into the pain," resting, and resuming walking improves the oxidative metabolic capacity of the muscle.
➤ Start slowly.
➤ Emphasize that it is not the speed or distance but the action of walking that is important.
➤ Assist client to set goals and the steps to achieve them.
  ➤ Will walk 10 minutes daily.
  ➤ Will walk 10 minutes daily and 20 minutes three times a week.
  ➤ Will walk 20 minutes daily.
  ➤ Will walk 30 minutes three times a week.
➤ Suggest a method to self-monitor progress (e.g., graph, checklist).

Rationale: A daily walking program improves the pumping action of the muscle, which enhances circulation.

6. Teach client the following:

➤ Avoid long car or plane rides (get up and walk around at least every hour, flex feet and bend knees while sitting).
➤ Keep dry skin lubricated (cracked skin eliminates the physical barrier to infection).
➤ Wear warm clothing during cold weather.
➤ Wear cotton or wool socks.
➤ Use gloves or mittens if hands are exposed to cold (including home freezers).
➤ Avoid dehydration in warm weather.
➤ Give special attention to feet and toes.
  ➤ Wash feet and dry well daily.
  ➤ Do not soak feet.
  ➤ Avoid harsh soaps or chemicals (including iodine) on feet.
  ➤ Keep nails trimmed and filed smooth.
➤ Inspect feet and legs daily for injuries and pressure points.
➤ Wear clean socks.
➤ Wear shoes that offer support and fit comfortably.
➤ Inspect the inside of shoes daily for rough lining.

Rationale: Immobility and venous stasis predispose to thrombus and embolus production. Daily foot care can reduce tissue damage and help prevent or detect early further injury and infection. Properly fitted shoes help prevent injury to skin and underlying tissue.

7. Briefly explain the relation of certain risk factors to the development of atherosclerosis.

➤ Smoking

Rationale: Causes vasoconstriction, decreased oxygenation of the blood, elevated blood pressure, increased lipidemia, and increased platelet aggregation.

➤ Hypertension

Rationale: Constant trauma of pressure causes damage to the vessel lining, which promotes plaque formation and narrowing.

➤ Sedentary lifestyle

Rationale: Immobility decreases muscle tone and strength and circulation.

➤ Excess weight

Rationale: Fatty tissue increases peripheral resistance and claudication.

8. Initiate referrals as indicated. Describe community resources available.

Rationale: Community resources can assist the client with weight loss, smoking cessation, diet, and exercise programs.

▼ Impaired Urinary Elimination

Definition

Impaired Urinary Elimination: State in which a person experiences or is at risk of experiencing urinary elimination problems.

Defining Characteristics

MAJOR (MUST BE PRESENT, ONE OR MORE)

Reports or experiences a urinary elimination problem, such as

Urgency
Bladder distention
Nocturia
Dribbling
Hesitancy
Incontinence
Frequency
Large residual urine volumes
Enuresis

Related Factors

PATHOPHYSIOLOGIC

Related to decreased bladder capacity or irritation to bladder secondary to

Infection
Carcinoma
Glucosuria
Urethritis
Trauma

Related to diminished bladder cues or impaired ability to recognize bladder cues secondary to

Cord injury/tumor/infection
Alcoholic neuropathy

Demyelinating diseases
Diabetic neuropathy
CVA
Parkinsonism
Brain injury/tumor/infection
Multiple sclerosis

TREATMENT-RELATED

Related to effects of surgery on bladder sphincter secondary to

Postprostatectomy
Extensive pelvic dissection

Related to diagnostic instrumentation
Related to decreased muscle tone secondary to

General or spinal anesthesia
Drug therapy (iatrogenic)

➤ Antihistamines
➤ Diuretics
➤ Sedatives
➤ Immunosuppressant therapy
➤ Anticholinergics
➤ Muscle relaxants
➤ Epinephrine
➤ Tranquilizers
➤ Postindwelling catheters

SITUATIONAL (PERSONAL, ENVIRONMENTAL)

Related to weak pelvic floor muscles secondary to

Obesity
Childbirth
Recent substantial weight loss
Aging

Related to inability to communicate needs
Related to bladder outlet obstruction secondary to fecal impaction/chronic constipation
Related to decreased bladder muscle tone secondary to dehydration
Related to decreased attention to bladder cues secondary to

Depression
Delirium
Confusion

Related to environmental barriers to bathroom secondary to

Distant toilets
Poor lighting
Bed too high
Siderails
Unfamiliar surroundings

Related to inability to access bathroom on time secondary to

Caffeine/alcohol use
Impaired mobility

MATURATIONAL

Child

Related to small bladder capacity
Related to lack of motivation

Impaired Urinary Elimination probably is too broad a diagnosis for effective clinical use. For this reason, the nurse should use a more specific diagnosis, such as Stress Incontinence, whenever possible. When the etiologic or contributing factors for incontinence have not be identified, the nurse could write a temporary diagnosis of Impaired Urinary Elimination related to unknown etiology, as evidenced by incontinence. The nurse performs a focus assessment to determine whether the incontinence is transient, in response to an acute condition (e.g., infection, medication side effects), or established in response to various chronic neural or genitourinary conditions (Miller, 2004). In addition, the nurse should differentiate the type of incontinence: functional, reflex, stress, urge, or total. The nurse should not use the diagnosis Total Incontinence unless all other types of incontinence have been ruled out. It is incorrect to write Impaired Urinary Elimination related to renal failure. This nursing diagnosis renames renal failure and is inappropriate. For this reason, the diagnosis Excess Fluid Volume related to acute renal failure also would be incorrect. Renal failure causes or contributes to various actual or potential nursing diagnoses, such as Risk for Infection and Risk for Imbalanced Nutrition, and collaborative problems, such as PC: Fluid/Electrolyte Imbalances and PC: Metabolic Acidosis. Impaired Urinary Elimination is currently not on the NANDA list but has been added by this author for clarity and usefulness. The physiologic effects of aging on the urinary tract system can influence functioning negatively when other risk factors (e.g., mobility problems, dehydration, side effects of medications, decreased awareness of bladder cues) also are present. This nursing diagnosis projects biased view of anticipated incontinence in an older adult, with associated use of indwelling catheters, incontinence briefs, and/or bed pads. When this equipment is used, the nurse is not treating incontinence but rather managing urine. The use of such equipment is a short-term solution.

> For these situations, Risk of Infection and Risk for Impaired Skin Integrity would apply. When an older adult has an incontinent episode, the nurse should proceed cautiously before applying the nursing diagnosis label of incontinence. If factors exist that increase the likelihood of recurrence and the client is motivated, the diagnosis Risk for Functional Urge Incontinence related to (specify, e.g., dehydration, mobility difficulties, decreased bladder capacity) could apply. This diagnosis would focus nursing interventions on preventing incontinence rather than expecting it as inevitable. For an older person with the combination of functional and urge incontinence, the nurse would focus on assisting him or her to increase bladder capacity and to reduce barriers to bathrooms, using the diagnosis Functional Urge Incontinence related to age-related effects on bladder capacity, self-induced fluid limitations, and unstable gait.

Key Concepts

GENERIC CONSIDERATIONS

> ➤ The three components of the lower urinary tract that assist to maintain continence are as follows (Porth, 2002):

1. Detrusor muscle in the bladder wall, which allows bladder expansion to increase with volume of urine;
2. Internal sphincter or proximal urethra, which, when contracted, prevents urine leakage;
3. External sphincter, which by voluntary control provides added support during stressed situations (e.g., overdistended bladder).

> ➤ Innervation of the bladder arises from the spinal cord at the levels of S2-S4. The bladder is under parasympathetic control. The cortex midbrain and medulla influence voluntary control over urination (Sampselle & DeLanccey, 1998).
> ➤ The female urethra is 3 to 5 cm long. The male urethra is approximately 20 cm long. The urethra primarily maintains continence, but the cerebral cortex is the principal area for suppression of the desire to micturate.
> ➤ Capacity of the normal bladder (without experiencing discomfort) is 250 to 400 ml. The desire to void occurs when 150 to 250 ml of urine is in the bladder.
> ➤ The sitting position for the female and the standing position for the male allow optimal relaxation of the external urinary sphincter and perineal muscles.
> ➤ Bladder tissue tone can be lost if the bladder is distended to 1,000 ml (atonic bladder) or continuously drained (Foley catheter).
> ➤ Mechanism to stimulate the voiding reflex or Crede's method may be ineffective if the bladder capacity is less than 200 ml.
> ➤ Alcohol, coffee, and tea have a natural diuretic effect and are bladder irritants.

➤ Injury to the spinal cords above S2-S4 produces a spastic or reflex bladder tone. Injury to the spinal cord below S2-S4 produces a flaccid or atonic bladder.

Infection

➤ Static or pooling of urine contributes to bacterial growth. Bacteria can travel up the urethra to the kidney (ascending infection).

➤ Recurrent bladder infections cause fibrotic changes in the bladder wall, with the resultant decrease in bladder capacity.

➤ Urinary stasis, infections, alkaline urine, and decreased urine volume contribute to the formation of urinary calculi.

Incontinence

➤ There are many effective corrective measures for the management of urinary tract disease in older adults, and a positive approach should be taken to minimize the incidence of urinary incontinence (Fanti et al., 1996).

➤ It is important to determine the natural history of the incontinent pattern. A new onset of incontinence is likely to be the result of a precipitating factor outside the urinary tract (e.g., medications, acute illness, inaccessible toilets, impaired mobility that prevents getting to the toilet on time), which can be easily corrected. Incontinence can be either transient (reversible) or established (controllable).

➤ Causes of transient incontinence include acute confusion, urinary tract infection, atrophic vaginitis, side effects of medications, metabolic imbalance, impaction, mobility problems, urosepsis, depression, and pressures sores.

➤ Controllable incontinence cannot be cured, but urine can be planned (Fanti, et al, 1996).

➤ Certain medications are associated with incontinence. Narcotics and sedatives diminish awareness of bladder cues. Adrenergic agents cause retention by increasing bladder outlet resistance. Anticholinergics (antidepressants, some antiparkinsonian medications, antispasmodics, antihistamines, antiarrhythmics, opiates) cause chronic retention with overflow. Diuretics rapidly increase urine volume and can cause incontinence if voiding cannot be delayed (Miller, 2004).

➤ People with diabetes mellitus, which can contribute to increased residual urine, frequency, and urgency, may have decreased awareness of bladder fullness.

➤ Social isolation of people with incontinence can be self-imposed because of fear and embarrassment or imposed by others because of odor and aesthetics.

➤ Depression can prevent the person from recognizing or responding to bladder cues and thus contributes to incontinence.

Intermittent Catheterization

➤ This method maintains the tonicity of the bladder muscle, prevents overdistention, and provides for complete emptying of the bladder.

➤ The initial removal of more than 500 ml of urine from a chronically distended bladder can cause severe hemorrhage, which results when bladder veins, previously compressed by the distended bladder, rapidly dilate and rupture when bladder pressure is abruptly released. (After the initial release of 500 ml of urine, alternate the release of 100 ml of urine with 15-minute catheter clamps.)

➤ The accumulation of more than 500 to 700 ml of urine in a bladder should not be permitted.

Total Incontinence

➤ A cognitively impaired person with total incontinence requires caregiver direct treatments. In institutional settings, indwelling catheters or disposable or washable incontinence briefs or pads are beneficial to the caregivers but detrimental to the incontinent person. Aids and equipment should be considered only after other means have been attempted. In the home setting, the caregiver's needs may take precedence over the cognitively impaired person's. Urinary incontinence is cited as the major reason for seeking institutional care for people living at home (Miller, 2004).

Geriatric Considerations

➤ Urinary incontinence affects 12% to 49% of older women and 7% to 22% of older men living in the community. Its prevalence increases to about 40% in hospitalized clients and 50% in institutionalized clients (Steeman & Defever, 1998). One of the major problems of incontinence in older adults is that it may be overlooked and not adequately evaluated by professionals; as a result, appropriate treatment is denied. Older clients may not admit to the problem because of attitudes about the inevitability of such complications.

➤ Age-related physiologic changes result in decreased bladder capacity, incomplete emptying, contractions during filling, and increased residual urine (Miller, 2004).

➤ Older adults can comfortably store 250 to 300 ml of urine, compared with a storage capacity of 350 to 400 ml in younger adults.

➤ The sensation to void is delayed in older adults, which shortens the interval between the initial perception of the urge and the actual need to void, resulting in urgency (Miller, 2004). Any factor that interferes with the older adult's perception to void (e.g., medications, depression, limited fluid intake, neurologic impairments) or delays his or her ability to reach the toilet can cause incontinence (e.g., problems walking).

➤ Other physiologic components of aging that contribute to incontinence are the diminished ability of kidneys to concentrate urine, decreased muscle tone of the pelvic floor muscles, and the inability to postpone urination.

➤ Frequent voiding out of habit or limiting liquids may contribute to urgency by impairing the neurologic mechanism that signals the need to void, because the bladder is rarely fully expanded.

➤ The diminished vision, impaired mobility, and decreased energy level that may accompany aging mean that increased time is needed to locate the toilet, which also requires the person to be able to delay urination.

➤ Older adults experience urgency because of the bladder's limited capacity and their decreased ability to inhibit bladder contractions.

FOCUS ASSESSMENT CRITERIA

Assess for subjective defining characteristics.

"Do you have a problem with controlling your urine (or going to the bathroom)?"
History of symptoms

➤ Lack of control
➤ Burning
➤ Urgency
➤ Onset and duration
➤ Restriction on lifestyle
➤ Social
➤ Role responsibilities
➤ Pain or discomfort
➤ Hesitancy
➤ Retention
➤ Dribbling
➤ Change in voiding pattern
➤ Frequency
➤ Sexual
➤ Occupational

Adult incontinence
History of incontinence

➤ Is degree of continence acceptable?
➤ Age of attainment of continence
➤ History of weak bladder
➤ Family history of incontinence
➤ Previous history of enuresis

Onset and duration (day, night, just certain times)

Factors that increase incidences

➤ Delay in getting to bathroom
➤ Excitement
➤ Turning in beds
➤ Coughing
➤ Standing
➤ Running
➤ Laughing
➤ Leaving bathroom

Perception of need to void

➤ Present
➤ Absent
➤ Diminished

Ability to delay urination after urge

➤ Present (how long?)
➤ Absent
➤ Diminished

Sensation before or during micturition

➤ Difficulty starting stream
➤ Lack of sensation to void
➤ Need to force urine out
➤ Painful straining (tenesmus)
➤ Difficulty stopping stream

Relief after voiding

➤ Complete
➤ Continued desire to void after emptying bladder

Objective

Urination stream

➤ Slow
➤ Starts and stops
➤ Dribble
➤ Sprays
➤ Drops
➤ Small
➤ Slow or hard to start

Urine

➤ Color, odor, appearance, specific gravity

➤ Negative or positive for glucose, red blood cells, bacteria, ketones, protein

Assess for related factors.

Subjective Data

Fluid intake pattern (type and amount, especially before bedtime)
Dehydration (self-imposed, overuse of diuretics, caffeine, alcohol)
Prostatic hypertrophy
Bladder, vaginal infections
Chronic illness (e.g., diabetes, alcoholism, Parkinson's disease, Alzheimer's disease, multiple sclerosis, CVA, vitamin B12 deficiency)
Metabolic disturbances (e.g., hypokalemia, hypercalcemia)
Fecal impaction/severe constipation
Certain medications (diuretics, anticholinergics, antihistamines, sedatives, acetaminophen, amitriptyline, barbiturates, chlorpropamide, clofibrate, fluphenazine, haloperidol, narcotic)
Multiple or difficult deliveries
Pelvic, bladder, or uterine surgeries, disorders
Environmental barriers
Location of bathroom within 40 feet
Stairs, narrow doorways
Dim lighting
Ability to locate bathroom in social settings

Objective Data

Voiding and fluid intake patterns

➤ Record for 2 to 4 days to establish a baseline

What is daily fluid intake?
When does incontinence occur?
Muscle tone

➤ Abdomen firm, or soft and pendulous?
➤ History of recent significant weight loss or gain?

Reflexes

➤ Presence or absence of cauda equine reflexes

Bladder

➤ Distention (palpable)
➤ Can it be emptied by external stimuli? (Crede's method, gentle suprapubic tapping, or warm water over the perineum, Valsalva maneuver, pulling of pubic hair, anal stretch)

➤ Capacity (at least 400 to 500 ml)
➤ Residual urine (none, present, in what amount)

Functional ability

➤ Get in/out of chair
➤ Manipulate clothing
➤ Walk alone to bathroom
➤ Maintain balance

Cognitive ability

➤ Ask to go to bathroom
➤ Expects to be incontinent
➤ Initiates toileting with reminders
➤ Aware of incontinence

Assess for any

➤ Constipation
➤ Mobility disorders
➤ Depression
➤ Dehydration
➤ Fecal impaction
➤ Sensory disorders

▾ Urinary Retention

Definition

Urinary Retention: State in which a person experiences a chronic inability to void followed by involuntary voiding (overflow incontinence).

Defining Characteristics

MAJOR (MUST BE PRESENT, ONE OR MORE)

Bladder distention (not related to acute reversible etiology)

or

Bladder distention with small frequent voids or dribbling (overflow incontinence)
100 ml or more residual urine

MINOR (MAY BE PRESENT)

Report that it feels like the bladder is not emptying after voiding

Related Factors

PATHOPHYSIOLOGIC

Related to sphincter blockage secondary to

Strictures
Prostatic enlargement
Ureterocele
Perineal indwelling
Bladder neck contractures

Related to impaired afferent pathways or inadequacy secondary to

Cord injury/tumor/infection
Demyelinating disease
Alcoholic neuropathy
Brain injury/tumor/infection
Multiple sclerosis
Tabes dorsalis
CVA
Diabetic neuropathy

TREATMENT-RELATED

Related to bladder outlet obstruction or impaired afferent pathways secondary to drug therapy (iatrogenic)

Antihistamines
Isoproterenol
Theophylline
Epinephrine
Anticholinergics

SITUATIONAL (PERSONAL, ENVIRONMENTAL)

Related to bladder outlet obstruction secondary to fecal impaction
Related to detrusor inadequacy secondary to

Deconditioned voiding
Association with stress or discomfort

 Carp's Cue

Urinary retention is a complex diagnosis that requires specialized interventions. As a beginning student, you should consult with your instructor before using it.

COLLABORATIVE PROBLEMS

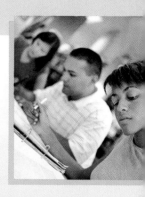

Section III presents 16 specific collaborative problems grouped under seven body system categories and one category relating to medication adverse effects. These problems were selected because they are useful and appropriate for a beginning nursing student. Information on each body system and adverse effect categories are presented under the following subheads:

> ➤ Physiologic Overview
> ➤ Carp's Cues (discussion of the problem to clarify its clinical use)

In addition, each of the 16 specific collaborative problems has the following information:

> ➤ Definition
> ➤ High-Risk Populations
> ➤ Skill Check (physical skills needed to monitor the client's status)
> ➤ Nursing Goals with Indicators
> ➤ Nursing Interventions with Rationale

These specifically direct the nurse to:

> ➤ Monitor for onset or early changes in condition
> ➤ Initiate physician-/advanced practice–prescribed interventions as indicated
> ➤ Initiate nurse-prescribed interventions as indicated

Prompts to consider an important point

Rationale: Explanation of why a sign/symptom is present or of the scientific reason for why an intervention is effective.

▼ Cardiac/Vascular System

Potential Complication (PC): Cardiovascular Dysfunction
PC: Hypovolemia
PC: Deep Vein Thrombosis

PHYSIOLOGIC OVERVIEW

The cardiovascular system consists of the heart, arteries, arterioles, veins, venules, capillaries, and lymphatic vessels. The hollow muscular heart pumps blood to tissues; blood supplies oxygen and other nutrients and carries away tissue waste products such as carbon dioxide back to the lungs. The liters per minute of blood pumped by the heart's ventricles during a given period—*cardiac output*—is affected by the amount of blood ejected with each heartbeat—*stroke volume.* Any change in circulatory blood volume and/or in heart rate affects cardiac output. Disorders of the heart or circulatory system can cause serious, even fatal, hypoxic states.

These three collaborative problems are useful to direct the nurse to monitor for changes in cardiovascular functioning of medical or surgical clients; the problems are appropriate for a first-year nursing student. Other collaborative problems in this category, for example: PC: Dysrhythmias, PC: Pulmonary Edema, are not addressed and are reserved for second-year students.

▼ PC: Cardiovascular Dysfunction

Definition

This collaborative problem is basic to all ill persons. At least every 8 hours in hospitals, every 24 hours in nursing homes, and with each home visit, the nurse will evaluate cardiac functioning and circulation of the person.

High-Risk Populations

Cardiac conditions
Hypertension
Hyperthermia
Posttrauma

Respiratory conditions
Postoperative
Hypothermia

Skill Check

Blood pressure measurement
Pulses (apical, radial, brachial, posterior tibial, dorsalis pedis)
Capillary refill
Use of pulse oximeter

NURSING GOALS

The nurse will detect early signs and symptoms of cardiovascular insufficiency and will intervene collaboratively to stabilize the client.

INDICATORS

Oxygen saturation > 90/60 (pulse oximeter)
Pulse regular rhythm, rate 60–100 beats
Capillary refill < 3 seconds
Peripheral pulses full, equal

Carp's Cue ▶ Compare your findings to the last recorded pulses. Consult with a nurse if rate is increased or decreased more than 10 beats. If person was just walking, wait 1 minute and take the pulse again.

NURSING INTERVENTIONS WITH RATIONALE

1. Obtain radial pulse at wrist. Determine the rate for 1 minute (or 30 seconds two times) or listen to the heart rate at the heart site on chest wall.

   ➤ Is the pulse rhythm regular or irregular?
   ➤ Is the rate between 60 and 100 beats?
   ➤ Is the radial pulse strong, weak, or unable to feel? Use four-point scale.

Four-point pulse force scale:
4+ bounding
3+ increased
2+ normal
1+ weak
0 Absent

➤ Document rate and rhythm (pulse, rhythm)

Rationale: Adult heart rates are usually between 60 and 100 beats per minute. Usually the rhythm is regular. Sometimes in healthy young adults, the rhythm can increase with breathing out (expiration). The strength of the pulse is related to the ability to pump. Using an apical pulse is necessary if peripheral pulses are irregular, weak, or very fast.

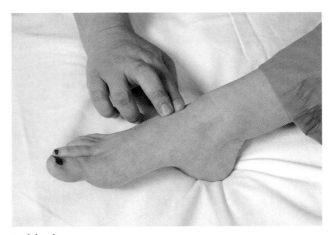

Pedal pulse.

2. Examine both feet.

➤ Obtain dorsalis pedis pulse.
➤ Are they warm and pink?
➤ Press the toenail down between thumb and third finger and then release (capillary refill).
➤ Does the color return before 3 seconds? (capillary refill time)
➤ Document: Capillary refill time greater than 3 seconds indicates inadequate tissue perfusion (circulation).

If the skin is cold or clammy (wet), notify a nurse immediately.

3. Use pulse oximetry if indicated.

➤ Document: pulse ox (-%)

Rationale: Pulse oximetry provides a noninvasive way to evaluate a person's arterial oxygen saturation. Pulse oximetry over 95% is normal.

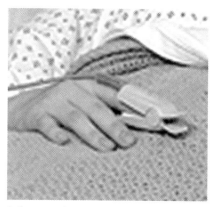

Oximeter pulse.

Pulse oximetry monitoring allows you to evaluate a person's ability to provide himself with enough oxygen during position changes, walking, suctioning, and physical therapy.

4. Take blood pressure. Compare with previous readings.

➤ Document: blood pressure (BP -). Evaluate pulse pressure.

Rationale: Normal blood pressure for adults is systolic more than 90 but less than 130 and diastolic more than 60 but less than 85. The systolic reading is written above the diastolic-systolic/diastolic. Blood represents the force that the blood exerts against the arterial wall. When the heart contracts and pulses blood into the aorta, the pressure on the walls is the highest, that is, systolic. When the heart relaxes after a contraction, the pressure in the walls is the lowest, that is, diastolic. Pulse pressure decreases with fluid loss.

If the systolic or diastolic number is different by 10 mm Hg, consult with a nurse.

▼ PC: Deep Vein Thrombosis

Definition

This problem describes a person with or at risk for deep vein thrombosis. Deep vein thrombosis is the presence of a clot in deep veins, usually in the legs. The clot is the result of slow blood flow, increased blood thickness, and blood vessel wall injury. Deep vein thrombosis may lead to a pulmonary embolism.

High-Risk Populations

Immobility
Obesity
Paralysis of legs
Cancer
Fractures
Heart failure
Orthopedic, urologic, or gynecologic surgery
Varicose veins
Cigarette smokers

Skill Check

Peripheral pulses (femoral, popliteal, dorsalis pedis, posterior tibial)
Auscultation of bruit
Capillary refill
Homan's sign
Application of antiembolic stockings
Urine specific gravity
Urine test for blood
Intake/output measurement
Weight
Isotonic leg exercises
Compression stockings

NURSING GOALS

The nurse will detect early signs and symptoms of deep vein thrombosis and will intervene collaboratively to stabilize the client.

INDICATORS

No leg pain
No leg edema
No pain with dorsiflexion of feet (Homan's sign)
Equal peripheral pulses

NURSING INTERVENTIONS WITH RATIONALE

1. Assess circulation of legs.

➤ Obtain femoral, popliteal, dorsalis pedis, and posterior tibial pulses on both legs.

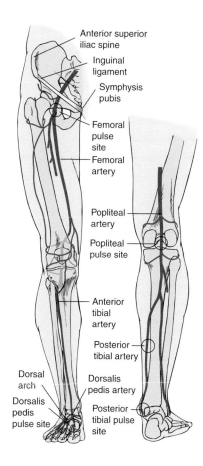

➤ Grade the force of the pulse on four-point scale.

4+ bounding
3+ increased
2+ normal
1+ weak
0 absent

➤ If pulse is weak or diminished, listen for a bruit.

When the flow of blood is partially occluded, the sound of blood hitting the vessel wall is called a bruit.

Rationale: Insufficient circulation will cause decreased pulse force.

2. Inspect for swelling. Measure leg 10 cm below and above the knee. Report if different swelling of one leg (unilateral).

Rationale: Inadequate venous circulation can cause swelling in affected leg.

3. Palpate temperature from feet to thigh comparing spots on one leg with another. Report an increase or decrease of temperature.

Rationale: Unusual warmth and redness are caused by inflammation. Coolness can indicate vascular obstruction.

4. Assess for Homan's sign. Document.

Ask person to quickly flex his foot toward the knee.

Rationale: If the person complains of calf pain, the Homan's sign is positive. It occurs in about 35% of cases of deep vein thrombosis.

5. Assess if leg pain is present.

Rationale: Leg pain results from decreased oxygen to muscle (hypoxia).

6. Evaluate hydration status with urine specific gravity, intake/output, and weight. Document.

Rationale: Decreased fluid volume will contribute to thrombosis formation.

7. Encourage to point toes forward, back, and make circles with foot and to move legs and bend knees to chest every hour.

Rationale: Movement increases venous return to the heart and prevents clots.

8. Instruct not to massage legs.

Rationale: Massage may dislodge clot.

9. If on bedrest, elevate legs above the heart. Do not use knee gatch.

Rationale: This position promotes venous drainage. The knee gatch position can decrease circulation by putting pressure on veins.

10. Encourage smoking cessation.

Rationale: Nicotine can cause vasospasms, which decrease circulation.

11. If prescribed, put on antiembolism stockings while person is lying down. Remove at night.

Rationale: Stockings prevent venous pooling.

12. Monitor for signs and symptoms of pulmonary embolism. Report to nurse.
   a. Symptoms

   ➤ Dyspnea
   ➤ Pleuric chest pain
   ➤ Anxiety/apprehension
   ➤ Cough
   ➤ Hemoptysis (blood in sputum)
   ➤ Diaphoresis (sweating)

   b. Signs

   ➤ Tachypnea (>16 breaths/min)
   ➤ Tachycardia (>100 beats/min)
   ➤ Fever (>99.5°F)
   ➤ Crackles, wheezes, ↓ breath sounds

Rationale: A clot in the leg can obstruct circulation by moving to the heart and lungs. These effects produce hypoxia with a tachypnea response. The local obstruction produces an inflammatory response (e.g., cough, fever, pain, and diaphoresis).

13. Instruct client to report any change in breathing or sudden feelings of apprehension immediately.

Rationale: These can be early symptoms of pulmonary embolism.

14. If on anticoagulant therapy, refer to your pharmacology book.

▼ PC: Hypovolemia

Definition

This problem describes a person with or at risk for decreased fluid volume. Decreased fluid volume can be caused by bleeding, shift of fluids from blood vessels to tissues, prolonged vomiting or diarrhea, high fevers, and extensive burns.

High-Risk Populations

Surgery
Shock
Trauma
Bleeding
Infants, children, elderly
Major burns
Uncontrolled diabetes mellitus

Skill Check

Blood pressure measurement
Capillary refill
Pulses (apical [heart], radial [wrist], dorsalis pedis [foot])
Use of pulse oximeter
Urine output measurement
Urine specific gravity
Adjustments in intravenous (IV) flow rate
IV intake calculation
Intake and output record

NURSING GOALS

The nurse will detect early signs and symptoms of hypovolemia and will intervene collaboratively to stabilize the client.

INDICATORS

Calm, alert, oriented
Pulse regular, rate 60–100 beats/min

Capillary refill < 3 seconds
Oxygen saturation > 95% (pulse oximeter)
Blood pressure > 90/60 < 140/90 mm Hg
Pulse pressure 30–40 mm difference between systolic and diastolic
  blood pressure
Peripheral pulses full, equal
Respirations 16–20 breaths/min
Skin warm, dry
Usual skin color
Urine output > 30 ml/h
Urine specific gravity 1.005–1.030

Inadequate blood volume will alert the body that it needs more oxygen. The body will respond by increasing heart rate, increasing respirations, decreasing urine output, and increasing urine concentration (increased specific gravity) (early signs). If fluid volume continues to decrease, the blood pressure will drop and the pulse pressure will decrease. The skin will become cool and clammy (wet).

NURSING INTERVENTIONS WITH RATIONALE

1. Obtain radial pulse at wrist. Determine the rate for 1 minute (or 30 seconds two times) or listen to the heart rate at the heart site on chest wall.

  ➤ Is the pulse rhythm regular or irregular?
  ➤ Is the rate between 60 and 100 beats?
  ➤ Is the radial pulse strong, weak, or unable to feel?
  ➤ Document rate and rhythm (pulse 85, regular)

Rationale: Adult heart rates are usually between 60 and 100 beats per minute. Usually the rhythm is regular. Sometimes in healthy young adults, the rhythm can increase with breathing out (expiration). The strength of the pulse is related to ability to pump. Using an apical pulse is necessary if peripheral pulses are irregular, weak, or very fast.

2. Examine both feet.

  ➤ Obtain dorsalis pedis pulse
  ➤ Are they warm and pink?
  ➤ Press the toenail between your thumb and third finger and then release (capillary refill).

> ➤ Does the color return before 3 seconds? (Capillary refill time)
> ➤ Document: Capillary refill time greater than 3 seconds indicates inadequate tissue perfusion (circulation).

If the skin is cold or clammy (wet), notify a nurse immediately.

3. Use pulse oximetry if indicated.

> ➤ Document: pulse ox (-%)

Rationale: Pulse oximetry provides a noninvasive way to evaluate a person's arterial oxygen saturation. Pulse oximetry over 98% is normal.

Pulse oximetry monitoring allows you to evaluate a person's ability to provide himself with enough oxygen during position changes, walking, suctioning, and physical therapy.

4. Take blood pressure. Compare with previous readings.

> ➤ Document: Blood pressure (BP -)

Rationale: Normal blood pressure for adults is systolic more than 90 but less than 130 and diastolic more than 60 but less than 85. The systolic reading is written above the diastolic. Blood represents the force that the blood exerts against the arterial wall. When the heart contracts and pulses blood into the aorta, the pressure in the walls is the highest, that is, systolic. When the heart relaxes after a contraction, the pressure in the walls is the lowest, that is, diastolic.

If the systolic or diastolic number is different by 10 mm Hg, consult with a nurse.

5. Monitor intake and output.

> ➤ Maintain urine output at least 30 ml/h
> ➤ Maintain urine specific gravity between 1.005 and 1.030
> ➤ Maintain and adjust intravenous fluid rates according to orders
> ➤ Document output

Rationale: Urine output is the best indicator of adequate fluid restriction.

6. Assess site of intravenous infusion for swelling, tenderness, or redness.

Rationale: Local complications of IV therapy are infiltration (swelling) and inflammation of the vein due to irritation (phlebitis).

7. Notify a nurse immediately if signs of a local complication are seen.

Rationale: Local complications of infiltration and phlebitis can be minimized if identified early.

8. Assess for restlessness, agitation, and change in mental status or orientation.

Rationale: Decreased oxygen to brain can cause restlessness and changes in mentation.

▼ PC: Neurovascular Compromise

Definition

This problem describes a person experiencing increased pressure in a limited space, such as a fascial envelope, which compromises circulation and function, usually in the forearm or leg (Bryant, 1998). Risk factors can either cause internal compression or external compression (Tumbarello, 2000).

High-Risk Populations

INTERNAL FACTORS

Fractures
Musculoskeletal surgery
Injuries (crush, electrical, vascular)
Allergic response (snake, insect bites)
Excessive edema
Thermal injuries
Vascular obstruction
Intramuscular bleeding

EXTERNAL FACTORS

Casts
Prolonged use of tourniquet
Tight dressings
Tight closure of fascial defects
Positioning during surgery
Lying on limb for extended periods

Skill Check

Intake measurement (oral, IV)
Urine output measurement
Urine specific gravity
Adjustments in IV flow rate
Intake/output record
Use of pulse oximeter
Blood pressure monitoring
Pulses (apical [heart], radial [wrist], dorsalis pedis [foot])
Capillary refill

NURSING GOALS

The nurse will monitor for early signs and symptoms of Neurovascular Compromise and will collaboratively intervene to stabilize client.

INDICATORS

Peripheral pulses: full, equal, strong
Sensation intact
No pain with passive dorsiflexion (calf and toes)
Mild edema
Pain relieved by analgesics
No tingling in legs
Can move legs
Capillary refill < 3 seconds

1. Examine the limb or limbs.

➤ Obtain radial or pedal pulse
➤ Is the skin warm and pink?
➤ Press the toenail (or fingernail) between your thumb and third finger and then release (capillary refill)
➤ Does the color return before 3 seconds? (normal capillary refill time)
➤ Document capillary refill time, skin condition, and presence of edema

Carp's Cue ▸ *If skin is cold or clammy (wet) or capillary refill is over 3 seconds, notify a nurse immediately.*

➤ Assess for edema. Document edema as none, mild, or pitting.

Press the tips of your fingers into the area, hold for 3 seconds, and then release. If the depression from your fingers does not rapidly refill, pitting edema is present.

2. Instruct client to report any changes however slight. Determine whether these changes are new and different.

Rationale: Neurovascular compromise often begins as minor sensations; early detection can enable prompt intervention to prevent serious complications (Bryant, 1998).

3. Assess ability to

➤ Move fingers and toes
➤ Feel sensations equally (e.g., both hands, both legs)

Rationale: Compression of nerves can impair the ability to move hands or feet and sense of touch.

 To evaluate light touch sensation, use a wisp of cotton to touch the client's hands, arms, legs, or feet. Have client close eyes and tell you if the sensation is equal.

4. Monitor for signs of Neurovascular Compromise.

Early signs

➤ Unrelieved or increased pain
➤ Pain with passive stretch movement or flexion of toes or fingers
➤ Mottled or cyanotic skin
➤ Delay in capillary refill
➤ Paresthesia
➤ Inability to move toes or fingers

Rationale: Pain and paresthesia indicate compression of nerves and increasing pressure within muscle compartment. Passive stretching of muscles decreases muscle compartment, thus increasing pain. Delayed capillary refill or mottled or cyanotic skin indicates obstructed capillary blood flow.

Late signs

➤ Pallor
➤ Diminished or absent pulse
➤ Cold skin

Rationale: Arterial occlusion produces these late signs.

Carp's Cue ▶ *The key to identifying Neurovascular Compromise before severe compression occurs is to carefully question the client. Ask if there are any new sensations (e.g., numbness). Always compare your previous findings with your present data.*

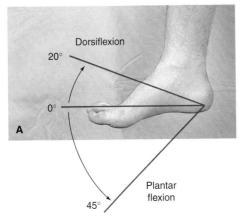

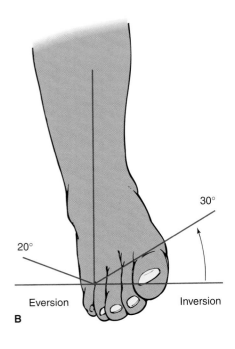

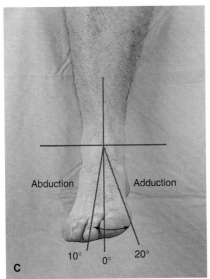

Normal range of motion of the feet and ankles: (*A*) dorsiflexion/plantar flexion; (*B*) eversion/inversion; (*C*) abduction/adduction. (Photos © B. Proud.)

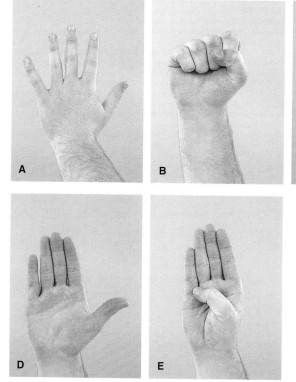

Normal range of motion of the fingers: (*A*) abduction, (*B*) adduction, (*C*) flexion-hyperextension, (*D*) thumb away from fingers, (*E*) thumb touching base of small finger. (© B. Proud.)

5. Report all changes (even slight) in assessment data to instructor.

Rationale: Early detection of signs and symptoms of obstructed blood flow and compression of nerves can prevent permanent tissue damage.

6. Before discharge, teach the following:

➤ How to monitor for circulatory or nerve impairments
➤ Cast care: Consult reference
➤ Skin care: Consult reference

Rationale: The person must continue to monitor for signs of Neurovascular Compromise. Cast and skin care is needed to prevent damage to cast and skin irritations.

▼ Respiratory System

PC: Respiratory Hypoxemia

PHYSIOLOGIC OVERVIEW

Respiratory functioning primarily depends on two systems: the oxygen conduction system and the respiratory center in the brainstem. Consisting of the upper airway (nose, nasal mucosa, pharynx, epiglottis) and lower airway (trachea, bronchi, bronchioles, alveolar ducts), the conducting system conducts and filters air, traps foreign bodies to be expectorated or swallowed, and warms and humidifies inspired air. The lungs consist of three lobes on the right side and two lobes on the left side. Oxygen (O_2) is exchanged for carbon dioxide (CO_2) across the alveolar capillary membrane by simple diffusion and wastes are removed by alveolar capillary membrane by simple diffusion, and wastes are removed by alveolar macrophages. Surfactant and phospholipids secreted by the alveoli prevent lung collapse by reducing surface tension of the lungs. Blood supply to the lungs consists of pulmonary circulation and bronchial circulation.

Located in the medulla oblongata in the brainstem, the respiratory center increases or decreases respiratory rate in response to CO_2 and hydrogen ion (H^+) concentration in the cerebrospinal fluid. The diaphragm is the major muscle of respiration. Additional respiratory muscles are the external intercostals, the scalene, and the sternocleidomastoid. Normally, expiration is passive. Diaphragmatic movement during inspiration and expiration changes the space in the thoracic cavity, allowing the lung to expand and deflate.

The right and the left pulmonary arteries transport deoxygenated blood from the right side of the heart to the lungs. The pulmonary veins transport oxygenated blood to the left side of the heart to be pumped through the body. The bronchial circulation supplies the lungs with oxygenated blood from the nutrition of the pulmonary nerves and the ganglia, arteries, and veins, pleura, and connective tissue.

The mechanism of respiration can be adversely affected by various factors, including foreign body obstruction, excessive or thickened secretions, edema, and poor positioning. Respiratory muscle movements may be impeded because of fatigue, mechanical ventilation, or depression of the respiratory center. Perfusion at the alveolar level can be impaired by compromised cardiac functioning, inadequate blood supply, inadequate oxyhemoglobin levels, or abnormalities in the alveoli (e.g., excessive mucus, tumor).

▼ PC: Respiratory Hypoxemia

 Carp's Cue▶ PC: Respiratory Hypoxemia is useful to direct you to monitor for changes in respiratory functioning of medical-surgical clients regardless of their medical diagnosis. In addition, PC: Pneumonia has been chosen because of its usefulness for a beginning student.

Definition

PC: Respiratory Hypoxemia: Describes a person experiencing or high risk to experience insufficient plasma oxygen saturation (Po_2) because of alveolar hypoventilation, pulmonary shunting or ventilation-perfusion inequality.

High-Risk Populations

Chronic obstructive pulmonary disease (COPD)
Pneumonia
Atelectasis
Pulmonary edema
Adult respiratory distress syndrome
Central nervous system depression
Spinal cord disorders
Guillain-Barré syndrome
Myasthenia gravis
Muscular dystrophy
Obesity
Compromised chest wall movement (e.g., trauma)
Drug overdose
Head injury
Near drowning
Multiple trauma
Immobile
Postoperative

Skill Check

Blood pressure measurement
Pulses (apical, radial)
Intake
Output
Use pulse oximeter (see page 491)

Respiratory rate, rhythm
Auscultation of lung sounds
Assessment of accessory muscles
Capillary refill
Oxygen therapy

 Carp's Cue ▶ *Respiratory function is directly affected by cardiovascular functioning and vice versa. These diagnoses are addressed separately in this book; therefore there is some repetition, for example, vital signs. Both diagnoses can be combined with PC: Cardiovascular/Respiratory Dysfunction. Consult with your instructor before combining these problems.*

NURSING GOALS

The nurse will detect early signs and symptoms of respiratory insufficiency and will intervene collaboratively to stabilize the client.

INDICATORS

Oriented, calm
Heart rate 60–100 beats/min
BP > 90/60, <140/90 mm Hg
Minimal change in pulse pressure
Respirations 16–20 breaths/min
Urine output >30 ml/h
Capillary refill < 3 seconds
Skin warm, no pallor, cyanosis, or grayness
Urine specific gravity 1.005–1.025
Blood urea nitrogen (BUN) 8–20 mg/dl
Carbon dioxide ($Paco_2$) 35–45 mm Hg
pH 7.35–7.45
Relaxed, regular, deep, rhythmic respirations
No rales, crackles, wheezing
Full, easy to palpate pulses
No seizure activity

NURSING INTERVENTIONS WITH RATIONALE

1. Obtain radial pulse at wrist. Determine the rate for 1 minute (or 30 seconds two times) or listen at the heart site on the chest wall.

➤ Is the pulse rhythm regular or irregular?
➤ Is the rate between 60 and 100 beats?
➤ Is the radial pulse strong, weak, or unable to feel? Use four-point scale

Five-point pulse force scale
   4+ bounding
   3+ increased
   2+ normal
   1+ weak
   0 absent

➤ Compare your findings to the last recorded pulse. Consult with a nurse if the rate is increased or decreased more than 10 beats.
➤ Document rate and rhythm (pulse _____, rhythm)

Rationale: Adult heart rates are usually between 60 and 100 beats per minute. Usually the rhythm is regular. Sometimes in healthy young adults, the rhythm can increase with the breathing out (expiration). The strength of the pulse is related to the ability to pump. With respiratory insufficiency the heart rate will initially increase.

2. Examine both feet.

➤ Obtain dorsalis pedis pulse
➤ Are they warm and pink?
➤ Press the toenail down between thumb and third finger and then release (capillary refill).
➤ Does the color return before 3 seconds? (Capillary refill time)
➤ Document: Capillary refill time greater than 3 seconds indicates inadequate tissue perfusion (circulation)

If the skin is cold or clammy (wet), notify a nurse immediately.

3. Use pulse oximetry if indicated.

➤ Document: pulse ox (_____%)

Rationale: Pulse oximetry provides a noninvasive way to evaluate a person's arterial oxygen saturation. Pulse oximetry over 95% is normal.
Refer to p. 491 to see oximeter.

Pulse oximetry monitoring allows you to evaluate a person's ability to provide himself with enough oxygen during position changes, walking, suctioning, and physical therapy.

4. Take blood pressure. Compare to previous readings.

➤ Document: blood pressure (BP -). Evaluate pulse pressure.

Rationale: Normal blood pressure for adults is systolic more than 90 but less than 130 and diastolic more than 60 but less than 85. The systolic reading is written above the diastolic, that is, systolic/diastolic. Blood represents the force that the blood exerts against the arterial wall. When the heart contracts and pulses the blood into the aorta, the pressure on the walls on the highest, that is, systolic. When the heart relaxes after a contraction, the pressure in the walls is the lowest, which is diastolic pressure. Pulse pressure decreases with fluid loss. Refer to PC: Cardiovascular dysfunction for more information on pulse pressure.

 Carp's Cue ➤ *If the systolic or diastolic number is different by 10 mm Hg, consult with a nurse.*

5. Assess respiratory rate.

➤ Normal 12–20 per min
➤ Tachypnea > 24 per min
➤ Bradypnea < 10 per min

Rationale: Respiratory rate will increase normally with fever, anxiety, and exercise and also with decreased circulating oxygen and pneumonia. Respiratory rate will decrease with medication-induced somnolence, diabetic coma, and neurologic trauma.

6. Assess respiratory pattern.

➤ Regular, easy rhythm
➤ Hypoventilation (diminished rate, diminished depth, irregular rhythm)
➤ Hyperventilation (increased rate, increased depth)
➤ Cheyne-Stokes (regular pattern with periods of rapid breathing alternating with periods of apnea)

Rationale: Hypoventilation occurs with overdose of narcotics or anesthetics. Hyperventilation can signify central nervous system dysfunction overdose of salicylate (aspirin) or severe anxiety.

7. Assess subjective respiratory data.

➤ Reports of difficulty breathing, at rest? When eating? Walking?
➤ Breathing pattern: relaxed, labored
➤ Presence of cough, sputum (amount, color)

Rationale: Subjective reports of dyspnea help establish baseline and present condition. Sputum color is usually white with colds. Yellow or green sputum are often associated with bacterial infections.

8. Auscultate breath sounds.

- ➤ Assess upper, middle, and lower lobes
- ➤ Compare right with left (equal?)
- ➤ Diminished? Absent?
- ➤ Presence of adventitious sounds? (crackles, wheezing)

Rationale: Evaluation of respiratory function will provide a baseline and criteria for subsequent assessments.

Auscultation of breath sounds is a skill that takes practice. Always practice auscultation on all your clients even if there is little risk of respiratory problem. Practice on your family and friends. Get to know what normal breath sounds sound like. When you are not sure, always ask another nurse for help.

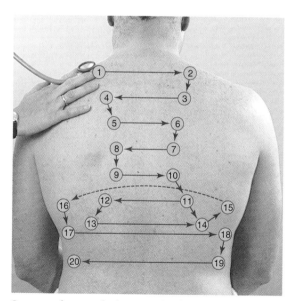

Sequence for auscultating posterior thorax.

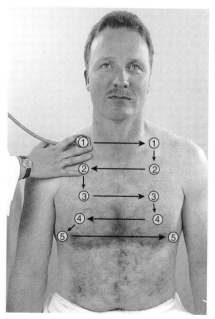

Sequence for auscultating anterior thorax.

9. Evaluate the position of person when breathing and use of accessory muscles (neck muscles)

Rationale: Persons with chronic obstructive lung disease usually lean forward with arms supporting weight to increase breathing capacity. The use of neck muscles is abnormal (other than after stressors like exercise for a short time) in an attempt to increase inspiration.

10. Monitor for signs of acid-base imbalance:

➤ Arterial blood gases analysis: pH < 7.35, $Paco_2 > 48$ mm Hg

Rationale: Arterial blood gases analysis helps evaluate gas exchange in the lungs. In mild to moderate COPD, the client may have a normal $Paco_2$ level as chemoreceptors in the medulla respond to increased $Paco_2$ by increasing ventilation. In severe COPD, however, the client cannot sustain this increased ventilation, and the $Paco_2$ value gradually increases.

➤ Increased and irregular pulse and increased respiratory rate initially, followed by decreased rate.

Rationale: Respiratory acidosis develops as a result of excessive CO_2 retention. A client with respiratory acidosis from chronic disease at first experiences increased heart rate and respirations in an attempt to compensate for decreased oxygenation. After a while, the client breathes more slowly and with prolonged expiration. Eventually, the respiration center may stop responding to the higher CO_2 levels, and breathing may stop abruptly.

➤ Changes in mentation (somnolence, confusion, irritability; changes in mentation result from cerebral tissue hypoxia)
➤ Decreased urine output (<5 ml/kg/h); cool, pale, or cyanotic skin.

Rationale: The compensatory response to decreased circulatory oxygen aims to increase blood oxygen by increasing heart and respiratory rates and to decrease circulation to the kidneys and extremities (marked by decreased pulses and skin changes).

Carp's Cue ➤ *Acid-base imbalance reflects changes in hydrogen ion concentration or the pH of the blood. These changes indicate acidosis (low pH) or alkalosis (high pH). Acidosis is a condition caused by metabolic problems such as renal impairment, diarrhea, diabetes, or inadequate respiratory exchange of oxygen and carbon dioxide (CO_2), resulting in CO_2 retention.*

Alkalosis is a condition caused by an increase in metabolic bases, such as in excess use of antacids, blood transfusions, and total parenteral nutrition, or by a decrease in acids, such as in prolonged vomiting, hypercortisolism, and hyperaldosteronism. Respiratory causes of alkalosis is the loss of carbon dioxide through hyperventilation.

11. Administer low flow (2 l/min) oxygen as needed through a mask or nasal cannula, if indicated.

Rationale: Oxygen therapy increases circulation oxygen levels. High flow rates increase CO_2 retention in people with COPD. Using a cannula rather than a mask may help reduce the client's fears of suffocation.

12. Evaluate the effects of positioning on oxygenation, using arterial blood gas values as a guide. Change client's position every 2 hours, avoiding positions that compromise oxygenation.

Rationale: This measure promotes optimal ventilation.

13. Instruct the client on the proper method of controlled coughing.

➤ Breathe deeply and slowly while sitting up as high as possible

Rationale: Use diaphragmatic breathing. Hold the breath for 3 to 5 seconds and then slowly exhale as much as possible through the mouth (the lower rib cage and abdomen should sink down). Take a second breath, hold, and cough from the chest (not from the back of the mouth or throat) using two short forceful coughs. Uncontrolled coughing is tiring and ineffective, leading to frustration. Sitting high shifts the abdominal organs away from the lungs, enabling grater expansion. Diaphragmatic breathing reduces the respiratory rate and increases the alveolar ventilation. Increasing the volume of air in lungs promotes expulsion of secretions.

14. Teach the client measures to reduce the viscosity of secretions.

➤ Maintain adequate hydration; increase fluid intake to 2 to 3 quarts a day if not contraindicated by decreased cardiac output or renal disease.
➤ Maintain adequate humidity of inspired air.

Rationale: Thick secretions are difficult to expectorate and can cause a mucous plug, which can lead to atelectasis.

15. Auscultate the lungs before and after the client coughs.

Rationale: This assessment helps to evaluate the effectiveness of the client's cough effort,

16. Encourage or provide good mouth care after coughing.

Rationale: Good oral hygiene promotes a sense of well-being and prevents mouth odor.

▼ Metabolic and Immune System

PHYSIOLOGIC OVERVIEW

Metabolic functioning influences all physical and chemical changes occurring within the body. Catabolism refers to the breakdown of ingested substances into simpler substances (e.g., food). Anabolism refers to the conversion of ingested substances to protoplasm for cellular activities and tissue growth and repair.

For proper metabolic functioning, adequate amounts of carbohydrates protein, fats, vitamins, electrolytes, minerals, and trace elements are needed. These nutrients are digested and absorbed into circulating blood and lymph.

Carbohydrates provide the preferred source of energy for cellular activity and are broken down into glucose, fructose, and galactose. Serum glucose levels are controlled primarily by the pancreatic hormones insulin and glucagon. Insulin facilitates glucose transport into cells. Glucagon, which stimulates the conversion of liver glycogen to glucose, is available for release when the blood glucose level falls below normal.

Proteins provide the structural basis of all lean body mass and are required for visceral functions, initiation of chemical reactions, transportation of apoproteins, preservation of immune function, and maintenance of osmotic pressure and blood neutrality (Porth, 2002). Proteins are broken down by gastric and pancreatic digestion into amino acids. Nitrogen remains after protein is metabolized and must be excreted by the kidneys.

Lipids or fats (fatty acids, triglycerides, phospholipids, cholesterol, cholesterol esters) are responsible for insulation and structure and temperature control. Endocrine glands, the pituitary, adrenals, thyroid, parathyroids, and parts of the pancreas secrete various hormones into the bloodstream. These hormones control metabolic functions such as rate of chemical reaction in cells, transport of substances across cell membranes, and growth and secretion. Chemical and neurologic stimuli regulate the release of hormones. Chemical control is accomplished by negative feedback (e.g., a rise or fall of the blood level of one hormone causes a corresponding rise or fall of the blood level of another hormone).

Body fluids contain water and dissolved substances; some are electrolytes. Electrolytes are substances that have positive or negative ions. Each fluid compartment (intracellular, interstitial, intravascular) has a particular composition of electrolytes. If a compartment has too little or too much of an electrolyte, normal functioning of the cells will be affected.

Allergic immune reactions are caused by allergens. Allergens can be inhaled (e.g., cleaning fluids), ingested (e.g., shellfish), or contact skin (e.g., makeup). An allergic reaction requires prior exposure to the allergen. The first exposure causes antibodies to be produced. The second exposure triggers inflammation. The inflammation can be local as edema or hives (urticaria) or systemic constriction of bronchial tissue and laryngeal edema.

These symptoms are very complex. As a beginning student your responsibilities are to assess for abnormal data. Even though you may not know why it is abnormal, it needs to be reported to your instructor or another nurse.

▼ PC: Hypo-/Hyperglycemia

Definition

PC: Hypo-/Hyperglycemia: Describes person experiencing or at high risk to experience a blood glucose level that is too low or too high for metabolic function.

High-Risk Populations

Diabetes mellitus
Parenteral nutrition
Sepsis
Enteral feedings
Corticosteroid therapy
Thermal injuries (severe)
Pancreatitis (hyperglycemia) cancer of pancreas
Addison's disease (hypoglycemia)
Adrenal gland hyper function
Liver disease (hypoglycemia)

 If a person is more at risk for hyperglycemia as with corticosteroid therapy, use PC: Hyperglycemia related to corticosteroid therapy. Remember "related to"'s are not usually needed for collaborative problems because this presence is obviously related to the medical diagnosis. Sometimes when it is not obvious, a "related to" is useful.

Skill Check

Vital signs
Glucometer
Urine analysis strip
IV therapy
Intake
Output
Capillary refill

NURSING GOALS

The nurse will monitor for early sign and symptoms of diabetic ketoacidosis, hyperosmolar hyperglycemia (nonketonic), hypoglycemia, and collaboratively intervene to stabilize the client.

INDICATORS

pH 7.35–7.45
Fasting blood glucose 70–115 mg/dl
No ketones in urine
Serum sodium 1.35–1.45 mEq/L
Serum phosphates, 1.8–2.6 mOsm/kg
Serum osmolarity, 280–295 mOsm/kg
BP < 90/160 or >140/190 mm Hg
Clear, oriented
Pulse 60–100 beats/min
Respirations 16–20 breaths/min
Capillary refill < 3 seconds
Warm dry skin

▼ PC: Hypoglycemia

NURSING INTERVENTION WITH RATIONALE

1. Monitor serum glucose level at the bedside before administering hypoglycemic agents and/or before meals and an hour before sleep.

Rationale: Serum glucose is a more accurate parameter than urine glucose, which is affected by renal threshold and renal function.

2. Monitor for signs and symptoms of hypoglycemia.

➤ Blood glucose < 70 mg/dl
➤ Pale, moist, cool skin
➤ Tachycardia, diaphoresis
➤ Jitteriness, irritability
➤ Incoordination
➤ Drowsiness
➤ Hypoglycemia unawareness

Rationale: Hypoglycemia may be caused by too much insulin, too little food, or physical activity. When blood glucose falls rapidly, the sympathetic system is stimulated to produce adrenaline, which causes diaphoresis, cool skin, tachycardia, and jitteriness (Porth, 2002).

Hypoglycemia unawareness is a defect in the body's defense system that impairs the ability to feel the warning symptoms usually associated with hypoglycemia. Such a client may progress from alertness to unconsciousness rapidly (Porth, 2002).

3. If blood glucose is under 70 mg/dl, report to instructor immediately. If client can swallow, give him or her 1/2 cup of orange juice, cola, or ginger ale every 15 minutes until blood glucose exceeds 69 mg/dl.

Rationale: Simple carbohydrates are metabolized quickly.

4. Consult with instructor or another nurse to administer glucagons hydrochloride subcutaneously or 50 ml of 50% glucose in water intravenously, according to protocol.

Rationale: Glucagon causes glycogenolysis in the liver when stores are adequate. In a client in critical condition who has been in a coma for some time, glycogen stores likely have already been used up, and IV glucose is the only effective treatment.

5. Recheck blood glucose level 1 hour after an initial blood glucose reading of greater than 69 mg/dl.

Rationale: Regular monitoring detects early signs of high or low levels.

6. If blood glucose drops during night, consult with a dietitian to provide a complex carbohydrate snack at bedtime.

Rationale: This measure can help prevent hypoglycemia during the night.

7. Teach signs and symptoms of hypoglycemia to client and family.
   a. Mild hypoglycemia

   ➤ Sudden plunges
   ➤ Tingling in hands, lips, and tongue
   ➤ Cold, clammy, pale skin
   ➤ Tachycardia/palpitations

   b. Moderate hypoglycemia < 50 mg/dl

   ➤ Uncooperative
   ➤ Irritable
   ➤ Often requires assistance

   c. Severe hypoglycemia (central nervous system): <40 mg/dl

   ➤ Incoherent speech
   ➤ Lack of motor coordination
   ➤ Mental confusion
   ➤ Seizure or coma/convulsions

Rationale: Early detection of hypoglycemia enables prompt intervention and may prevent serious complications. Insulin reaction, insulin shock, and hypoglycemia are all synonymous with low blood glucose < 70 mg/dl. Hypoglycemia may result from too much insulin, too little food, or too vigorous activity. Low BG may occur just before meal times, during or after exercise, and/or when insulin is at its peak action.

    8. Teach client to prevent hypoglycemia.

➤ Routine BG monitoring
➤ Scheduled meal plan
➤ BG monitoring before exercise or strenuous activity
➤ Guidelines for decreasing insulin or increasing food before exercise
➤ Awareness of changes in daily routines that may precipitate hypoglycemia
➤ Need to carry some form of glucose for emergencies
➤ Need to plan food intake carefully when drinking alcohol (one to two drinks only)
➤ Need to wear diabetes identification

Rationale: Regular BG monitoring may help to minimize fluctuations in BG levels. Emergency treatment must be available all the time. Diabetes identification is very important to alert others when the person is confused or unconscious.

    9. Teach person and family the signs and symptoms of hypoglycemia and the treatment (e.g., ½ cup fruit juice, ½ cup regular soda, six to seven lifesavers).

Rationale: Quick-acting carbohydrates are needed to increase blood glucose quickly.

    10. If severe hypoglycemia, teach family member how to prepare and administer commercial glucagons (e.g., glucose gels, liquid or injectable glucagon).

Rationale: Gels and liquid are treatments of choice for semiconscious person. Injectable glucagon is indicated for a confused or unconscious person.

The teaching under this problem is limited. All persons with diabetes mellitus will also have the nursing diagnosis: High risk for ineffective therapeutic regimen management related to insufficient knowledge of diabetes, monitoring of BG, medications, meal planning, treatment of hypoglycemia, weight control, sick day management, exercise routine, foot care, risk of complications. Refer to another reference for the specific teaching needed.

➤ Document vital signs, blood glucose reading. Abnormal signs/ symptoms, treatment. Response, teaching.

▼ PC: Hyperglycemia

1. Monitor for signs/symptoms of diabetic ketoacidosis.

➤ Recent illness/infection
➤ BG > 300 mg/dl
➤ Moderate/large ketones
➤ Anorexia, nausea, vomiting, abdominal pain
➤ Kussmaul's respiration (deep, nonlabored)
➤ pH < 7.35
➤ Decreased sodium, potassium, phosphates
➤ Dehydration

Rationale: When insulin is not available, BG levels rise and the body metabolizes fat for energy-producing ketone bodies. Excessive ketone bodies cause headaches, nausea, vomiting, and abdominal pain. Increased respiratory rate and depth CO_2 exertion and reduces acidosis. Glucose inhibits water reabsorption in the renal glomerulus, leading to osmotic diuresis with loss of water, sodium, potassium, and phosphates. Diabetic ketoacidosis occurs in type 1 diabetes (Porte & Sherwin, 1997).

Diabetic ketoacidosis occurs when there is severe insulin deficiency and excess levels of ketones, glucose, fatty acids, and hydrogen ions. When there is insufficient insulin, the body metabolizes fat, which causes ketone bodies to accumulate and increases hydrogen ions, resulting in acidemia. The increased glucose blood levels cause a shift of fluid into the blood stream, causing tissue dehydration and electrolyte imbalances.

2. Consult with instructor or another nurse for assistance in fluid/electrolyte intravenous replacement and insulin and glucose replacement.

Rationale: Diabetic ketoacidosis is a medical emergency. Careful replacement of fluids is needed to prevent congestive heart failure. Hypoglycemia can occur if insulin treatment is not supplemented with glucose.

3. Careful monitoring as prescribed at least every 30 minutes.

➤ Vital signs
➤ Intravenous input
➤ Blood glucose levels
➤ Serum electrolytes
➤ Urine output, specific gravity

Rationale: Accurate assessments are needed during the acute stage (first 10–12 hours) to prevent overhydration or underhydration.

4. Monitor cardiac function and circulatory status and evaluate the following:

➤ Rate, rhythm (cardiac, respiratory)
➤ Skin color, temperature
➤ Capillary refill time, central venous pressure
➤ Peripheral pulses
➤ Serum potassium

Rationale: Severe dehydration can cause reduced cardiac output and compensatory vasoconstriction. Cardiac dysrhythmias can result from potassium imbalances. Document findings.

5. Document mental status, intake, output, blood glucose results, and vital signs.
6. Monitor for signs and symptoms of infection.

➤ Cough
➤ Urinary frequency, burning
➤ Abdominal pain
➤ Purulent vaginal discharge
➤ Red, painful edema/lesions

7. Teach person early signs of hyperglycemia.

➤ Nausea, weakness
➤ Blurred vision
➤ Excessive thirst
➤ Excessive urination
➤ Document presence of any of the above signs or symptoms.

Rationale: Increased glucose in epidermis and urine promotes bacterial growth. The early diagnosis and treatment of infection in a patient with diabetes is necessary because infection is a leading cause of metabolic abnormalities (Guthrie & Guthrie, 1997). Early symptoms of hyperglycemia if treated can prevent ketoacidosis. Instruct person to increase fluids and to seek immediate treatment if blood glucose is above 300 mg/dl.

 ## Renal/Urinary Systems

PHYSIOLOGIC OVERVIEW

The kidneys and urinary system have related functions but also very distinct purposes. The kidneys regulate fluid and electrolyte balance, acid-base balance, and excretion of metabolic waste products. They also regulate arterial blood pressure, erythropoiesis, and vitamin D metabolism. Highly vascular, the kidneys receive the entire circulatory volume 20 times each hour to regulate body fluid composition. Factors affecting renal clearance include age, fluid volume, renal blood flow, glomerular membrane permeability, blood pressure, and cardiac output. The urinary system (ureters, bladder, urethra) serves as a reservoir and conduit for urine from the kidney to elimination through urination. Factors that can affect this function are infections, prostate enlargement, neurogenic bladder, renal calculi (stones), and tumors.

The kidneys are very sensitive to acute problems in circulation or oxygen transport. Decreased urine output is an earlier sign of low blood oxygen than changes in pulse or BP. Remember to carefully monitor hourly urine output in all clients with a risk for bleeding (e.g., postsurgery). You do not need a physician order for hourly urine monitoring. It is a nursing judgment. Persons with severe renal insufficiency are too complex for a beginning nursing student. Consult with your instructor for assistance.

▼ PC: Acute Urinary Retention

Definition

PC: Acute Urinary Retention: Describes a person experiencing or at high risk to experience an acute abnormal accumulation of urine in the bladder and the inability to void due to a temporary situation (e.g., postoperative status) or to a condition reversible with surgery (e.g., prostatectomy) or medications.

High-Risk Populations

Postoperative status (e.g., surgery of the perineal area, lower abdomen)
Anxiety
Prostate enlargement, prostatitis
Medication side effects (e.g., atropine, antidepressants, antihistamines)
Postarteriography status
Bladder outlet obstruction (infection, tumor)

Skill Check (side-bar)

Hourly urine output
Specific gravity
Palpation of suprapubic area
Percussion of full bladder
Urinary catheterization

NURSING GOALS

The nurse will monitor for early signs and symptoms of urinary retention and will intervene collaboratively to stabilize the client.

INDICATORS

Urine output > 30 ml/h
No bladder distention
No difficulty voiding

NURSING INTERVENTIONS WITH RATIONALE

1. Monitor a postoperative client for urinary retention.

Rationale: Trauma to the detrusor muscle and injury to the pelvic nerves during surgery can inhibit bladder function. Anxiety and pain can cause spasms of the reflex sphincters. Bladder neck edema also can cause retention. Sedatives and narcotics can affect the central nervous system and effectiveness of smooth muscles (Porth, 2002).

2. Measure urinary output every hour.

Rationale: Urinary output less than 30 to 40 ml may indicate retention or renal insufficiency.

3. Palpate for a distended bladder. If the bladder is palpable, percuss the suprapubic area.

Rationale: Normally, the bladder is not palpable unless distended. A distended bladder is smooth, round, and firm. If distended, percussion sounds will be dull.

4. Instruct client to report bladder discomfort or inability to void.

Rationale: Bladder discomfort and failure to void may be early signs of urinary retention.

5. Monitor for signs of urinary retention.

➤ Bladder distention
➤ Voiding small amounts

Rationale: Anesthesia produces muscle relaxation, affecting the bladder. As muscle tone returns, spasms of the bladder sphincter prevent urine outflow, causing bladder distention. When urine retention increases the intravesical pressure, the sphincter releases urine and control of flow is regained. Small amounts (30–60 ml) of urine every 15–30 minutes indicate overflow.

6. After the first voiding postdelivery or postsurgery, continue to monitor and to encourage client to void again in 1 hour or so. The first voiding usually does not empty the bladder completely.
7. If the client does not void within 8 to 10 hours after surgery or complains of bladder discomfort, do the following:

➤ Warm the bedpan.
➤ Encourage client to get out of bed to use the bathroom if possible.
➤ Instruct a male client to stand when urinating if possible.
➤ Run water in the sink as client attempts to void.
➤ Pour warm water over the client's perineum.

Rationale: These measures may help to promote relaxation of the urinary sphincter and facilitate voiding.

8. If the client cannot still void after 10 hours, follow protocols for straight catheterization, as ordered by physician/advanced practice nurse.

Rationale: Straight catheterization is preferable to indwelling catheterization because it carries less risk of urinary tract infections from ascending pathogens.

9. If person is voiding small amounts, consult with instructor regarding possible straight catheterization to determine postvoid residual amount.

Rationale: A postvoid residual amount > 200 ml may require an indwelling urinary catheter.

10. If person has chronic urinary retention, see the nursing diagnosis Urinary Retention in Section I.

➤ Document: palpation/percussion findings, c/o discomfort, urine output, intake, catheterization with amount of urine collected

▼ PC: Renal Insufficiency

Definition

PC: Renal Insufficiency: Describes a person experiencing or at high risk to experience a decrease in glomerular filtration rate that results in oliguria or anuria.

High-Risk Populations

Excessive diuretic use
Pulmonary embolism
Burns
Renal infections
Peritonitis
Sepsis
Hypovolemia
Hypotension
Congestive heart failure
Myocardial infarction
Diabetes mellitus
Transfusion reaction
Postsurgical
Renal tubular necrosis from toxicity (e.g., nonsteroidal antiinflammatory
     drugs, certain street drugs, insecticides)

Skill Check

Palpation for edema
Weights
Urine output, urine specific gravity
Intake, output records
IV monitoring

NURSING GOALS

The nurse will detect early signs and symptoms of renal insufficiency and will
intervene collaboratively to stabilize the client.

INDICATORS

Oriented, calm
Urine output > 30 ml/h
Urine specific gravity 1.005–1.025
BUN 8–20 mg/dl
Creatinine 0.6–1.2 mg/dl
Potassium 3.5–5.0 mEq/l
Magnesium 1.84–3.0 mEq/l
Sodium 135–145 mEq/l
Calcium 8.5–10.5 mg/dl

NURSING INTERVENTIONS WITH RATIONALE

1. Monitor fluid status. Evaluate the following:

➤ Intake (parenteral, oral)
➤ Urine output
➤ Other losses (drainage, bleeding, vomiting, diarrhea)

Rationale: If the losses are greater than the input, hypovolemia and renal insufficiency can occur.

2. Monitor urine output hourly. Report if amount is less than 30 ml/h.

Rationale: Urine output less than 30 ml/h indicates hypovolemia and/or renal insufficiency.

3. Weigh the client daily at a minimum; more often, if indicated. Ensure accurate findings by weighing at the same time each day, on the same scale, and with the client wearing the same amount of clothing. (Daily weights and intake and output records help evaluate fluid balance and guide fluid intake recommendations.)

4. Monitor for early signs and symptoms of renal insufficiency: Report any signs.

➤ Sustained insufficient urine output (<5 ml/kg/h), elevated blood pressure
➤ Sustained elevated urine specific gravity
➤ Elevated BUN, serum creatinine, potassium, phosphorus, and ammonia; decrease creatinine clearance
➤ Dependent edema (periorbital, pedal, pretibial, sacral)
➤ Nocturia
➤ Lethargy
➤ Itching
➤ Nausea/vomiting

(Hypovolemia and hypotension activate the renin-angiotensin system, increasing renal vasculature resistance, which decreases renal plasma flow and glomerular filtration rate. Decreased glomerular filtration rate eventually causes insufficient urine output and stimulates renin production, elevating the blood pressure in an attempt to increase blood flow to the kidney. Decreased excretion of urea and creatinine in the urine elevates BUN and creatinine levels. Dependent edema results from increased plasma hydrostatic pressure, salt and water retention, and/or decreased colloid osmotic pressure from the plasma protein losses [Porth, 2002]).

5. Distribute fluid intake fairly evenly throughout the entire day and night. Maintaining a constant fluid balance, without major fluctuations, is essential. Allowing toxins to accumulate because of poor hydration can cause complications such as nausea and sensorium changes.

6. If the person is also at risk for hypovolemia, refer to PC: Hypovolemia in this section.

➤ Document: urine output, other fluid losses, urine specific gravity, intake (oral, IV), all client complaints

▼ PC: Renal Calculi

Definition

PC: Renal Calculi: Describes a person with or at high risk for development of a solid concentration of mineral salts in the urinary tract.

High-Risk Populations

History of renal calculi
Urinary infection
Urinary stasis, obstruction
Immobility
Hypercalcemia (dietary)
Conditions that cause hypercalcemia
Hyperparathyroidism
Renal tubular acidosis
Myeloproliferative disease (leukemia, polycythemia vera, multiple myeloma)
Excessive excretion of uric acid
Inflammatory bowel disease
Gout
Dehydration

Skill Check

Urine output
Urine bedside analysis (e.g., red blood cell, specific gravity)
Straining urine

NURSING GOALS

The nurse will detect early signs/symptoms of renal calculi and urinary tract infections and collaboratively intervene to stabilize the client.

INDICATORS

Temperature 98–99.5°F
Urine specific gravity 0.005–0.030
Urine output > 30 ml/min
Clear urine
Prealbumin 20–50 ml/dl
No flank pain

NURSING INTERVENTIONS WITH RATIONALE

1. Monitor for signs and symptoms of calculi.

➤ Increased or decreased urine output
➤ Sediment in urine
➤ Flank or loin pain
➤ Hematuria
➤ Abdominal pain, distention, nausea, diarrhea

Rationale: Stones in the urinary tract can cause obstruction, infection, and edema, manifested by loin/flank pain, hematuria, and dysuria. Stones in the renal pelvis may increase urine production. Calculi-stimulating renointestinal reflexes can cause gastrointestinal (GI) symptoms.

2. Send urine for culture and sensitivity as ordered; send 24-hour urine for calcium oxalate, phosphorus, and uric acid.

Rationale: Tests are needed to determine type of stone and infection.

3. Strain urine to obtain a stone sample; send samples to the laboratory for analysis.

Rationale: Acquiring a stone sample confirms stone formation and enables analysis of stone constituents.

4. If the client complains of pain, consult with the physician or advanced practice nurse for aggressive therapy (e.g., narcotics, antispasmodics).

Rationale: Calculi can produce severe pain from spasms and proximity of the nerve plexus.

5. Track the pain by documenting the location, any radiation, duration, and intensity (using a rating scale of 0 to 10).

Rationale: This measure helps evaluate movement of the calculi.

6. Instruct the client to increase fluid intake, if not contraindicated.

Rationale: Increased fluid intake promotes increased urination, which can help facilitate stone passage and flush bacteria and blood from the urinary tract.

7. Prepare person for KUB x-ray and/or renal ultrasound.

Rationale: X-ray of the kidney, ureter, and bladder or ultrasound will be ordered to evaluate presence and location of the stone.

8. Monitor for signs and symptoms of pyelonephritis.
   ➤ Fever, chills
   ➤ Costovertebral angle pain (a dull constant backache below the 12th rib)
   ➤ Leukocytosis
   ➤ Bacteria, blood, and pus in the urine
   ➤ Dysuria, frequency

Rationale: Urinary stasis or irritation of tissue by calculi can cause urinary tract infections. Signs and symptoms reflect various mechanisms. Bacteria can act as pyrogen, which may be mediated through prostaglandins. Chills can occur when the temperature set-point of the hypothalamus changes rapidly. Costovertebral angle pain results from distention of the renal capsule. Leukocytosis reflects increased leukocytes to fight infection through phagocytosis. Bacteria and pus in urine indicate a urinary tract infection. Bacteria can irritate bladder tissue, causing spasms and frequency (Porth, 2002).

9. Monitor for early signs and symptoms of renal insufficiency. (Refer to PC: Renal Insufficiency.)

10. When stone constituents are known, consult with physician or nurse practitioner for a referral to a nutritionist. (Specific dietary restrictions may be indicated e.g., low calcium, low sodium, and low protein).

➤ Document: Intake, urine output, results of bedside urinalysis, pain assessment (0 to 10 scale), relief from analgesics (0 to 10 scale)

Carp's Cue ➤ *Pain is a subjective experience. Use a scale of 0 (no pain) to 10 (worst pain experienced ever) to assess pain. After a pain relief measure (e.g., medication) ask person to rate pain again (0–10). Ask person what level he/she can tolerate. If reported pain level is higher than reported tolerable number, consult with physician or nurse practitioner.*

▼ Neurologic System

PC: Increased Intracranial Pressure
PC: Seizures

PHYSIOLOGIC OVERVIEW

The neurologic system, in conjunction with the endocrine system, controls all body functions. Composed of the brain and spinal cord, the central nervous system is divided into three major functional units: the spinal cord, the lower brain level, and the higher brain level or cortical function.

The brain contains four major structures. The cerebrum is divided into two hemispheres with four lobes in each (frontal, parietal, temporal, and occipital). Its functions include maintaining consciousness and controlling memory, mental processes, sensations, emotions, and voluntary movements. Included in these functions are speech, auditory recognition of written and spoken language, and vision. Located under the occipital lobe, the cerebellum controls balance and coordination. The diencephalon consists of the right and left thalamus, which function as conducting pathways for sensory impulses to the cerebral cortex, and the hypothalamus, which controls the autonomic nervous system, body temperature, and water balance and influences appetite and wakefulness.

Brainstem structures include the midbrain, pons, and medulla. The midbrain serves as a nerve pathway of the cerebral hemispheres and the lower brain. All but two of the cranial nerves originate from the brainstem. Cranial nerves III and IV originate from the midbrain; V, VI, VII, and VIII originate from the pons; and nerves IX, X, XI, and XII originate from the medulla. The medulla contains the vasomotor center controlling heart rate and blood pressure. Respiratory centers are located throughout the brainstem (Hickey, 2002).

Consisting of 31 segments, the spinal cord provides conduction pathways to and from the brain and serves as the center for reflex actions. In the peripheral nervous system, cranial and spinal nerves and ganglia control movements (descending pathways) and sensations (ascending pathways). The autonomic nervous system controls involuntary functions through the sympathetic and parasympathetic nervous systems. Sympathetic system responses include increased cardiovascular response, vasodilation, papillary dilatation, decreased peristalsis, temperature regulation, blood glucose increases, rectal and bladder sphincter contraction, and increased secretion of sweat glands and thick saliva. The parasympathetic nervous system acts to constrict blood vessels, constrict pupils, slow heart rate, increase peristalsis, increase secretion of thin saliva, and relax rectal and bladder sphincters.

As a beginning student you will be responsible for monitoring basic neurologic functions such as orientation, vital signs, pupils, eye movements, and use of arms and legs (strength, movement). If a person is at risk for several types of neurologic problems you can use PC: Neurologic Deficits. You will learn more advanced neurologic assessments in later courses.

▼ PC: Increased Intracranial Pressure

Definition

PC: Increased Intracranial Pressure: Describes a person experiencing or at high risk to experience increased pressure (>15 mm Hg) exerted by cerebrospinal fluid within the brain's ventricles or the subarachnoid space.

High-Risk Populations

Intracerebral mass (lesions, hematomas, tumors, abscesses)
Blood clots
Blockage of venous outflow
Head injuries
Meningitis
Post cerebral vascular accident (stroke)
Cranial surgery

Skill Check

Vital signs
Pupil assessment
Swallowing reflex assessment
Range of motion of limbs
Pulse oximeter
Use of penlight

NURSING GOALS

The nurse will detect early signs and symptoms of increased intracranial pressure (ICP) and collaboratively intervene to stabilize client.

INDICATORS

Respirations: quiet, regular, unlabored
Respirations 16–20 per minute
BP>90/60 <140/90
Pulse 60–100 per minute
Temperature 98–99.5°F
Alert, oriented
Pupils equal, reactive to light
Intact motor function
Clear speech
Swallowing reflex intact
Full range of motion in upper/lower limbs
Urine output >30 ml/h
Oxygen saturation (Sao_2) 95–100 mm Hg (pulse oximetry)

NURSING INTERVENTIONS WITH RATIONALE

1. Monitor level of consciousness. Call the person's name and evaluate response: Report any change immediately.

➤ Alert: opens eyes, looks at you, responds appropriately
➤ Lethargy: opens eyes, answers questions, falls back asleep
➤ Obtunded: opens eyes to loud voice, is confused
➤ Stupor: wakes to vigorous shake but returns to unresponsive sleep
➤ Coma: remains unresponsive with eyes closed

Rationale: Cortical functioning can be assessed by evaluating eye opening and motor response. No response may indicate damage to the midbrain.

2. Assess vital signs.

➤ Pulse changes: slowing rate to 60 or below or increasing rate to 100 or above
➤ Respiratory irregularities: slowing of rate with lengthening periods of apnea
➤ Rising blood pressure or widening pulse pressure

Rationale: These vital signs changes may reflect increasing ICP.

➤ Changes in pulse may indicate brainstem pressure by being slowed at first and then increasing to compensate for hypoxia.

➤ Respiratory patterns vary with impairments at various sites. Cheyne-Stokes breathing (a gradual increase followed by a gradual decrease then a period of apnea) points to damage in both cerebral hemispheres, midbrain, and upper pons. Ataxic breathing (irregular with random sequence of deep and shallow breaths) indicates medullar dysfunction.

➤ Blood pressure and pulse pressure changes are late signs indicating severe hypoxia.

Remember pulse pressure is the difference between the diastolic and systolic blood pressure reading. Determine what the client's usual pulse pressure is and use this as the baseline.

3. Assess pupillary responses.

➤ Inspect the pupils with and without a flashlight to evaluate size, configuration, and reaction to light. Compare both eyes for similarities and differences.

➤ Evaluate gaze to determine whether it is conjugated (paired, working together) or if eye movements are abnormal

Rationale: Pupillary changes indicate pressure on oculomotor or optic nerves

➤ Pupil reactions are regulated by the oculomotor nerve (cranial nerve III) in the brainstem.

➤ Conjugate eye movements are regulated from parts of the cortex and brainstem.

Measure pupils size using pupil gauge. To evaluate pupil response to light, darken room. Cover one eye and test the other. Repeat with other eye.

Pupil Gauge (mm)

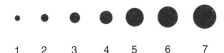

Pupillary gauge measures pupils (dilation or constriction) in millimeters (mm).
(© B. Proud.)

➤ Some hospitals use a preestablished scale to evaluate cerebral function. One scale is the Glasgow Coma Scale. If this is true, consult with your instructor for help on using it.

4. Assess limb function movement.

➤ Ask person to move arms, then legs; assess strength
➤ Ask person to squeeze your hands both at the same time
➤ Ask to kick your hands
➤ Sensation
  ➤ Lightly brush a tissue over arms, right then left, and then legs, right then left.

Rationale: Assessment of movement, strength, and sensation can be used to evaluate cerebral and cerebellar function.

5. Evaluate the equalness and quality of strength and equalness of perception of touch.

Rationale: The comparison of right to left is important to evaluate cerebral function on left and right side.

➤ Note the presence of the following:
  ➤ Vomiting
  ➤ Headache (constant, increasing in intensity, or aggravated by movement or straining)
  ➤ Subtle changes (e.g. lethargy, restlessness, forced breathing, purposeless movements, and changes in mentation)

Rationale: Vomiting results from pressure on the medulla that stimulates the brain's vomiting center. Compression of neural tissue movement increases ICP and increases pain. These changes may be early indicators of ICP changes.

6. Report immediately any changes in assessment data
7. Elevate the head of the bed 15 to 30 degrees unless contraindicated. Avoid changing position rapidly.

Rationale: Slight head elevation can aid venous drainage to reduce cerebrovascular congestion.

8. Avoid the following:

➤ Carotid massage
➤ Neck flexion or rotation > 45 degrees
➤ Digital anal stimulation
➤ Breath holding, straining
➤ Extreme flexion of hips and knees

Rationale: These situations or maneuvers can increase ICP.

➤ Carotid massage slows heart rate and reduces systemic circulation; this is followed by a sudden increase in circulation.

➤ Neck flexion or extreme rotation disrupts cerebrospinal fluid and venous drainage from intracranial cavity

➤ These activities initiate Valsalva's maneuver, which impairs venous return by constricting the jugular veins and increases ICP.

9. Consult the physician for stool softeners if needed.

Rationale: Stool softeners prevent constipation and straining that initiate Valsalva's maneuver.

10. Maintain a quiet, calm, soft environment. Plan activities to minimize ICP.

Rationale: These measures promote rest and decrease stimulation, helping decrease ICP. Suctioning, positioning changes, and neck flexion in succession will markedly increase cranial pressure.

11. Teach to exhale during position change.

Rationale: This prevents the Valsalva's maneuver, which can impair venous return.

12. Avoid sequential performance of activities that increase ICP (e.g. coughing, suctioning, repositioning, bathing).

Rationale: Research has validated that such sequential activities can cause a cumulative increase in ICP (Thelan et al., 1998).

➤ Document vital signs, pupil assessment, muscle movement, muscle strength, light touch sensation, level of consciousness

▼ PC: Seizures

Definition

PC: Seizures: Describes a person experiencing or at high risk to experience paroxysmal episodes of involuntary muscular contraction (tonus) and relaxation (clonus).

High-Risk Populations

Family history of seizure disorder
Cerebral cortex lesions
Head injury

Infectious disorder (e.g., meningitis)
Cerebral circulatory disturbance (e.g., cerebral palsy, stroke)
Brain tumor
Alcohol overdose or withdrawal
Drug overdose or withdrawal (e.g., Theophylline)
Electrolyte imbalances (e.g., hypocalcemia, pyridoxine deficiency)
Hypoglycemia
High fever
Poisoning (mercury, lead, carbon monoxide)

Skill check

Vital signs
Suctioning
O_2 (nasal catheter)
IV monitoring
Intake/output measurement

NURSING GOALS

The nurse will detect early signs/symptoms of seizures and status epilepticus and collaboratively intervene to stabilize the client.

INDICATORS

Respirations 16–20 breaths/min
Heart rate 60–100 beats/min
BP > 90/60, <140/90 mm Hg
No seizure activity
Serum pH 7.35–7.45
Serum P_{CO_2} 35–45 mm Hg
Pulse oximetry (Sa_{O_2}) > 95

NURSING INTERVENTIONS WITH RATIONALE

1. Determine whether the client senses an aura before onset of seizure activity. If so, reinforce safety measures to take during an aura (e.g., call the nurse and lie down).

Rationale: Injury from falling may be prevented.

2. If seizure activity occurs, observe and document the following (Hickey, 2002):

➤ Where seizure began
➤ Type of movements, parts of body involved
➤ Changes in pupil size or position
➤ Urinary or bowel incontinence
➤ Duration
➤ Unconsciousness (duration)
➤ Behavior after seizure
➤ Weakness, paralysis after seizure
➤ Sleep after seizure (postictal period)

Rationale: Progression of seizure activity may assist in identifying its anatomic focus.

3. Provide privacy during and after seizure activity. This will protect the client from embarrassment.
4. During seizure activity, take measures to ensure adequate ventilation (e.g., loosen clothing). Do not try to force an airway or tongue blade through clenched teeth.

Rationale: Strong clonic/tonic movements can cause airway occlusion. Forced airway insertion can cause injury.

5. During seizure activity, gently guide movements to prevent injury. Do not attempt to restrict movements.

Rationale: Physical restraint could result in musculoskeletal injury.

6. If the client is sitting when activity occurs, ease him or her to the floor and place something under his or her head.

Rationale: These measures help prevent injury.

7. After seizure activity subsides, position client on the side.

Rationale: This position helps prevent aspiration of secretions. Allow person to sleep after seizure activity; reorient on awakening. The person may experience amnesia; reorientation can help him or her regain a sense of control and can help reduce anxiety.

8. If the person continues to have generalized convulsions, notify physician or advanced practice nurse and access a nurse to

➤ Establish airway
➤ Suction PRN
➤ Administer oxygen through nasal catheter
➤ Initiate an IV line

Rationale: Status epilepticus is a medical emergency with a 10% mortality rate. Impaired respiration can cause system and cerebral hypoxia. IV administration of a rapid-acting anticonvulsant (e.g., Diazepam) is indicated (Hickey, 2002).

9. Keep the bed in a low position with the side rails up and pad the side rails with blankets.

Rationale: These precautions help prevent injury from fall or trauma.

10. If the client's condition is chronic, evaluate the need for teaching self-management techniques. Use the nursing diagnosis Risk for Ineffective Therapeutic Regimen Management related to insufficient knowledge of condition, medication regimen, safety measures, and community resources (see Section II).

 Should you witness a seizure, stay with person and call for help or ring emergency button in bathroom.

➤ Document: Seizure (see intervention 21), vital signs, treatment

 ## Gastrointestinal/Hepatic System

PHYSIOLOGIC OVERVIEW

A tube extending from the mouth to anus, the GI system also includes the esophagus, stomach, and small and large intestines. Its functions include ingesting and breaking down food particles into small molecules for digestion, absorbing the small molecules into the bloodstream, and eliminating undigested and unabsorbed foodstuffs and other body wastes. Specific hormones (e.g., gastrin, secretin) and enzymes (e.g., pepsin, hydrochloric acid) as well as large volumes of fluid are needed for digestion, absorption, and elimination. Blood supply to the GI tract, through the thoracic and abdominal arteries, comprises about 20% of the total cardiac output, more after eating.

The body's largest gland, the liver, performs various regulatory, digestive, and other biochemical functions. Important functions include carbohydrate metabolism, fat metabolism, protein metabolism, phagocytosis (Kupffer cells), bile formation, vitamin storage (A, D, B complex), iron storage, and formulation of coagulation factors (fibrinogen, prothrombin, acceleration globulin, and factor VII). About 75% of the blood that perfuses the liver comes from the portal vein; this blood is rich with nutrients from the GI tract. The remaining hepatic blood supply comes from the hepatic artery and is oxygen-rich. The hepatic vein provides the only exit pathway. Hepatic dysfunction can involve local enlargement and portal hypertension as well as systemic effects, such as altered blood coagulation and nutritional and metabolic problems.

A small pear-shaped organ attached to the liver's inferior surface, the gall-bladder stores bile for release into the intestines, where it acts in fat emulsification. The hepatic duct from the liver and the cystic duct from the gallbladder join to form the common bile duct to the duodenum.

These three systems are grouped together for convenience in this book. Clinically, you can use either PC: Gastrointestinal, PC: Hepatic, or PC: Biliary to specify the individual system.

▼ PC: Paralytic Ileus

Definition

PC: Paralytic Ileus: Describes a person experiencing or at high risk to experience diminished or absent peristalsis that can cause a bowel obstruction.

High-Risk Populations

Postoperative status (bowel, retroperitoneal, or spinal cord injury)
Hypokalemia
Postshock status
Hypovolemia
Posttrauma (e.g., spinal cord injury)
Strangulated hernias
Uremia
Spinal cord lesion

This collaborative problem is present in all persons after surgery and in all persons after trauma. Early detection can prevent bowel obstructions. Practice auscultation of bowel sounds on all your assigned clients even if they are not at risk. To gain expertise in assessment, practice cardiac, circulatory, respiratory, and bowel auscultation on every assigned client. In fact, practice on your friends and family.

Skill Check

Vital signs
Auscultation of bowel sounds
Intake/output measurement
Urine specific gravity

NURSING GOALS

The nurse will monitor for early signs and symptoms of paralytic ileus and will intervene collaboratively to stabilize the client.

INDICATORS

Bowel sounds present
No nausea and vomiting
No abdominal distention

NURSING INTERVENTIONS WITH RATIONALE

1. Assess bowel sounds in all four quadrants. Consult with a nurse for frequency and report findings to nurse.

➤ Frequency
➤ Intensity

Rationale: Normal sounds are soft and occur a rate of 5–30 per minute. Hypoactive bowel sounds indicate diminished bowel motility, normal after surgery. Absent bowel sounds signify the absence of bowel motility associated with paralytic ileus.

2. In a postoperative client, monitor bowel function, looking for the following:

➤ Bowel sounds in all four quadrants, returning within 24 to 48 hours of surgery
➤ Flatus and defecation resuming by the second or third postoperative day

Rationale: Surgery and anesthesia decrease innervation of the bowel, reducing peristalsis and possibly leading to transient paralytic ileus (Gillenwater et al., 1996).

3. Do not allow client any fluids until bowel sounds are present. When indicated, begin with small amounts as ordered. Monitor client's response to resumption of fluid and food intake, and note the nature and amount of any emesis or stools.

Rationale: The client will not tolerate any fluids until bowel sounds resume.

4. Monitor for signs of paralytic ileus.

➤ Primarily pain, typically localized, sharp, and intermittent
➤ Hiccups
➤ Nausea/vomiting
➤ Constipation
➤ Distended abdomen
➤ Rebound tenderness

Rationale: Intraoperative manipulation of abdominal organs and the depressive effects of narcotics and anesthetics on peristalsis can cause paralytic ileus, typically developing between the third and fifth postoperative day.

5. If paralytic ileus is related to hypovolemia, refer to PC: Hypovolemia for more information and specific interventions.

➤ Document: Bowel sounds, present and number per minute, intake, output, abnormal findings or complaints (distended abdomen, nausea, vomiting, hiccups), pain (location, 0–10 scale)

▼ PC: GI Bleeding

Definition

PC: GI Bleeding: Describes a person experiencing or at high risk to experience GI bleeding.

High-Risk Populations

Disorders of GI, hepatic, and biliary systems
Transfusion of 5 U (or more) of blood
Recent stress (e.g., trauma, sepsis), prolonged mechanical ventilation
Esophageal varices
Peptic ulcer
Colon cancer
Platelet deficiency
Coagulopathy
Shock, hypotension

Major surgery (>3 hours)
Severe vascular disease
Burns (>35% of body)
Daily use of aspirin or nonsteroidal antiinflammatory drugs

Skill Check

Vital signs
Bedside hematocrit
Occult blood test for gastric fluid
pH monitoring of gastric fluid

NURSING GOALS

The nurse will detect early signs/symptoms of GI bleeding and collaboratively intervene to stabilize the client.

INDICATORS

Respiratory rate 16–20 breaths/min
Normal breath sounds, no adventitious sounds
Normal, relaxed, quiet, even breathing
Pulse 60–100 beats/min
Blood pressure > 90/60, <140/90 mm Hg
Calm, oriented
No nausea or vomiting
Bowel sounds present in all quadrants
Stool occult blood, negative
No abdominal pain
Vitamin B12 130–785 pg/ml
Folate 2.5–20 ng/ml
Hemoglobin
   Males 13.18 g/dl
   Females 12.16 g/dl

NURSING INTERVENTIONS WITH RATIONALE

1. Monitor for early signs and symptoms of GI bleeding.

➤ Nausea
➤ Hematemesis
➤ Blood in stool, black stools

➤ Decreased hematocrit or hemoglobin
➤ Diarrhea or constipation
➤ Anorexia (decreased appetite)

(Clinical manifestations depend on the amount and duration of GI bleeding. Early detection enables prompt intervention to minimize complications. Black stools may indicate upper GI bleeding. Blood seen in the stool indicates a problem in rectum or lower colon.)

2. Instruct client to report any changes in the color of their stool and symptoms of nausea or anorexia.

Rationale: The client will be able to report changes to the nurse if explained.

Persons on iron therapy will have dark stools but will test negative for occult blood in stools.

3. Monitor gastric pH every 2 to 4 hours as ordered.

➤ Use pH paper that has a range from 0 to 7.5. Use good light to interpret the color on the pH paper.
➤ Position client on the left side lying down,
➤ Use two syringes (>30 ml) to obtain the aspirate. Aspirate a gastric sample and discard. Use aspirate in second syringe for testing.

Rationale: Maintenance of gastric pH < 5 has decreased bleeding complications by 89% (Thelan et al., 1998). The left side down allows the tip of the nasogastric (NG) or gastrostomy tube to move into the greater curvature of the stomach and usually below the level of gastric fluid. The first aspirate clears the tube of antacids and other substances that can alter the pH of the sample.

4. Evaluate for other factors that affect the pH reading.

➤ Medications (e.g., cimetidine)
➤ Tube feedings
➤ Irrigations

Rationale: False-positive and false-negative findings can result when aspirate contains certain substances. Most investigators recommend a range of 3.5 to 5.0 (Thelan et al., 1998).

5. Monitor vital signs often, particularly blood pressure and pulse.

Rationale: Careful monitoring can detect early changes in blood volume.

6. Consult with physician or advanced practice nurse for the specific prescription for titration ranges of pH and antacid administration.

7. If NG intubation is prescribed, request assistance and follow protocols for insertion and client care.

Rationale: An NG tube can remove irritating gastric secretions, blood, and clots and can reduce abdominal distention.

8. Follow the protocol for gastric lavage, if ordered. Lavage provides local vasoconstriction and may help control GI bleeding.

➤ Monitor hemoglobin, hematocrit, red blood cell count and platelets. These values reflect the value of therapy.

➤ If hypovolemia occurs, refer to PC: Hypovolemia for more information and specific interventions.

➤ Prepare for transfusion per physician/advanced practice nurse order.

Rationale: Consult with instructor for assistance. Doing so can reestablish volume status.

➤ Document: Vital signs, stool color, stool occult blood results, gastric pH results, gastric lavage, NG insertion, intake and output, c/o nausea, vomiting, diarrhea, constipation, anorexia

PC: GI Bleeding focuses on monitoring high-risk persons for early signs of GI bleeding, not the hypovolemia that this bleeding may cause. If hypovolemia is also a risk or is occurring, see also PC: Hypovolemia for interventions.

▼ PC: Hepatic Dysfunction

Definition

PC: Hepatic Dysfunction: Describes a person experiencing or at high risk to experience liver dysfunction.

High-Risk Populations (Thelan et al., 1998)

INFECTIONS

Hepatitis A, B, C, D, E, non-A, non-B, non-C
Herpes simplex virus (types 1 and 2)
Epstein-Barr virus
Varicella zoster
Dengue fever virus
Rift Valley fever virus

DRUGS/TOXINS

Industrial substances
Amanita phalloides (poisonous mushrooms)
Aflatoxin (isoniazid, rifampin, halothane, methyldopa, tetracycline, valproic acid, monoamine oxidase inhibitors, phenytoin, nicotinic acid, tricyclic antidepressants, isoflurane, ketoconazole, cotrimethoprim, sulfasalazine, pyrimethamine, octreotide)
Acetaminophen toxicity
Cocaine
Alcohol
Ingestion of raw contaminated fish

HYPOPERFUSION

Venous obstructions
Veno-occlusive disease
Ischemia

METABOLIC DISORDERS

Hyperbilirubinemia
Heat stroke
Nutritional deficiencies

SURGERY

Jejunoileal bypass
Partial hepatectomy
Liver transplant failure

Skill Check

Skin assessment
Stool color
Stool occult test

NURSING GOALS

The nurse will detect early signs/symptoms of hepatic dysfunction and collaboratively intervene to stabilize the client.

INDICATORS

Blood glucose < 140 2 hours after eating
Prothrombin time 11–12.5 seconds
Partial prothrombin time 60–70 seconds
Aspartate aminotransferase
   Male 7–21 U/l
   Female 6–18 U/l
Alanine aminotransferase 5–35 U/l
Alkaline phosphatase 30–150 U/l
BUN 5–25 mg/dL
Serum electrolytes (refer to laboratory values in institution)
Prealbumin 20–50 mg/dl
Alert, oriented
Pulse 60–100 beats/min
BP > 90/60, <140/90
Temperature 98–99.5°F
Respiration 16–20 per minute

NURSING INTERVENTIONS WITH RATIONALE

1. Assess eyes and skin for signs of liver dysfunction.

➤ Presence of jaundice (yellowed skin, yellowed sclera)
➤ Presence of pruritis (itching)
➤ Presence of petechiae
➤ Ecchymosis (white of eyes).

Rationale: Jaundice of skin and sclera is caused by excess bilirubin production. Petechiae and ecchymosis of the skin are caused by impaired synthesis of clotting factors. Pruritus is caused by an accumulation of bile salts under the skin.

Petechiae (pronounces P-Tee-Kee-I) are small (1–2 mm) round red or purple macular (not a raised) lesion. They are caused by bleeding caused by clotting problems. Ecchymosis (pronounced Ek-a-mo-sis) are larger, round or irregular macular lesions. They are caused by bleeding under the skin caused by trauma or clotting problems. The color can be varied from black, yellow, and greenish hues. If pruritus is present, refer also to Altered Comfort.

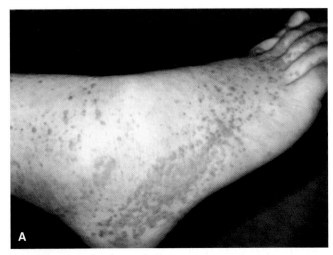

Petechiae. (Dermik Laboratories.)

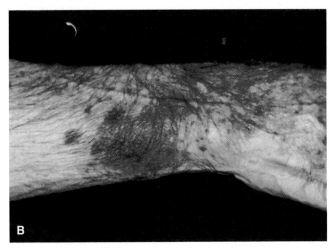

Purpura (hemorrhagic disease that produces ecchymoses and petechiae). (Syntex Laboratories, Inc.)

2. Monitor for signs and symptoms of liver dysfunction.

➤ Anorexia, indigestion
➤ Clay-colored stools
➤ Elevated liver function tests (e.g., serum bilirubin, serum transaminase)
➤ Prolonged prothrombin time

Rationale: Circulatory toxins cause anorexia and indigestion. Decrease in bile in stools cause light-colored stools. Elevated liver function tests indicate liver inflammation.

3. With hepatic dysfunction, monitor for hemorrhage in urine and stool. Refer to PC: Hypovolemia. The liver has a central role in hemostasis. Decreased platelet count results from impaired production of new platelets from the bone marrow. Decreased clearance of old platelets by the reticuloendothelial system also results. In addition, synthesis of coagulation factors (II, V, VII, IX, and X) is impaired, resulting in bleeding. The most frequent site is the upper GI tract. Other sites include the nasopharynx, lungs, retroperitoneum, kidneys, and intracranial and skin puncture sites (Porth, 2002).

4. Monitor for signs/symptoms of (refer to the index under each electrolyte for specific signs and symptoms; Thelan et al., 1998).

➤ Hypoglycemia
➤ Hypokalemia
➤ Hypophosphatemia

Rationale: Hypoglycemia is caused by loss of glycogen stores in the liver from damaged cells and decreased serum concentrations of glucose, insulin, and growth hormones. Potassium losses occur from vomiting, NG suctioning, diuretics, or excessive renal losses. The loss of potassium ions causes the proportional loss of magnesium ions. Increased phosphate loss, transcellular shifts, and decreased phosphate intake contribute to hypophosphatemia.

5. Assess for side effects of medications. Consult with instructor before administering narcotics, sedatives, and tranquilizers and exposing the client to ammonia products.

Rationale: Liver dysfunction results in decreased metabolism of certain medications (e.g., opiates, sedatives, tranquilizers), increasing the risk of toxicity from high drug blood levels. Ammonia products should be avoided because of the client's already high serum ammonia level.

6. Monitor for signs and symptoms of renal failure. (Refer to PC: Renal Failure for more information.)

Rationale: Obstructed hepatic blood flow results in decreased blood to the kidneys, impairing glomerular filtration and leading to fluid retention and decreased urinary output.

7. Monitor for hypertension. (Fluid retention and fluid overload can cause hypertension.)

8. Teach client and family to report signs and symptoms of complications, such as

➤ Increased abdominal girth
➤ Rapid weight loss or gain
➤ Bleeding
➤ Tremors
➤ Confusion

Rationale: Increased abdominal girth may indicate an accumulation of fluid (ascites) caused by increased portal pressure. Weight loss points to negative nitrogen balance; weight gain points to fluid retention. Unusual bleeding indicates decreased prothrombin time and clotting factors. Tremors can result from impaired neurotransmission because of failure of the liver to detoxify enzymes that act as false neurotransmitters. Confusion can result from cerebral hypoxia caused by high serum ammonia levels resulting from the liver's impaired ability to convert ammonia to urea.

➤ Document: vital signs, skin color, sclera color, presence of petechiae and/or ecchymosis, color of stools, stool occult results, presence of blood in urine, complaints of bleeding, nausea, itching

▽ Musculoskeletal System

PHYSIOLOGIC OVERVIEW

Providing the support structure for the body and housing all the body systems, the skeletal system contains 206 bones as well as ligaments (which provide stability to joints) and tendons (which connect bone to muscle). Besides their structural function, bones also provide a site for red blood cell production and mineral—especially calcium—storage. Joints, the unions between two or more bones, are classified as fibrous (e.g., distal tibiofibular junction), cartilaginous (e.g., symphysis pubis), or synovial (e.g., wrist bones). Cartilage, a connective tissue, provides support and facilitates movement in joints, while also absorbing shock.

Skeletal muscles serve important functions in movement, posture, and heat production. Each skeletal muscle is composed of many elongated multinucleated muscle fibers, through which run slender protein threads known as myofibrils. Motor impulses transmitted from the brain through peripheral motor nerves trigger neurochemical mechanisms—acetylcholine release, calcium release, adenosine triphosphate release—that in turn control muscle traction and relaxation.

Musculoskeletal injuries are common and range from mild to severe. Although not usually life threatening, disorders of this system, especially when chronic, can adversely affect a person's ability to perform all activities of daily living.

Fractures from trauma are not collaborative problems but rather a condition that has collaborative problems like PC: Neurovascular Compromise, PC: Fat Embolism, or PC: Bleeding. There are also associated nursing diagnoses as Acute Pain, Self-Care Deficit, and Risk for Impaired Self Integrity. Do not use PC: Fractures. Pathologic fractures are

not caused by trauma but by defects in the bone structure as osteoporosis or cancer. PC: Pathologic Fractures is correct as a collaborative problem. As a beginning student, this may be too advanced for you. Consult with your instructor.

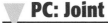 # PC: Joint Dislocation

Definition

PC: Joint Dislocation: Describes a person experiencing or at high risk to experience displacement of a bone from its position in a joint.

High-Risk Populations

Total hip replacement
Total knee replacement
Fractured hip, knee, shoulder

Skill Check

Correct positioning of joint postsurgery
Use of abduction pillows for turning

NURSING GOALS

The nurse will detect early signs and symptoms of dislocation (hip, knee) and will collaboratively intervene to stabilize the client.

INDICATORS

Hip in abduction or neutral rotation
Legs' length even
Knee in neutral position

NURSING INTERVENTIONS WITH RATIONALE

1. Maintain correct positioning (Altizer, 1998).

   ➤ Hip: Maintain the hip in abduction, neutral rotation, or slight external rotation.

➤ Hip: Avoid hip flexion over 60 degrees.
➤ Knee: Slightly elevated from hip; avoid using bed knee gatch or placing pillows under the knee (to prevent flexion contractures). Place pillows under the calf.

Rationale: Specific positions are used to prevent prosthesis dislocation.

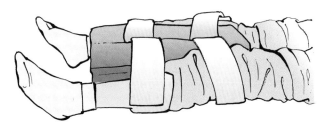

An abduction pillow may be used after a total hip replacement to prevent dislocation of the prosthesis.

2. Assess for signs of joint (hip, knee) dislocation.

➤ Hip
  ➤ Acute groin pain in operative hip
  ➤ Shortening of leg with external rotation
➤ Hip, knee, shoulder
  ➤ "Popping" sound heard by client
  ➤ Bulge at surgical site
  ➤ Inability to move
  ➤ Pain with mobility

Rationale: As the surrounding muscles and joint capsule heal, joint dislocation may occur if positioning exceeds the limits of the prosthesis, as in flexing or hyperextending the knee or abducting the hip > 45 degrees.

3. Immediately report any signs of dislocation.

Rationale: Dislocation will put pressure on nerves and blood vessels, which can cause Neurovascular Compromise. Refer to PC: Neurovascular Compromise if indicated.

4. Maintain bed rest as ordered. Keep the affected joint in neutral position with rolls, pillows, or specified devices. (Bed rest typically is ordered for 1 to 3 days after surgery to allow stabilization of the prosthesis.)
5. Help to turn toward either side unless contraindicated. Always maintain an abduction pillow when turning; limit the use of the Fowler's position.

Rationale: If proper positioning is maintained, including the abduction pillow, clients may safely be turned toward the operative and nonoperative side. This promotes circulation and decreases the potential for pressure ulcer formation as a result of immobility. A prolonged Fowler's position can dislocate the prosthesis (Salmond, 1996).

6. Monitor for shoulder joint dislocation/subluxation.

Rationale: Total shoulder arthroplasty has a higher risk of joint dislocation/subluxation because the shoulder is capable of movement in three planes (flexion/extension, abduction/adduction, internal/external rotation; Altizer, 1998).

➤ Document: Positions of joint, complaints of acute pain, changes at joint, inability to move, changes in leg lengths.

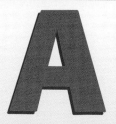

appendix

A

Nursing Admission Database

Date _____ Arrival Time _____ Contact Person _____ Phone _____

ADMITTED FROM: _____ Home alone _____ Home with relative _____ Long-term care facility

_____ Homeless _____ Home with _____

(Specify)

_____ ER _____ Other _____

MODE OF ARRIVAL: _____ Wheelchair _____ Ambulance _____ Stretcher

REASON FOR HOSPITALIZATION: _____

_____

_____

LAST HOSPITAL ADMISSION: Date _____ Reason _____

PAST MEDICAL HISTORY: _____

_____

MEDICATION (Prescription/Over-the-Counter)	DOSAGE	LAST DOSE	FREQUENCY

HEALTH MAINTENANCE-PERCEPTION PATTERN

USE OF:

Tobacco: _____ None _____ Quit (date) _____ Pipe _____ Cigar _____ <1 pk/day

_____ 1–2 pks/day _____ >2 pks/day Pks/year history _____

Alcohol: _____ Date of last drink _____ Amount/type

_____ No. of days in a month when alcohol is consumed

Other Drugs: _____ No _____ Yes Type _____ Use _____

Allergies (drugs, food, tape, dyes): _____ Reaction _____

Exercise _____ None _____ Specify _____

ACTIVITY-EXERCISE PATTERN

SELF-CARE ABILITY:

0 = Independent 1 = Assistive device 2 = Assistance from others

3 = Assistance from person and equipment 4 = Dependent/Unable

	0	1	2	3	4
Eating/Drinking					
Bathing					
Dressing/Grooming					
Toileting					
Bed Mobility					
Transferring					
Ambulating					
Stair Climbing					
Shopping					
Cooking					
Home Maintenance					

ASSISTIVE DEVICES: _____ None _____ Crutches _____ Bedside commode _____ Walker

_____ Cane _____ Splint/Brace _____ Wheelchair _____ Other

Side One

NUTRITION–METABOLIC PATTERN

Special Diet/Supplements _____

Previous Dietary Instruction: _____ Yes _____ No

Appetite: _____ Normal _____ Increased _____ Decreased _____ Decreased taste sensation
_____ Nausea _____ Vomiting

Weight Fluctuations Last 6 Months: _____ None _____ lbs. Gained/lost

Swallowing difficulty: _____ None _____ Solids _____ Liquids

Dentures: _____ Upper (_ Partial _ Full) _____ Lower (_ Partial _ Full) _____ None
With Person _____ Yes _____ No

History of Skin/Healing Problems: _____ None _____ Abnormal Healing _____ Rash
_____ Dryness _____ Excess Perspiration _____ Latex Allergy

ELIMINATION PATTERN

Bowel Habits: _____ # BMs/day _____ Date of last BM _____ Within normal limits
_____ Constipation _____ Diarrhea _____ Incontinence
_____ Ostomy: Type: _____ Appliance _____ Self-care _____ Yes _____ No

Bladder Habits: _____ WNL _____ Frequency _____ Dysuria _____ Nocturia _____ Urgency
_____ Hematuria _____ Retention

Incontinence: _____ No _____ Yes _____ Total _____ Daytime _____ Nighttime
_____ Occasional _____ Difficulty delaying voiding
_____ Difficulty reaching toilet

Assistive Devices: _____ Intermittent catheterization
_____ Indwelling catheter _____ External catheter
_____ Incontinent briefs _____ Penile implant type _____

SLEEP–REST PATTERN

Habits: _____ hrs/night _____ AM nap _____ PM nap
Feel rested after sleep _____ Yes _____ No

Problems: _____ None _____ Early waking _____ Insomnia _____ Nightmares

COGNITIVE–PERCEPTUAL PATTERN

Mental Status: _____ Alert _____ Receptive aphasia _____ Poor historian
_____ Oriented _____ Confused _____ Combative _____ Unresponsive

Speech: _____ Normal _____ Slurred _____ Garbled _____ Expressive aphasia
Spoken language _____ Interpreter _____

Language spoken: _____ English _____ Spanish _____ Other _____

Ability to Read English: _____ Yes _____ No _____

Ability to Communicate: _____ Yes _____ No _____

Ability to Comprehend: _____ Yes _____ No _____

Level of Anxiety: _____ Mild _____ Moderate _____ Severe _____ Panic

Interactive Skills: _____ Appropriate _____ Other _____

Hearing: _____ WNL _____ Impaired (_ Right _Left) _____ Deaf (_ Right _Left)
_____ Hearing Aid

Vision: _____ WNL _____ Eyeglasses _____ Contact lens
_____ Impaired _____ Right _____ Left
_____ Blind _____ Right _____ Left
_____ Prosthesis _____ Right _____ Left

Vertigo: _____ Yes _____ No Memory intact _____ Yes _____ No

Discomfort/Pain: _____ None _____ Acute _____ Chronic _____ Description _____

Pain Management: _____

COPING–STRESS TOLERANCE/SELF-PERCEPTION/SELF-CONCEPT PATTERN

Major concerns regarding hospitalization or illness (financial, self-care): _____
_____

Major loss/change in past year: _____ No _____ Yes _____

Fear of violence _____ Yes _____ No Who _____

Outlook on future _____ (rate 1–poor to 10–very optimistic)

SEXUALITY–REPRODUCTIVE PATTERN

LMP: _____ Gravida _____ Para _____

Menstrual/Hormonal Problems: _____ Yes _____ No _____

Last Pap Smear: _____ Hx of Abnormal Pap _____

Monthly Self-Breast/Testicular Exam: _____ Yes _____ No Last Mammogram: _____

Sexual Concerns: _____

ROLE–RELATIONSHIP PATTERN

Marital Status: _____

Occupation: _____

Employment Status: _____ Employed _____ Short-term disability
_____ Long-term disability _____ Unemployed

Support System: _____ Spouse _____ Neighbors/Friends _____ None
_____ Family in same residence _____ Family in separate residence
_____ Other _____

Family concerns regarding hospitalization: _____

VALUE–BELIEF PATTERN

Religion: _____

Religious Restrictions: _____ No _____ Yes (Specify) _____

Request Chaplain Visitation at This Time: _____ Yes _____ No

PHYSICAL ASSESSMENT (Objective)

1. CLINICAL DATA

Age _____ Height _____ Weight _____ (Actual/Approximate)

Temperature _____

Pulse: _____ Strong _____ Weak _____ Regular _____ Irregular

Blood Pressure: _____

2. RESPIRATORY/CIRCULATORY

Rate _____

Quality: _____ WNL _____ Shallow _____ Rapid _____ Labored _____ Other _____

Cough: _____ No _____ Yes/Describe _____

Auscultation

Upper rt lobes _____	WNL _____	Decreased _____	Absent _____	Abnormal sounds _____
Upper lt lobes _____	WNL _____	Decreased _____	Absent _____	Abnormal sounds _____
Lower rt lobes _____	WNL _____	Decreased _____	Absent _____	Abnormal sounds _____
Lower lt lobes _____	WNL _____	Decreased _____	Absent _____	Abnormal sounds _____

Right Pedal Pulse: _____ Strong _____ Weak _____ Absent

Left Pedal Pulse: _____ Strong _____ Weak _____ Absent

3. METABOLIC–INTEGUMENTARY

SKIN:

Color: _____ WNL _____ Pale _____ Cyanotic _____ Ashen _____ Jaundice _____ Other _____

Temperature: _____ WNL _____ Warm _____ Cool

Turgor: _____ WNL _____ Poor

Edema: _____ No _____ Yes/Description/location _____

Lesions: _____ None _____ Yes/Description/location _____

Bruises: _____ None _____ Yes/Description/location _____

Reddened: _____ No _____ Yes/Description/location _____

Pruritus: _____ No _____ Yes/Description/location _____

Tubes: _____ Specify _____

Changes _____ None, If Yes/Description/location _____

MOUTH:

Gums: _____ WNL _____ White plaque _____ Lesions _____ Other _____

Teeth: _____ WNL _____ Other _____

ABDOMEN:

Bowel Sounds: _____ Present _____ Absent

4. NEURO/SENSORY

Pupils: _____ Equal _____ Unequal

Left: • • • • • • ● ●

Right: • • • • • • ● ●

Reactive to light:

Left: _____ Yes _____ No/Specify _____

Right: _____ Yes _____ No/Specify _____

Eyes: _____ Clear _____ Draining _____ Reddened _____ Other _____

5. MUSCULAR–SKELETAL

Range of Motion: _____ Full _____ Other _____

Balance and Gait: _____ Steady _____ Unsteady

Hand Grasps: _____ Equal _____ Strong _____ Weakness/Paralysis (__ Right __Left)

Leg Muscles: _____ Equal _____ Strong _____ Weakness/Paralysis (__ Right __Left)

DISCHARGE PLANNING

Lives: Alone _____ With _____ No known residence _____

Intended Destination Post-Discharge: _____ Home _____ Undetermined _____ Other _____

Previous Utilization of Community Resources:

_____ Home care/Hospice _____ Adult day care _____ Church groups _____ Other _____

_____ Meals on Wheels _____ Homemaker/Home health aide _____ Community support group

Post-discharge Transportation:

_____ Car _____ Ambulance _____ Bus/Taxi

_____ Unable to determine at this time

Anticipated Financial Assistance Post-discharge?: _____ No _____ Yes _____

Anticipated Problems with Self-care Post-discharge?: _____ No _____ Yes _____

Assistive Devices Needed Post-discharge?: _____ No _____ Yes _____

Referrals: (record date)

Discharge Coordinator _____ Home Health _____

Social Service _____ V.N.A. _____

Other Comments: _____

_____

SIGNATURE/TITLE _____ Date _____

This care plan (Level I) presents nursing diagnoses and collaborative problems that commonly apply to clients (and their significant others) undergoing hospitalization for any medical disorder. Nursing diagnoses and collaborative problems specific to a disorder are presented in the care plan (Level II) for that disorder.

DIAGNOSTIC CLUSTER

Collaborative Problems

PC: Cardiovascular Dysfunction

PC: Respiratory Insufficiency

Nursing Diagnoses

Anxiety related to unfamiliar environment, routines, diagnostic tests, treatments, and loss of control

Risk for Injury related to unfamiliar environment and physical and mental limitations secondary to condition, medications, therapies, and diagnostic tests

Risk for Infection related to increased microorganisms in environment, risk of person-to-person transmission, and invasive tests and therapies

(Specify) Self-Care Deficit related to sensory, cognitive, mobility, endurance, or motivation problems

Risk for Imbalanced Nutrition: Less Than Body Requirements related to decreased appetite secondary to treatments, fatigue, environment, and changes in usual diet and to increased protein and vitamin requirements for healing

Risk for Constipation related to change in fluid and food intake, routine, and activity level; effects of medications; and emotional stress

Risk for Impaired Skin Integrity R/T prolonged pressure on tissues associated with decreased mobility, increased fragility of the skin associated with dependent edema, decreased tissue perfusion, malnutrition, and urinary/fecal incontinence

Disturbed Sleep Pattern related to unfamiliar noisy environment, change in bedtime ritual, emotional stress, and change in circadian rhythm

Risk for Spiritual Distress related to separation from religious support system, lack of privacy, or inability to practice spiritual rituals

Interrupted Family Processes related to disruption of routines, change in role responsibilities, and fatigue associated with increased workload and visiting hour requirements

Risk for Ineffective Therapeutic Regimen Management related to complexity and cost of therapeutic regimen, complexity of health care system, shortened length of stay, insufficient knowledge of treatment and barriers to comprehension secondary to language barriers, cognitive deficits, hearing and/or visual impairment, anxiety, and lack of motivation

Discharge Criteria

Specific discharge criteria vary depending on the client's condition. Generally, all diagnoses in the above diagnostic cluster should be resolved before discharge.

Collaborative Problems

PC: Cardiovascular Dysfunction

PC: Respiratory Insufficiency

Nursing Goal

The nurse will detect early signs and symptoms of (a) cardiovascular dysfunction and (b) respiratory insufficiency and will intervene collaboratively to stabilize the client.

Indicators

➤ Calm, alert, oriented (a, b)
➤ Respirations 16–20 beats/min (b)
➤ Respirations relaxed and rhythmic (b)
➤ Breath sounds present all lobes (b)
➤ No rales or wheezing (b)
➤ Pulse 60–100 beats/min (a, b)
➤ BP >90/60, <140/90 mm Hg (a, b)
➤ Capillary refill < 3 seconds (a)
➤ Peripheral pulses full, equal (a)
➤ Skin warm and dry (a, b)
➤ Temperature 98.5–99°F (a, b)

Interventions	Rationales
1. Monitor cardiovascular status	1. Physiologic mechanisms governing cardiovascular function are very sensitive to any changes in body function, making changes in cardiovascular status important clinical indicators.
a. Radial pulse (rate and rhythm)	a. Pulse monitoring provides data to detect cardiac dysrhythmias, blood volume changes, and circulatory impairment.
b. Apical pulse (rate and rhythm)	b. Apical pulse monitoring is indicated if the client's peripheral pulses are irregular, weak, or extremely rapid.
c. Blood pressure	c. Blood pressure represents the force that the blood exerts against the arterial walls. Hypertension (systolic pressure > 140 mm Hg, diastolic pressure > 85 mm Hg) may indicate increased peripheral resistance, cardiac output, blood volume, or blood viscosity. Hypotension can result from significant blood or fluid loss, decreased cardiac output, and certain medications.
d. Skin (color, temperature, moisture) and temperature	d. Skin assessment provides information evaluating circulation, body temperature, and hydration status.
e. Pulse oximetry	

2. Monitor respiratory status
   a. Rate
   b. Rhythm
   c. Breath sounds
	2. Respiratory assessment provides essential data for evaluating the effectiveness of breathing and detecting adventitious or abnormal sounds, which may indicate airway moisture, narrowing, or obstruction.

Related Physician-Prescribed Interventions

Dependent on the underlying pathology

Documentation

Flow records
  Pulse rate and rhythm
  Blood pressure
  Respiratory assessment
Progress notes
  Abnormal findings
  Interventions

Nursing Diagnoses

Anxiety Related to Unfamiliar Environment, Routines, Diagnostic Tests, Treatments, and Loss of Control

Goal

The client will communicate feelings regarding the condition and hospitalization.

Indicators

➤ Verbalize, if asked, what to expect regarding routines and procedures.
➤ Explain restrictions.

Interventions	Rationales
1. Introduce yourself and other members of the health care team, and orient the client to the room (e.g., bed controls, call bell, bathroom).	1. A smooth professional admission process and warm introduction can put a client at ease and set a positive tone for his or her hospital stay.
2. Explain hospital policies and routines. a. Visiting hours b. Mealtimes and availability of snacks c. Vital sign monitoring d. Availability of newspapers e. Television rental and operation f. Storage of valuables g. Telephone use h. Smoking policy i. Policy for off-unit trips	2,3. Providing accurate information can help decrease the client's anxiety associated with the unknown and unfamiliar.

(continued)

Interventions	**Rationales**

3. Determine the client's knowledge of his or her condition, its prognosis, and treatment measures. Reinforce and supplement the physician's explanations as necessary.

4. Explain any scheduled diagnostic tests, covering the following:
   a. Description
   b. Purpose
   c. Pre-test routines
   d. Who will perform the procedure and where
   e. Expected sensations
   f. Post-test routines
   g. Availability of results

5. Discuss all prescribed medications:
   a. Name and type
   b. Purpose
   c. Dosage
   d. Special precautions
   e. Side effects

6. Explain any prescribed diet:
   a. Purpose
   b. Duration
   c. Allowed and prohibited foods

7. Provide the client with opportunities to make decisions about his or her care, whenever possible.

8. Provide reassurance and comfort. Spend time with the client, encourage him or her to share feelings and concerns, listen attentively, and convey empathy and understanding.

Rationales

4–6. Teaching the client about tests and treatment measures can help decrease his or her fear and anxiety associated with the unknown and improve his or her sense of control over the situation.

7. Participating in decision making can help give a client a sense of control, which enhances his or her coping ability. Perception of loss of control can result in a sense of powerlessness, then hopelessness.

8. Providing emotional support and encouraging sharing may help a client clarify and verbalize his or her fears, allowing the nurse to get realistic feedback and reassurance.

(continued)

Interventions	**Rationales**
9. Correct any misconceptions and inaccurate information the client may express.	9. A common contributing factor to fear and anxiety is incomplete or inaccurate information; providing adequate accurate information can help allay client fears.
10. Allow the client's support people to share their fears and concerns, and encourage them in providing meaningful and productive support.	10. Supporting the client's support people can enhance their ability to help the client.

Documentation

> Progress notes
> > Unusual responses or situations
> > Client's knowledge/information provided related to diagnosis, treatment, and hospital routine

Risk for Injury Related to Unfamiliar Environment and Physical or Mental Limitations Secondary to the Condition, Medications, Therapies, and Diagnostic Tests

Goal

The client will not injure self during hospital stay.

Indicators

> ➤ Identify factors that increase risk of injury.
> ➤ Describe appropriate safety measures.

Interventions	**Rationales**
1. Orient the client to his or her environment (e.g., location of bathroom, bed controls, call bell). Leave a light on in the bathroom at night.	1. Orientation helps provide familiarity; a light at night helps the client find his or her way safely.
2. Instruct the client to wear slippers with nonskid soles and to avoid newly washed floors.	2. These precautions can help prevent foot injuries and falls from slipping.

(continued)

Interventions	Rationales
3. Teach him or her to keep the bed in the low position with side rails up at night.	3. The low position makes it easier for the client to get in and out of bed.
4. Make sure that the telephone, eyeglasses, and frequently used personal belongings are within easy reach.	4. Keeping objects at hand helps prevent falls from overreaching and overextending.
5. Instruct the client to request assistance whenever he needs it.	5. Getting needed help with ambulation and other activities reduces a client's risk of injury.
6. Explain the hospital's smoking policy.	6. The hospital is a nonsmoking institution.
7. For an uncooperative high-risk client, consult with the physician for a 24-hour sitter or restraints, as indicated.	7. In some cases, extra measures are necessary to ensure a client's safety and prevent injury to him or her and others.

Documentation

Progress notes
Multidisciplinary client education record
Client teaching
Response to teaching

Risk for Infection Related to Increased Microorganisms in the Environment, Risk of Person-to-Person Transmission, and Invasive Tests or Therapies

Goal

The client will describe or demonstrate appropriate precautions to prevent infection.

Interventions	Rationales
1. Teach the client to wash his or her hands regularly, especially before meals and after toileting.	1. Proper handwashing deters the spread of microorganisms.
2. Teach the client to avoid coughing, sneezing, or breathing on others and to use disposable tissues.	2. These techniques help prevent infection transmission through airborne droplets.

(continued)

Interventions	Rationales
3. Follow institutional policies for IV and indwelling urinary catheter insertion and care.	3. Proper insertion and care reduce the risk of inflammation and infection.
4. Teach a client undergoing IV therapy not to bump or disturb the IV catheterization site.	4. Movement of the device can cause tissue trauma and possible inflammation.

5. Teach a client with an indwelling catheter in place to do the following:
  a. Avoid pressure on the catheter.
  b. Wipe from front to back after a bowel movement.
	5. Catheter movement can cause tissue trauma, predisposing to inflammation. Feces can readily contaminate an indwelling catheter.

6. Instruct the client to watch for and report immediately any signs and symptoms of inflammation.
  a. Redness or pain at the catheter insertion site
  b. Bladder spasms and cloudy urine, for a client with an indwelling urinary catheter
  c. Feelings of warmth and malaise
	6. Nosocomial infections occur in 5–6% of all hospitalized clients. Early detection enables prompt intervention to prevent serious complications and a prolonged hospital stay.

Documentation

Flow records
  Catheter and insertion site care
Progress notes
  Abnormal findings

(Specify) Self-Care Deficit Related to Sensory, Cognitive, Mobility, Endurance, or Motivational Problems

Goal

The client will perform self-care activities (feeding, toileting, dressing, grooming, bathing) with assistance as needed.

Indicators

➤ Demonstrate optimal hygiene after care is provided.
➤ Describe restrictions or precautions needed.

Interventions	Rationales
1. Promote the client's maximum involvement in self-feeding.	1–4. Enhancing a client's self-care abilities can increase his or her sense of control and independence, promoting overall well-being.
a. Determine the client's favorite foods and provide them, when possible.	
b. As feasible, arrange for meals to be served in a pleasant, relaxed, familiar setting without too many distractions.	
c. Ensure good oral hygiene before and after meals.	
d. Encourage the client to wear his or her dentures and eyeglasses when eating, as appropriate.	
e. Have the client sit upright in a chair at a table, if possible. If not, position him or her as close to upright as he can be.	
f. Provide some social contact during meals.	
g. Encourage a client who has trouble handling utensils to eat "finger foods" (bread, sandwiches, fruit, nuts).	
h. Provide needed adaptive devices for eating such as a plate guard, suction device under the plate or bowl, padded-handle utensils, wrist or hand splints with clamp, special drinking cup.	
i. Assist with meal setup as needed—open containers, napkins, and condiment packages, cut meat, and butter bread.	
j. Arrange foods so the client can eat them easily.	

(continued)

Interventions	Rationales

2. Promote the client's maximum involvement in bathing.
   a. Encourage and help set up a regular schedule for bathing.
   b. Keep the bathroom and bath water warm.
   c. Ensure privacy.
   d. Provide needed adaptive equipment, such as bath board, tub chair or stool, washing mitts, hand-held shower spray.
   e. Make sure the call bell is within easy reach of a client bathing alone.
3. Promote or provide assistance with grooming and dressing.
   a. Deodorant application
   b. Cosmetic application
   c. Hair care: shampooing and styling
   d. Shaving and beard care
   e. Nail and foot care
4. Promote the client's maximum involvement in toileting activities.
   a. Evaluate his or her ability to move to and use the toilet unassisted.
   b. Provide assistance and supervision only as needed.
   c. Provide needed adaptive devices, e.g., commode chair, spill-proof urinal, fracture bedpan, raised toilet seat, support rails.
   d. Whenever possible, encourage a regular elimination routine using the toilet and avoiding a bedpan or urinal.

Documentation

Flow records
Assistance needed for self-care

Risk for Imbalanced Nutrition: Less Than Body Requirements Related to Decreased Appetite Secondary to Treatments, Fatigue, Environment, and Changes in Usual Diet and to Increased Protein and Vitamin Requirements for Healing

Goal

The client will ingest daily nutritional requirements in accordance with activity level, metabolic needs, and restrictions.

Indicators

➤ Relate the importance of good nutrition.
➤ Relate restrictions if any.

Interventions	Rationales
1. Explain the need for adequate consumption of carbohydrates, fats, protein, vitamins, minerals, and fluids.	1. During illness, good nutrition can reduce the risk of complications and speed recovery.
2. Consult with a nutritionist to establish appropriate daily caloric and food type requirements for the client.	2. Consultation can help ensure a diet that provides optimal caloric and nutrient intake.
3. Discuss with the client possible causes of his or her decreased appetite.	3. Factors such as pain, fatigue, analgesic use, and immobility can contribute to anorexia. Identifying a possible cause enables interventions to eliminate or minimize it.
4. Encourage the client to rest before meals.	4. Fatigue further reduces an anorexic client's desire and ability to eat.
5. Offer frequent small meals instead of a few large ones.	5. Even distribution of total daily caloric intake throughout the day helps prevent gastric distention, possibly increasing appetite.
6. Restrict liquids with meals and avoid fluids 1 hour before and after meals.	6. These fluid restrictions help prevent gastric distention.
7. Encourage and help the client to maintain good oral hygiene.	7. Poor oral hygiene leads to bad odor and taste, which can diminish appetite. *(continued)*

Interventions	Rationales
8. Arrange to have high-calorie and high-protein foods served at the times that the client usually feels most like eating.	8. This measure increases the likelihood of the client's consuming adequate calories and protein.
9. Take steps to promote appetite. a. Determine the client's food preferences and arrange to have those foods provided, as appropriate. b. Eliminate any offensive odors and sights from the eating area. c. Control any pain or nausea before meals. d. Encourage the client's support persons to bring allowed foods from home, if possible. e. Provide a relaxed atmosphere and some socialization during meals.	9. These measures can improve appetite and lead to increased intake.
10. Give the client printed materials outlining a nutritious diet that includes the following: a. High intake of complex carbohydrates and fiber b. Decreased intake of sugar, simple carbohydrates, salt, cholesterol, total fat, and saturated fats c. Alcohol use only in moderation d. Proper caloric intake to maintain ideal weight e. Approximately 10 cups of water daily, unless contraindicated	10. Today, diet planning focuses on avoiding nutritional excesses. Reducing fats, salt, and sugar can reduce the risk of heart disease, diabetes, certain cancers, and hypertension.

Documentation

Flow records
  Dietary intake
  Daily weight
  Diet instruction
  Use of assistive devices

Risk for Constipation Related to Change in Fluid or Food Intake, Routine, or Activity Level; Effects of Medications; and Emotional Stress

Goal

The client will maintain prehospitalization bowel patterns.

Indicators

➤ State importance of fluids, fiber, and activity.
➤ Report difficulty promptly.

Interventions	Rationales
1. Auscultate bowel sounds.	1. Bowel sounds indicate the nature of peristaltic activity.
2. Implement measures to promote a balanced diet that promotes regular elimination. a. Encourage increased intake of high-fiber foods, such as fresh fruit with skin, bran, nuts and seeds, whole-grain breads and cereals, cooked fruits and vegetables, and fruit juices. (Note: If the client's diet is low in fiber, introduce fiber slowly to reduce irritation to the bowel.) b. Discuss the client's dietary preferences and plan diet modifications to accommodate them, whenever possible. c. Encourage the client to eat approximately 800 grams of fruits and vegetables—the equivalent of about four pieces of fresh fruit and a large salad—daily to promote regular bowel movements.	2. A well-balanced diet high in fiber content stimulates peristalsis and regular elimination.
3. Promote adequate daily fluid intake. a. Encourage intake of at least 2 liters (8 to 10 glasses) per day, unless contraindicated.	3. Adequate fluid intake helps maintain proper stool consistency in the bowel and aids regular elimination.

(continued)

Interventions	**Rationales**

b. Identify and accommodate fluid preferences, whenever possible.

c. Set up a schedule for regular fluid intake.

4. Establish a regular routine for elimination.

   a. Identify the client's usual elimination pattern before the onset of constipation.

   b. Review the client's daily routine to find an optimal time for elimination, and schedule adequate time.

   c. Suggest that he attempt defecation about 1 hour following meals; instruct him or her to remain on the toilet for a sufficient length of time.

4. Devising a routine for elimination based on the body's natural circadian rhythms can help stimulate regular defecation.

5. Attempt to simulate the client's home environment for elimination.

   a. Have the client use the toilet rather than a bedpan or commode, if possible. Offer a bedpan or commode only when necessary.

   b. Assist the client into proper position on the toilet, bedpan, or commode, as necessary.

   c. Provide privacy during elimination attempts—close the bathroom door or draw curtains around the bed, play the television or radio to mask sounds, use a room deodorizer.

   d. Provide adequate comfort, reading material as a diversion, and a call bell for safety reasons.

5. A sense of normalcy and familiarity can help reduce embarrassment and promote relaxation, which may aid defecation.

(continued)

Interventions	Rationales
6. Teach the client to assume an optimal position on the toilet or commode (sitting upright, leaning forward slightly) or bedpan (head of bed elevated to put the client in high Fowler's position or at permitted elevation); assist him or her in assuming this position as necessary.	6. Proper positioning takes full advantage of abdominal muscle action and the force of gravity to promote defecation.
7. Explain how physical activity affects daily elimination. Encourage and, as necessary, assist with regular ambulation, unless contraindicated.	7. Regular physical activity aids elimination by improving abdominal muscle tone and stimulating appetite and peristalsis.

Documentation

Flow records
   Bowel movements
   Bowel sounds
   Instructions for obtaining regular elimination pattern

Risk for Impaired Skin Integrity Related to Prolonged Pressure on Tissues Associated with Decreased Mobility, Increased Fragility of the Skin Associated with Dependent Edema, Decreased Tissue Perfusion, Malnutrition, Urinary/Fecal Incontinence

Goal

The client will maintain present intact skin/tissue.

Indicators

➤ No redness (erythema)
➤ Relate risk factors to skin/tissue trauma.

Interventions	Rationales
1. Skin assessment a. *Assessment.* All clients will be assessed upon admission for risk factors that predispose to skin breakdown. These risk factors include,	1. To prevent pressure ulcers, individuals at risk must be identified so that risk factors can be reduced through intervention.

(continued)

Interventions	Rationales

but are not limited to, the
following:
- Altered level of
  consciousness
- Poor nutrition/hydration
- Impaired mobility
- Impaired sensation
  (paralysis)
- Incontinence
- Multisystem failure
- Steroid or immunosuppres-
  sive therapy
- Age over 65

b. *Inspection.* Upon admission,
bony prominences and skin
folds will be inspected for evidence of redness or skin
breakdown.

c. *Documentation.* Within
8 hours of admission, document the following infor-
mation on skin section of
Nursing Admission History:
- Describe existing areas of
  breakdown and indicate
  location on body.

2. Prevention protocol
   a. Pressure relief
      - Change client's position
        when in bed at least every
        2 hours around the clock.
        Use large and small shifts
        of weight.

      - Post position change
        schedule ("turn clock") at
        bedside.

      - Utilize prevention mode on
        specialty beds.
      - Use foam with cushion in
        chair; no donuts.

Rationales column:

- The critical time period for tissue
  changes due to pressure is
  between 1 and 2 hours, after
  which irreversible changes
  can occur.
- The "turn clock" alerts caregiver
  to recommended position
  changes and appropriate time
  intervals for turning.

- The risk of developing a pressure
  ulcer can be diminished by reducing the mechanical loading on the
  tissue. This can be accomplished

(continued)

Interventions	Rationales
	by using pressure-reducing devices. Donuts are known to cause venous congestion and edema. A study of at-risk clients found that ring cushions are more likely to cause pressure ulcers than prevent them. The donut relieves pressure in one area but increases pressure in the surrounding areas.
b. Limit shearing forces/friction • Keep head of bed at or below 30 degrees whenever possible.	• Clinically, shear is exerted on the body when the head of the bed is elevated. In this position, the skin and superficial fascia remain fixed against the bed linens while the deep fascia and skeleton slide down toward the foot of the bed. As a result of shear, blood vessels in the sacral area are likely to become twisted and distorted and tissue may become ischemic and necrotic.
• Avoid dragging client in bed. Use lift sheet or overhead trapeze.	• Friction injuries to the skin occur when it moves across a coarse surface such as bed linens. Most friction injuries can be avoided by using appropriate techniques when moving individuals so that their skin is never dragged across the linens.
• Use elbow protectors. Remove to inspect every shift. • Apply transparent film dressing (Tegaderm) over bony prominences as appropriate.	• Voluntary and involuntary movements by the individuals themselves can lead to friction injuries, especially on elbows and heels. Any agent that eliminates this contact or decreases the friction between the skin and the linens will reduce the potential for injury.
c. Nutritional assessment • Monitor intake and consider consultation with	c. Nutritional deficit is a known risk factor for the development of pressure ulcers. Poor gen-

(continued)

Interventions	Rationales
physician/dietary if the client: Eats less than 50% of meals for 3 or more days Is NPO or on a clear liquid diet for 5 days Has a serum albumin of <3.5 • Place on intake and output. If intake is less than 2,000 cc/24 hours, force fluids unless contraindicated. • Record actual weight on admission and weekly thereafter. • Request multivitamin/ mineral supplement and/or dietary supplements (Burnshakes, Ensure) if indicated. • Assess lab values: CBC Albumin Hemoglobin/hematocrit	eral nutrition is frequently associated with loss of weight and muscle atrophy. The reduction in subcutaneous tissue and muscle reduces the mechanical padding between the skin and underlying bony prominences and increases susceptibility to pressure ulcers. Poor nutrition also leads to decreased resistance to infection and interferes with wound healing.
d. Skin care • Inspect skin at least daily during bath for reddened areas or breakdown. Check bony prominences for redness with each position change.	• Skin inspection is fundamental to any plan for preventing pressure ulcers. Skin inspection provides the information essential for designing interventions to reduce risk and for evaluating the outcomes of those interventions.
• Keep skin clean and dry. Gently apply moisturizers such as Eucerin, Lubriderm, or Sween Cream as needed.	• For maximum skin vitality, metabolic wastes and environmental contaminants that accumulate on the skin should be removed frequently. It is prudent to treat clinical signs and symptoms of dry skin with a topical moisturizer.
• Avoid massage over bony prominences.	• There is research evidence to suggest that massage over bony prominences may be harmful.

(continued)

Interventions	Rationales
e. Incontinence care • Assess the cause of incontinence: History of incontinence Change in medications Antibiotic therapy Client disoriented at night • Maintain skin as dry as possible. Have call light within reach. Check client for incontinence every 1–2 hours. Take client to bathroom or offer bed pan every 2 hours while awake and h.s. If diapers are used, check every 2 hours and PRN for wetness. If chux are used, place chux inside lift sheet, never in direct contact with the client's skin. Cleanse perineal area after each incontinent episode, followed by the application of a moisture barrier ointment (Desitin, Vaseline, A & D Ointment, BAZA).	• Moist skin due to incontinence leads to maceration; which can make the skin more susceptible to injury. Moisture from incontinence of urine or feces also reduces the resistance of the skin to bacteria. Bacteria and toxins in the stool increase the risk of skin breakdown. Chux hold moisture next to the skin. They are not absorbent and serve only as "bed protectors." Never use chux unless they are covered with smooth linen to absorb moisture. A moisture barrier is a petrolatum-based ointment that repels urine and fecal material and moisturizes the skin to assist in healing reddened, irritated areas resulting from incontinence.

Disturbed Sleep Pattern Related to an Unfamiliar Noisy Environment, a Change in Bedtime Ritual, Emotional Stress, and a Change in Circadian Rhythm

Goal

The client will report a satisfactory balance of rest and activity.

Indicators

➤ Complete at least four sleep cycles (100 minutes) undisturbed.
➤ State factors that increase or decrease the quality of sleep.

Interventions	Rationales
1. Discuss the reasons for differing individual sleep requirements, including age, lifestyle, activity level, and other possible factors.	1. Although many believe that a person needs 8 hours of sleep each night, no scientific evidence supports this. Individual sleep requirements vary greatly. Generally, a person who can relax and rest easily requires less sleep to feel refreshed. With age, total sleep time usually decreases—especially stage IV sleep—and stage I sleep increases.

2. Institute measures to promote relaxation.
  a. Maintain a dark quiet environment.
  b. Allow the client to choose pillows, linens, and covers as appropriate.
  c. Provide a regular bedtime ritual.
  d. Ensure good room ventilation.
  e. Close the door, if desired.
	2. Sleep is difficult without relaxation. The unfamiliar hospital environment can hinder relaxation.

3. Schedule procedures to minimize the times you need to wake the client at night. If possible, plan for at least 2-hour periods of uninterrupted sleep.	3. To feel rested, a person usually must complete an entire sleep cycle (70 to 100 minutes) four or five times a night.
4. Explain the need to avoid sedative and hypnotic drugs.	4. These medications begin to lose their effectiveness after a week of use, requiring increased dosages and leading to the risk of dependence.
5. Assist with usual bedtime routines as necessary, such as personal hygiene, snack, or music for relaxation.	5. A familiar bedtime ritual may promote relaxation and sleep.

6. Teach the client sleep-promoting measures.
  a. Eating a high-protein snack (such as cheese or milk) before bedtime
  b. Avoiding caffeine
	6. These practices may help promote sleep.
	  a. Digested protein produces tryptophan, which has a sedative effect.
	  b. Caffeine stimulates metabolism and deters relaxation.

(continued)

Interventions	Rationales
c. Attempting to sleep only when feeling sleepy	c. Frustration may result if the client attempts to sleep when not sleepy or relaxed.
d. Trying to maintain consistent nightly sleep habits	d. Irregular sleeping patterns can disrupt normal circadian rhythms, possibly leading to sleep difficulties.
7. Explain the importance of regular exercise in promoting good sleep.	7. Regular exercise not only increases endurance and enhances the ability to tolerate psychological stress, but also promotes relaxation.

Documentation

Progress notes
Reports of unsatisfactory sleep

Risk for Spiritual Distress Related to Separation from Religious Support System, Lack of Privacy, or Inability to Practice Spiritual Rituals

Goal

The client will maintain usual spiritual practices not detrimental to health.

Indicators

➤ Ask for assistance as needed.
➤ Relate support from staff as needed.

Interventions	Rationales
1. Explore whether the client desires to engage in an allowable religious or spiritual practice or ritual. If so, provide opportunities for him or her to do so.	1. For a client who places a high value on prayer or other spiritual practices, these practices can provide meaning and purpose and can be a source of comfort and strength.
2. Express your understanding and acceptance of the importance of the client's religious or spiritual beliefs and practices.	2. Conveying a nonjudgmental attitude may help reduce the client's uneasiness about expressing his or her belief and practices.

(continued)

Interventions	Rationales
3. Provide privacy and quiet for spiritual rituals, as the client desires and as practicable.	3. Privacy and quiet provide an environment that enables reflection and contemplation.
4. If you wish, offer to pray with the client or read from a religious text.	4. The nurse—even one who does not subscribe to the same religious beliefs or values of the client—can still help him or her meet his or her spiritual needs.
5. Offer to contact a religious leader or hospital clergy to arrange for a visit. Explain available services, e.g., hospital chapel, Bible.	5. These measures can help the client maintain spiritual ties and practice important rituals.
6. Explore whether any usual hospital practices conflict with the client's beliefs, e.g., diet, hygiene, treatments. If so, try to accommodate the client's beliefs to the extent that policy and safety allow.	6. Many religions prohibit certain behaviors; complying with restrictions may be an important part of the client's worship.

Documentation

Progress notes
Spiritual concerns

Interrupted Family Processes Related to Disruption of Routines, Changes in Role Responsibilities, and Fatigue Associated with Increased Workload, and Visiting Hour Requirements

Goal

The client and family members will verbalize feelings regarding the diagnosis and hospitalization.

Indicators

➤ Identify signs of family dysfunction.
➤ Identify appropriate resources to seek when needed.

Interventions	Rationales
1. Approach the family and attempt to create a private and supportive environment.	1. Approaching a family communicates a sense of caring and concern.

(continued)

Interventions	Rationales
2. Provide accurate information, using simple terms.	2. Moderate or high anxiety impairs the ability to process information. Simple explanations impart useful information most effectively.
3. Explore the family members' perceptions of the situation.	3. Evaluating family members' understanding can help identify any learning needs they may have.
4. Assess their current emotional response—guilt, anger, blame, grief—to the stresses of hospitalization.	4. A family member's response to another member's illness is influenced by the extent to which the illness interferes with his or her goal-directed activity, the significance of the goal interfered with, and the quality of the relationship.
5. Observe the dynamics of client–family interaction during visitations. Evaluate the following: a. Apparent desire for visit b. Effects of visit c. Interactions d. Physical contact	5. These observations provide information regarding family roles and interrelationships and the quality of support family members provide for each other.
6. Determine whether the family's current coping mechanism is effective.	6. Illness of a family member may necessitate significant role changes, putting a family at high risk for maladaptation.
7. Promote family strengths: a. Involve family members in caring for the client. b. Acknowledge their assistance. c. Encourage a sense of humor and perspective.	7. These measures may help maintain an existing family structure, allowing it to function as a supportive unit.
8. As appropriate, assist the family in reorganizing roles at home, resetting priorities, and reallocating responsibilities.	8. Reordering priorities may help reduce stress and maintain family integrity.
9. Warn family members to be prepared for signs of depres-	9. Anticipatory guidance can alert family members to impending

(continued)

Interventions	Rationales
sion, anxiety, anger, and dependency in the client and other family members.	problems, enabling intervention to prevent the problems from occurring.
10. Encourage and help the family to call on their social network (friends, relatives, church members) for support.	10. Adequate support can eliminate or minimize family members' feelings that they must "go it alone."
11. Emphasize the need for family members to address their own physical and psychological needs. To provide time for this, suggest measures such as these: a. Taking a break and having someone else visit the client for a change b. Calling the unit for a status report rather than traveling to the hospital every day	11. A family member who ignores his or her own needs for sleep, relaxation, or nutrition and changes his or her usual health practices for the worse impairs his or her own effectiveness as a support person.
12. If the family becomes overwhelmed, help them to prioritize their duties and problems and to act accordingly.	12. Prioritizing can help a family under stress focus on and problem-solve those situations requiring immediate attention.
13. At the appropriate time, have family members list perceived problems and concerns. Then develop a plan of action to address each item.	13. Addressing each problem separately allows the family to identify resources and reduce feelings of being overwhelmed.
14. Encourage the family to continue their usual method of decision making, including the client when appropriate.	14. Joint decision making reduces the client's feelings of dependency and reinforces that continued support is available.
15. As possible, adjust visiting hours to accommodate family schedules.	15. This measure may help promote regular visitation, which can help maintain family integrity.
16. Identify any dysfunctional coping mechanisms. a. Substance abuse b. Continued denial c. Exploitation of one or more family members d. Separation or avoidance	16. Families with a history of unsuccessful coping may need additional resources. Families with unresolved conflicts prior to a member's hospitalization are at high risk.

(continued)

Interventions	Rationales

e. Assess for domestic abuse/violence
- Definition of domestic abuse/violence
  Any person who has been physically, emotionally, or sexually abused by an intimate partner or former intimate partner
  Involves infliction or threat of infliction of any bodily injury; harmful physical contact; the destruction of property or threat thereof as a method of coercion, control, revenge, or punishment
- Subcategories of domestic abuse/violence
  Physical
  Sexual
  Harassment
  Intimidation of a dependent
  Interference with personal liberty or willful deprivation
- High risk indicators for suspected abuse: Should you notice any of the following indicators in combination with each other, it may warrant a referral to either the Medical Social Work Department (clients admitted to medical units) or Crisis Intervention.

  Physical indicators:
  Physician's exam reveals that the client has injuries the spouse/

(continued)

Interventions	**Rationales**

intimate partner/client
had not divulged

Too many "unexplained"
injuries or explanations
inconsistent with
injuries

Over time, explanations
for injuries become
inconsistent

Prolonged interval
between trauma or ill-
ness and presentation
for medical care

Conflicting or implausible
accounts regarding
injuries or incidents

History of MD shopping or
ER shopping

Social indicators:

Age

Young (chronologically or
developmentally)

Older

Spouse/intimate partner
is forced by circum-
stances to care for client
who is unwanted

Spouse/intimate partner
inappropriately will not
allow you to interview
client alone despite
explanation

Client/spouse/intimate
partner socially isolated
or alienated

Client/spouse/intimate
partner demonstrates
poor self-image

Financial difficulties

Client claims to have been
abused

(continued)

Interventions	Rationales
Behavioral indicators: Client/spouse/intimate partner presents vague explanation regarding injuries with implausible stories Client/spouse/intimate partner is very evasive in providing explanations Client has difficulty maintaining eye contact and appears shameful about injuries Client appears very fearful, possibly trembling Client expresses ambivalence regarding relationship with spouse/intimate partner Client quickly blames himself/herself for injuries Client is very passive or withdrawn Spouse/intimate partner appears "overprotective" Client appears fearful of spouse/intimate partner Refer for counseling if necessary.	
17. Direct the family to community agencies and other sources of emotional and financial assistance, as needed.	17. Additional resources may be needed to help with management at home.
18. As appropriate, explore whether the client and family have discussed end-of-life decisions; if not, encourage them to do so.	18. Intense stress is experienced when families and health care providers are faced with decisions regarding either initiation or discontinuation of life-support systems or other medical interventions that prolong life, e.g., nasogastric tube feeding.

(continued)

Interventions	**Rationales**
	If the client's wishes are unknown, additional conflicts arise—especially if the family disagrees with decisions made by the health care providers, or vice versa.
19. When appropriate, instruct the client or family members to provide the following information:	19. During an episode of acute illness, these discussions may not be appropriate. Clients and families should be encouraged to discuss their directions to be used to guide future clinical decisions, and their decisions should be documented. One copy should be given to the person designated as the decision maker in the event the client becomes incapacitated or incompetent, with another copy retained in a safe deposit box and one copy on the chart.
a. Person to contact in the event of emergency	
b. Person whom the client trusts with personal decisions	
c. Decision whether to maintain life support if the client were to become mentally incompetent	
d. Any preference for dying at home or in the hospital	
e. Desire to sign a living will	
f. Decision on organ donation	
g. Funeral arrangements; burial, cremation	

Documentation

Progress notes
  Interactions with family
Assessment of family functioning
End-of-life decisions, if known
  Advance directive in chart

Risk for Ineffective Therapeutic Regimen Management Related to Complexity and Cost of Therapeutic Regimen, Complexity of Health Care System, Insufficient Knowledge of Treatment, and Barriers to Comprehension Secondary to Language Barriers, Cognitive Deficits, Hearing and/or Visual Impairment, Anxiety, and Lack of Motivation

Goal

The client or primary caregiver will describe disease process, causes and factors contributing to symptoms, and the regimen for disease or symptom control.

Indicators

➤ Relate the intent to practice health behaviors needed or desired for recovery from illness/symptom management and prevention of recurrence or complications.

➤ Describe signs and symptoms that need reporting.

Interventions	Rationales
1. Determine the client's knowledge of his condition, prognosis, and treatment measures. Reinforce and supplement the physician's explanations as necessary.	1. Assessing the client's level of knowledge will assist in the development of an individualized learning program. Providing accurate information can decrease the client's anxiety associated with the unknown and unfamiliar.
2. Identify factors that influence learning.	2. The client's ability to learn will be affected by a number of variables that need to be considered. Denial of illness, lack of financial resources, and depression may affect the client's ability and motivation to learn. Cognitive changes associated with this might influence the client's ability to learn new information.
3. Provide the client and family with information about how to utilize the health care system (billing and payment, making appointments, follow-up care, resources available, etc.).	3. Information on how to "work the system" will help the client and family to feel more comfortable and more in control of client's health care. This will positively influence compliance with the health care regimen.
4. Explain and discuss with client and family/caregiver (when possible): a. Disease process b. Treatment regimen (medications, diet, procedures, exercises, equipment use) c. Rationale for regimen d. Side effects of regimen	4. Depending on client's physical and cognitive limitations, it may be necessary to provide the family/caregiver with the necessary information for managing the treatment regimen. To assist the client with post-discharge care, the client needs information about the disease process,

(continued)

Interventions	Rationales

e. Lifestyle changes needed
f. Follow-up care needed
g. Signs or symptoms of complications
h. Resources, support available
i. Home environment alterations needed

treatment regimen, symptoms of complications, etc., as well as resources available for assistance.

5. Promote a positive attitude and active participation of the client and family.
   a. Solicit expression of feelings, concerns, and questions from client and family.
   b. Encourage client and family to seek information and make informed decisions.
   c. Explain responsibilities of client/family and how these can be assumed.

5. Active participation in the treatment regimen helps the client and family feel more in control of the illness, which enhances the effective management of the therapeutic regimen.

6. Ensure that the client with visual and/or hearing impairments has glasses and a hearing aid available and uses them during teaching sessions. Provide adequate lighting and a quiet place for teaching sessions. Provide written teaching materials in the client's first language when possible.

6. Vision and hearing aids, adequate lighting, written materials in client's primary language, etc., will help to compensate for barriers to learning. Decreasing external stimuli will assist the client to correctly perceive what is being said.

7. Explain that changes in lifestyle and needed learning will take time to integrate.
   a. Provide printed material (in client's primary language when possible).
   b. Explain whom to contact with questions.
   c. Identify referrals or community services needed for follow-up.

7. Explaining that changes are expected to take time to integrate will provide reassurance for the client that he or she does not have to make changes all at once. Support and reassurance will assist the client with compliance. Providing information about available resources also helps the client to feel supported in his or her efforts.

Documentation

Progress notes
   Specific discharge needs and plans
Discharge instructions
   Referrals made
   Client and family teaching about disease, plan of treatment, referrals,
   etc.

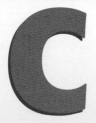

Generic Care Plan for the Surgical Client

KATHLEEN M. KILLMAN, RN, C, MS

This care plan presents nursing diagnoses and collaborative problems that commonly apply to clients (and their significant others) experiencing all types of surgery. Nursing diagnoses and collaborative problems specific to a surgical procedure are presented in the care plan for that procedure.

Time Frame

Preoperative and postoperative periods

DIAGNOSTIC CLUSTER

Preoperative

Nursing Diagnosis

➤ Anxiety/Fear related to surgical experience, loss of control, unpredictable outcome, and insufficient knowledge of preoperative routines, postoperative exercises and activities, and postoperative changes and sensations

Postoperative

Collaborative Problems

PC: Hemorrhage
PC: Hypovolemia/Shock
PC: Evisceration/Dehiscence
PC: Paralytic Ileus
PC: Infection (Peritonitis)
PC: Urinary Retention
PC: Thrombophlebitis

Nursing Diagnoses

➤ Risk for Ineffective Respiratory Function related to immobility secondary to postanesthesia state and pain
➤ Risk for Infection related to a site for organism invasion secondary to surgery

➤ Acute Pain related to surgical interruption of body structures, flatus, and immobility

➤ Risk for Imbalanced Nutrition: Less Than Body Requirements related to increased protein and vitamin requirements for wound healing and decreased intake secondary to pain, nausea, vomiting, and diet restrictions

➤ Risk for Constipation related to decreased peristalsis secondary to immobility and the effects of anesthesia and narcotics

➤ Activity Intolerance related to pain and weakness secondary to anesthesia, tissue hypoxia, and insufficient fluid and nutrient intake

➤ Risk for Ineffective Therapeutic Regimen Management related to insufficient knowledge of care of operative site, restrictions (diet, activity), medications, signs and symptoms of complications, and follow-up care

Discharge Criteria

Before discharge, the client and/or family will

1. Describe any at-home activity restrictions.
2. Describe at-home wound and pain management.
3. Discuss fluid and nutritional requirements for proper wound healing.
4. List the signs and symptoms that must be reported to a health care professional.
5. Describe necessary follow-up care.

Preoperative: Nursing Diagnosis

Anxiety/Fear Related to Surgical Experience, Loss of Control, Unpredictable Outcome, and Insufficient Knowledge of Preoperative Routines, Postoperative Exercises and Activities, and Postoperative Changes and Sensations

Goal

The client will communicate feelings regarding the surgical experience.

Indicators

➤ Verbalize, if asked, what to expect regarding routines, environment, and sensations.

➤ Demonstrate postoperative exercises, splinting, and respiratory regimen.

Interventions	Rationales
1. Provide reassurance and comfort: stay with client, encourage her or him to share his feelings and concerns, listen attentively, and convey a sense of empathy and understanding.	1. Providing emotional support and encouraging client to share allows her or him to clarify fears and provides opportunities for nurse to provide realistic feedback and reassurance.

(continued)

Interventions	Rationales
2. Correct any misconceptions and inaccurate information that the client has about the procedure.	2. Modifiable contributing factors to anxiety include incomplete and inaccurate information. Providing accurate information and correcting misconceptions may help to eliminate fears and reduce anxiety.
3. Determine if client desires spiritual support (e.g., visit from clergy or other spiritual leader, religious article, or ritual). Arrange for this support if necessary.	3. Many clients need spiritual support to enhance coping ability.
4. Allow and encourage family members and significant others to share their fears and concerns. Enlist their support for the client, but only if it is meaningful and productive.	4. Effective support from family members, other relatives, and friends can help client to cope with surgery and recovery.
5. Notify physician if client exhibits severe or panic anxiety.	5. Immediate notification enables prompt assessment and possible pharmacologic intervention.

6. Notify physician if client needs any further explanations about the procedure; beforehand, the physician should explain the following:
  a. Nature of the surgery
  b. Reason for and expected outcome of surgery
  c. Any risks involved
  d. Type of anesthetic to be used
  e. Expected length of recovery and any postoperative restrictions and instructions
	6. The physician is responsible for explaining the surgery to the client and family; the nurse, for determining their level of understanding and then notifying the physician of the need to provide more information.

7. Involve family members or significant others in client teaching whenever possible.	7. Knowledgeable family members or significant others can serve as "coaches" to remind client of postoperative instructions and restrictions.
8. Provide instruction (bedside or group) on general information	8. Preoperative teaching provides client with information; this

(continued)

Interventions	Rationales
pertaining to the need for active participation, preoperative routines, environment, personnel, and postoperative exercises.	can help to decrease anxiety and fear associated with the unknown and enhance client's sense of control over the situation.
9. Present information or re-inforce learning using written materials (e.g., books, pamphlets, instruction sheets) or audiovisual aids (e.g., videotapes, slides, posters).	9. Simultaneous stimulation of multiple senses augments the learning process. Written materials can be retained and used as a reference after discharge. These materials may be especially useful for caregivers who did not participate in client teaching sessions.
10. Explain the importance and purpose of all preoperative procedures.	10. This information can help to relieve anxiety and fear associated with lack of knowledge of necessary preoperative activities and routines.
a. Enemas	a. Enemas are sometimes given to empty the bowel of fecal material; this can help to reduce risk of postoperative bowel obstruction as peristalsis resumes.
b. Nothing-by-mouth (NPO) status	b. Eliminating oral fluids preoperatively reduces risk of aspiration postoperatively.
c. Skin preparation	c. Tests and studies establish baseline values and help to detect any abnormalities before surgery.
d. Laboratory studies	d. Preoperative sedatives reduce anxiety and promote relaxation that increase the effectiveness of anesthesia and decrease secretions in response to intubation.
11. Discuss expected intraoperative procedures and sensations. a. Appearance of operating room and equipment	11. Client's understanding of expected procedures and sensations can help to ameliorate fears.

(continued)

Interventions	Rationales
b. Presence of surgical staff	
c. Administration of anesthesia	
d. Appearance of postanesthesia recovery room	
e. Recovery from anesthesia	
12. Explain all expected postoperative routines and sensations.	12. Explaining what the client can expect, why the procedures are done, and why certain sensations may occur can help to reduce fears associated with the unknown and unexpected.
a. Parenteral fluid administration	a. Parenteral fluids replace fluids lost from NPO state and blood loss.
b. Vital sign monitoring	b. Careful monitoring is needed to determine status and track any changes.
c. Dressing checks and changes	c. Until wound edges heal, wound must be protected from contaminants.
d. Nasogastric (NG) tube insertion and care	d. An NG tube promotes drainage and reduces abdominal distention and tension on the suture line.
e. Indwelling (Foley) catheter insertion and care	e. A Foley catheter drains the bladder until muscle tone returns as anesthesia is excreted.
f. Other devices such as intravenous (IV) lines, pumps, and drains	
g. Symptoms including nausea, vomiting, and pain	g. Nausea and vomiting are common side effects of preoperative medications and anesthesia; other contributing factors include certain types of surgery, obesity, electrolyte imbalance, rapid position changes, and psychological and environmental factors. Pain commonly occurs as medications lose their effectiveness.

(continued)

Interventions	Rationales
h. The availability of analgesics and antiemetics if needed	
13. As applicable, teach client (using return demonstration to ensure understanding and ability) how to do the following: a. Turn, cough, and deep breathe. b. Support the incision site while coughing. c. Change position in bed every 1 to 2 hours. d. Sit up, get out of bed, and ambulate as soon as possible after surgery (prolonged sitting should be avoided).	13. Client's understanding of postoperative care measures can help to reduce anxiety associated with the unknown and promote compliance. Teaching the client about postoperative routines before surgery ensures that her or his understanding is not impaired postoperatively by the continuing effects of sedation.
14. Explain the importance of progressive activities postoperatively including early ambulation and self-care as soon as client is able.	14. Activity improves circulation and helps to prevent pooling of respiratory secretions. Self-care promotes self-esteem and can help to enhance recovery.
15. Explain important hospital policies to family members or significant others (e.g., visiting hours, number of visitors allowed at one time, location of waiting rooms, how physician will contact them after surgery).	15. Providing family members and significant others with this information can help to reduce their anxiety and allow them to better support the client.
16. Evaluate client's and family's or significant others' abilities to achieve preset, mutually planned learning goals.	16. This assessment identifies the need for any additional teaching and support.

Documentation

Flow records
Progress notes
Unusual interactions
Preoperative teaching

Postoperative: Collaborative Problems

Potential Complication: Hemorrhage

Potential Complication: Hypovolemia/Shock

Potential Complication: Evisceration/Dehiscence

Potential Complication: Paralytic Ileus

Potential Complication: Infection (Peritonitis)

Potential Complication: Urinary Retention

Potential Complication: Thrombophlebitis

Nursing Goal

The nurse will monitor for early signs and symptoms of (a) hemorrhage; (b) hypovolemia/shock; (c) evisceration/dehiscence; (d) paralytic ileus; (e) infection; (f) urinary retention; and (g) thrombophlebitis and will intervene collaboratively to stabilize the client.

Indicators

➤ Calm, alert, oriented (a, b)
➤ Respirations 16–20 beats/min (a, b)
➤ Respirations relaxed and rhythmic (a, b)
➤ Breath sound present all lobes (a, b)
➤ No rales or wheezing (a, b)
➤ Pulse 60–100 breaths/min (a, b)
➤ BP > 90/60, <140/90 mm Hg (a, b)
➤ Capillary refill < 3 seconds (a, b)
➤ Peripheral pulses full, equal (a, b)
➤ Skin warm and dry (a, b)
➤ Temperature 98.5–99°F (a, b, e)
➤ Urine output > 30 ml/h (a, b)
➤ Usual skin color (a, b)
➤ Surgical wound intact (c, e)
➤ Minimal drainage serosanguinous (e)
➤ Bowel sounds present (b, d)
➤ No nausea and vomiting (b, d)
➤ No abdominal distention (b, d)
➤ Decreasing abdominal tenderness (c, e)
➤ Decreasing wound tenderness (c, e)
➤ No bladder distension (f)
➤ No difficulty voiding (f)
➤ Negative Homans sign (no pain with dorsiflexion of foot) (g)
➤ No calf tenderness, warmth, edema (g)
➤ White blood cells 4,000–10,000 mm^3 (e)

➤ Hemoglobin (a)
  ➢ Male 14–18 g/dl
  ➢ Female 12–16 g/dl
➤ Hematocrit (a)
  ➢ Male 42–52%
  ➢ Female 37–47%
➤ Oxygen saturation (SaO_2) > 95% (a, b)

Interventions	Rationales

1. Monitor for signs and symptoms of hemorrhage/shock and promptly report changes to surgeon.
  a. Increased pulse rate with normal or slightly decreased blood pressure
  b. Urine output < 30 ml/h
  c. Restlessness, agitation, decreased mentation
  d. Increased capillary refill over 3 seconds
  e. Decreased oxygen saturation < 95% (pulse oximetry)
  f. Increased respiratory rate
  g. Diminished peripheral pulses
  h. Cool, pale, or cyanotic skin
  i. Thirst
	1. The compensatory response to decreased circulatory volume aims to increase blood oxygen through increased heart and respiratory rates and decreased peripheral circulation (manifested by diminished peripheral pulses and cool skin). Decreased oxygen to the brain results in altered mentation.

2. Monitor fluid status; evaluate the following:
  a. Intake (parenteral and oral)
  b. Output and other losses (urine, drainage, and vomiting)
	2. Fluid loss during surgery and as a result of NPO status can disrupt fluid balance in a high-risk client. Stress can cause sodium and water retention.

3. Teach client to splint the surgical wound with a pillow when coughing, sneezing, or vomiting.	3. Splinting reduces stress on the suture line by equalizing pressure across the wound.
4. Monitor surgical site for bleeding, dehiscence, and evisceration.	4. Careful monitoring enables early detection of complications.
5. If dehiscence or evisceration occurs, contact surgeon immediately and do the following:	5. Rapid interventions can reduce severity of complications.

(continued)

Interventions	Rationales
a. Place client in low Fowler's position.	a. Low Fowler's position uses gravity to minimize further tissue protrusion.
b. Instruct client to lie still and quiet.	b. Lying still and quiet also minimizes tissue protrusion.
c. Cover protruding viscera with a wet sterile dressing.	c. A wet sterile dressing helps to maintain tissue viability.
6. Do not initiate fluids until bowel sounds are present; begin with small amounts. Monitor client's response to resumption of fluids and foods and note the nature and amount of any emesis.	6,7. Intraoperative manipulation of abdominal organs and the depressive effects of narcotics and anesthetics on peristalsis can cause paralytic ileus usually between the third and fifth postoperative day. Pain typically is localized, sharp, and intermittent.
7. Monitor for signs of paralytic ileus. a. Absent bowel sounds b. Nausea, vomiting c. Abdominal distention	
8. Monitor for signs and symptoms of infection/sepsis. a. Increased temperature b. Chills c. Malaise d. Elevated white blood cell (WBC) count e. Increasing abdominal tenderness f. Wound tenderness, redness, or edema	8. Microorganisms can be introduced into the body during surgery or through the incision. Circulating pathogens trigger the body's defense mechanisms: WBCs are released to destroy some pathogens, and the hypothalamus raises the body temperature to kill others. Wound redness, tenderness, and edema result from lymphocyte migration to the area.
9. Monitor for signs of urinary retention. a. Bladder distention b. Urine overflows (30 to 60 ml or urine every 15 to 30 minutes)	9. Anesthesia produces muscle relaxation, affecting the bladder. As muscle tone returns, spasms of the bladder sphincter prevent urine outflow, causing bladder distention. When urine retention increases the intravesical pressure, the sphincter releases urine and control of flow is regained.

(continued)

Interventions	Rationales
10. Instruct client to report bladder discomfort or inability to void.	10. Bladder discomfort and failure to void may be early signs of urinary retention.

11. If client does not void within 8 to 10 hours after surgery or complains of bladder discomfort, do the following:
  a. Warm the bedpan.
  b. Encourage client to get out of bed to use the bathroom if possible.
  c. Instruct a male client to stand when urinating if possible.
  d. Run water in the sink as client attempts to void.
  e. Pour warm water over client's perineum.
	11. These measures may help to promote relaxation of the urinary sphincter and facilitate voiding.

12. If client still cannot void, follow protocols for straight catheterization as ordered.	12. Straight catheterization is preferable to indwelling catheterization because it carries less risk of urinary tract infection from ascending pathogens.

13. Monitor for signs and symptoms of thrombophlebitis.
  a. Positive Homans' sign (pain on dorsiflexion of the foot, due to insufficient circulation)
  b. Calf tenderness, unusual warmth, or redness
	13. Vasoconstriction due to hypothermia decreases peripheral circulation. Anesthesia and immobility reduce vasomotor tone, resulting in decreased venous return with peripheral blood pooling. In combination, these factors increase risk of thrombophlebitis.

14. Apply antiembolic hose as ordered.	14. They apply even compression, enhance venous return, and reduce venous pooling.
15. Remind client to move and flex legs every hour.	15. This will increase circulation.
16. Encourage client to perform leg exercises. Discourage placing pillows under the knees, use of a knee gatch, crossing the legs, and prolonged sitting. Use TED hose/compression boots as appropriate.	16. These measures help to increase venous return and prevent venous stasis.

Related Physician-Prescribed Interventions

Medications.
Preoperative: Sedatives, narcotic analgesics, anticholinergics
Postoperative: Narcotic analgesics, antiemetics

Intravenous Therapy. Fluid and electrolyte replacement

Laboratory Studies. Complete blood count, urinalysis, chemistry profile

Diagnostic Studies. Chest x-ray film, electrocardiography

Therapies. Indwelling catheterization, incentive spirometry, wound care, liquid diet progressed to full diet as tolerated, preoperative NPO status, antiembolic hose, pulse oximetry

Documentation

Flow records
Vital signs (pulses, respirations, blood pressure, temperature)
Circulation (color, peripheral pulses)
Intake (oral, parenteral)
Output (urinary, tubes, specific gravity)
Bowel function (bowel sounds, defecation, distention)
Wound (color, drainage)
Progress notes
Unusual complaints or assessment findings
Interventions
Postoperative teaching

Postoperative: Nursing Diagnoses

Risk for Ineffective Respiratory Function Related to Immobility Secondary to Postanesthesia State and Pain

Goal

The client will exhibit clear lung fields.

Indicators

➤ Breath sounds present in all lobes
➤ Relaxed rhythmic respirations

Interventions	Rationales
1. Auscultate lung fields for diminished and abnormal breath sounds.	1. Presence of rales indicates retained secretions. Diminished breath sounds may indicate atelectasis.

(continued)

Interventions	Rationales
2. Take measures to prevent aspiration. Position client on side with pillows supporting the back and with knees slightly flexed.	2. In the postoperative period, decreased sensorium and hypoventilation contribute to increased risk of aspiration.
3. Reinforce preoperative client teaching about the importance of turning, coughing, and deep breathing and leg exercises every 1 to 2 hours.	3. Postoperative pain may discourage compliance; reinforcing the importance of these measures may improve compliance.
4. Promote the following as soon as client returns to unit. 　a. Deep breaths 　b. Coughing (except if contraindicated) 　c. Frequent turning 　d. Incentive spirometry if indicated 　e. Early ambulation	4. Exercises and movement promote lung expansion and mobilization of secretions. Incentive spirometry promotes deep breathing by providing a visual indicator of the effectiveness of the breathing effort. Coughing assists to dislodge mucous plugs. Coughing is contraindicated in people who have had a head injury, intracranial surgery, eye surgery, or plastic surgery because it increases intracranial and intraocular pressure and tension on delicate tissues (plastic surgery)
5. Encourage adequate oral fluid intake as indicated.	5. Adequate hydration liquefies secretions, which enables easier expectoration and prevents stasis of secretions that provide a medium for microorganism growth. It also helps to decrease blood viscosity, which reduces risk of clot formation.

Documentation

Flow record
　　Temperature
　　Respiratory rate and rhythm
　　Breath sounds
　　Respiratory treatments and client's response
Progress notes
　　Unsatisfactory response to respiratory treatments

Risk for Infection Related to a Site for Organism Invasion Secondary to Surgery

Goal

The client will demonstrate healing of wound.

Indicators

➤ No abnormal drainage
➤ Intact approximated wound edges

Interventions	Rationales

1. Monitor for signs and symptoms of wound infection.
  a. Increased swelling and redness
  b. Wound separation
  c. Increased or purulent drainage
  d. Prolonged subnormal temperature or significantly elevated temperature
	1. Tissue responds to pathogen infiltration with increased blood and lymph flow (manifested by edema, redness, and increased drainage) and reduced epithelialization (marked by wound separation). Circulating pathogens trigger the hypothalamus to elevate the body temperature; certain pathogens cannot survive at higher temperatures.

2. Monitor wound healing by noting the following:
  a. Evidence of intact approximated wound edges (primary intention)
  b. Evidence of granulation tissue (secondary and tertiary intention)
	2. A surgical wound with edges approximated by sutures usually heals by primary intention. Granulation tissue is not visible and scar formation is minimal. In contrast, a surgical wound with a drain or an abscess heals by secondary intention or granulation and has more distinct scar formation. A restructured wound heals by third intention and results in a wider and deeper scar.

3. Teach client about factors that can delay wound healing.
  a. Dehydrated wound tissue
	3.
	  a. Studies report that epithelial migration is impeded under dry crust; movement is three times faster over moist tissue.

b. Wound infection	b. The exudate in infected wounds impairs epithelialization and wound closure.

(continued)

Interventions	Rationales
c. Inadequate nutrition and hydration	c. To repair tissue, the body needs increased protein and carbohydrate intake and adequate hydration for vascular transport of oxygen and wastes.
d. Compromised blood supply	d. Blood supply to injured tissue must be adequate to transport leukocytes and remove wastes.
e. Increased stress or excessive activity	e. Increased stress and activity result in higher levels of chalone, a mitotic inhibitor that depresses epidermal regeneration.
4. Take steps to prevent infection. a. Wash hands before and after dressing changes. b. Wear gloves until wound is sealed. c. Thoroughly clean area around drainage tubes. d. Keep tubing away from incision. e. Discard unused irrigation solutions after 24 hours.	4. These measures help to prevent introduction of microorganisms into the wound; they also reduce the risk of transmitting infection to others.
5. Explain when a dressing is indicated for wounds healing by primary intention and by secondary intention.	5. A wound healing by primary intention requires a dressing to protect it from contamination until the edges seal (usually by 24 hours). A wound healing by secondary intention requires a dressing to maintain adequate hydration; the dressing is not needed after wound edges seal.
6. Minimize skin irritation by the following means: a. Using a collection pouch, if indicated b. Changing saturated dressings often	6. Preventing skin irritation eliminates a potential source of microorganism entry.

(continued)

Interventions	Rationales

7. Protect wound and surrounding skin from drainage by these methods:
  a. Using a collection pouch if indicated
  b. Applying a skin barrier
	7. Protecting skin can help to minimize excoriation by acid drainage. A semipermeable skin barrier provides a moist environment for healing and prevents bacteria entry.

8. Teach and assist client in the following:
  a. Supporting the surgical site when moving
  b. Splinting the area when coughing, sneezing, or vomiting
  c. Reducing flatus accumulation
	8. A wound typically requires 3 weeks for strong scar formation. Stress on the suture line before this occurs can cause disruption.

9. Consult with an enterostomal or a clinical nurse specialist for specific skin care measures.	9. Management of a complex wound or impaired healing requires expert nursing consultation.

Documentation

    Progress notes
      Signs and symptoms of infection
    Flow records
      Temperature
      Status of wound

Acute Pain Related to Surgical Interruption of Body Structures, Flatus, and Immobility

Goal

A client will report progressive reduction of pain and an increase in activity.

Indicators

   ➤ Relate factors that increase pain.
   ➤ Report effective interventions.

Interventions	Rationales
1. Collaborate with client to determine effective pain relief interventions.	1. A client experiencing pain may feel a loss of control over his body and his life. Collaboration can help minimize this feeling.

(continued)

Interventions	Rationales
2. Express your acceptance of client's pain. Acknowledge the pain's presence, listen attentively to client's complaints, and convey that you are assessing the pain because you want to understand it better, not because you are trying to determine whether it really exists.	2. A client who feels the need to convince health care providers that she or he actually is experiencing pain is likely to have increased anxiety that can lead to increased pain.
3. Reduce client's fear and clear up any misinformation by doing the following: a. Teaching what to expect; describing the sensation as precisely as possible including how long it should last b. Explaining pain relief methods such as distraction, heat application, and progressive relaxation	3. A client who is prepared for a painful procedure with a detailed explanation of the sensations that he or she will feel usually experiences less stress and pain than a client who receives vague or no explanations.
4. Explain the differences between involuntary physiologic responses and voluntary behavioral responses regarding drug use. a. Involuntary physiologic responses: • Drug tolerance is a physiologic phenomenon in which, after repeated doses, the prescribed dose begins to lose its effectiveness. • Physical dependence is a physiologic state that results from repeated administration of a drug. Withdrawal is experienced if the drug is abruptly discontinued. Tapering the drug dosage helps to manage withdrawal symptoms.	4. Many clients and families are misinformed regarding the nature and risks of drug addiction and consequently may be reluctant to request pain medication.

(continued)

Interventions	Rationales
b. Voluntary behavioral responses: • Drug abuse is the use of a drug in any manner that deviates from culturally acceptable medical and social uses (McCafferty, 1989). Addiction is a behavioral pattern of drug use characterized by overwhelming involvement with use of the drug and securing its supply and the high tendency to relapse after withdrawal.	
5. Provide client with privacy for his or her pain experience (e.g., close curtains and room door, ask others to leave the room).	5. Privacy allows client to express pain in his or her own manner, which can help to reduce anxiety and ease pain.
6. Provide optimal pain relief with prescribed analgesics.	6.
a. Determine preferred administration route—by mouth, intramuscular, intravenous, or rectal. Consult with physician or advanced practice nurse.	a. The proper administration route optimizes efficacy of pain medications. The oral route is preferred in most cases; for some drugs, the liquid dosage form may be given to a client who has difficulty swallowing. If frequent injections are necessary, the intravenous (IV) route is preferred to minimize pain and maximize absorption; however, IV administration may produce more profound side effects than other routes.
b. Assess vital signs—especially respiratory rate—before and after administering any narcotic agent.	b. Narcotics can depress the respiratory center of the brain.
c. Consult with a pharmacist regarding possible adverse interactions between the	c. Some medications potentiate the effects of narcotics; identifying such medications

(continued)

Interventions	**Rationales**

prescribed drug and other medications the client is taking (e.g., muscle relaxants, tranquilizers).

d. Take a preventive approach to pain medication, i.e., administer medication before activity (e.g., ambulation) to enhance participation (but be sure to evaluate the hazards of sedation); instruct client to request pain medication as needed before pain becomes severe.

e. After administering pain medication, return in ½ hour to evaluate its effectiveness.

7. Explain and assist with noninvasive and nonpharmacologic pain relief measures.
   a. Splinting the incision site
   b. Proper positioning
   c. Distraction
   d. Breathing exercises
   e. Massage
   f. Heat and cold application
   g. Relaxation techniques

8. Assist client in coping with the aftermath of the pain experience.
   a. If indicated, inform client that the painful procedure is completed and that the pain should soon subside.
   b. Encourage client to discuss the experience.

before administration can prevent excessive sedation.

d. The preventive approach may reduce the total 24-hour dose as compared with the PRN approach; it also provides a more constant blood drug level, reduces the client's craving for the drug, and eliminates the anxiety associated with having to ask for and wait for PRN relief.

e. Each client responds differently to pain medication; careful monitoring is needed to assess individual response. For example, too often every surgical client is expected to respond to 50 mg of meperidine (Demerol) every 3 to 4 hours regardless of body size, type of surgery, or previous experiences.

7. These measures can help to reduce pain by substituting another stimulus to prevent painful stimuli from reaching higher brain centers. In addition, relaxation reduces muscle tension and may help increase client's sense of control over pain.

8. These measures can help to reduce anxiety and help client to regain the sense of control altered by the painful experience.

(continued)

Interventions	**Rationales**

c. Clarify any misconceptions the client still may have.
 d. Praise the client for her or his endurance and behavior.
 9. Teach client to expel flatus by the following measures:
   a. Walking as soon as possible after surgery
   b. Changing positions regularly as possible (e.g., lying prone, assuming the knee–chest position)
	9. Postoperatively, sluggish peristalsis results in accumulation of nonabsorbable gas. Pain occurs when unaffected bowel segments contract in an attempt to expel gas. Activity speeds the return of peristalsis and the expulsion of flatus; proper positioning helps gas rise for expulsion.

Documentation

Medication administration record
  Type, route, and dosage schedule of all prescribed medications
Progress notes
  Unsatisfactory relief from pain-relief measures

Risk for Imbalanced Nutrition: Less Than Body Requirements Related to Increased Protein and Vitamin Requirements for Wound Healing and Decreased Intake Secondary to Pain, Nausea, Vomiting, and Diet Restrictions

Goal

The client will resume ingestion of the daily nutritional requirements.

Indicators

➤ Selections from the four basic food groups
➤ 2,000 to 3,000 ml of fluids
➤ Adequate fiber, vitamins, and minerals

Interventions	**Rationales**

1. Explain the need for an optimal daily nutritional intake including these items:
   a. Increased protein and carbohydrate intake
   b. Increased intake of vitamins A, B, B_{12}, C, D, and E, and niacin
	1. Understanding the importance of optimal nutrition may encourage client to comply with the dietary regimen.

(continued)

Interventions	Rationales
c. Adequate intake of minerals (zinc, magnesium, calcium, copper)	
2. Take measures to reduce pain.	2. Pain causes fatigue, which can reduce appetite.
a. Plan care so that painful or unpleasant procedures are not scheduled before mealtimes.	
b. Administer pain medication as ordered.	
c. Position for optimal comfort.	
3. Explain the possible causes of the client's nausea and vomiting.	3. Client's understanding of the source and normalcy of nausea and vomiting can reduce anxiety, which may help to reduce symptoms.
a. Side effect of preoperative medications and anesthesia	
b. Surgical procedure	
c. Obesity	
d. Electrolyte imbalance	
e. Gastric distention	
f. Too-rapid or strenuous movement	
Reassure client that these symptoms are normal.	
4. Take steps to reduce nausea and vomiting.	4.
a. Restrict fluids before meals and large amounts of fluids at any time; instead, encourage client to ingest small amounts of ice chips or cool clear liquids (e.g., dilute tea, Jell-O water, flat ginger ale, or cola) frequently, unless vomiting persists.	a. Gastric distention from fluid ingestion can trigger the vagal visceral afferent pathways that stimulate the medulla oblongata (vomiting center).
b. Teach client to move slowly.	b. Rapid movements stimulate the vomiting center by triggering vestibulocerebellar afferents.
c. Reduce or eliminate unpleasant sights and odors.	c. Noxious odors and sights can stimulate the vomiting center.
d. Provide good mouth care after client vomits.	d. Good oral care reduces the noxious taste.

(continued)

Interventions	Rationales
e. Teach deep-breathing techniques.	e. Deep breaths can help to excrete anesthetic agents.
f. Instruct client to avoid lying down flat for at least 2 hours after eating. (A client who must rest should sit or recline with head at least 4 inches higher than feet.)	f. Pressure on the stomach can trigger vagal visceral afferent stimulation of the vomiting center in the brain.
g. Ensure patency of any NG tube.	g. A malfunctioning NG tube can cause gastric distention.
h. Teach client to practice relaxation exercises during episodes of nausea.	h. Concentrating on relaxation activities may help to block stimulation of the vomiting center.
5. Maintain good oral hygiene at all times.	5. A clean refreshed mouth can stimulate appetite.
6. Administer an antiemetic agent before meals if indicated.	6. Antiemetics prevent nausea and vomiting.

Documentation

Flow record
    Intake (amount, type, time)
    Vomiting (amount, description)

Risk for Constipation Related to Decreased Peristalsis Secondary to Immobility and the Effects of Anesthesia and Narcotics

Goal

The client will resume effective preoperative bowel function.

Indicators

➤ No bowel distention
➤ Bowel sounds in all quadrants

Interventions	Rationales
1. Assess bowel sounds to determine when to introduce liquids. Advance diet as ordered.	1. Presence of bowel sounds indicates return of peristalsis.

(continued)

Interventions	Rationales
2. Explain the effects of daily activity on elimination. Assist with ambulation when possible.	2. Activity influences bowel elimination by improving abdominal muscle tone and stimulating appetite and peristalsis.
3. Promote factors that contribute to optimal elimination. a. Balanced diet: • Review a list of foods high in bulk (e.g., fresh fruits with skins, bran, nuts and seeds, whole grain breads and cereals, cooked fruits and vegetables, and fruit juices). • Discuss dietary preferences. • Encourage intake of approximately 800 g of fruits and vegetables (about four pieces of fresh fruit and a large salad) for normal daily bowel movement. b. Adequate fluid intake: • Encourage intake of at least 8 to 10 glasses (about 2,000 ml) daily unless contraindicated. • Discuss fluid preferences. • Set up a regular schedule for fluid intake. c. Regular time for defecation: • Identify the normal defecation pattern before the onset of constipation. • Review daily routine. • Include time for defecation as part of the regular daily routine. • Discuss a suitable time based on responsibilities, availability of facilities, and so on. • Suggest that client attempt defecation about 1 hour	3. a. A well-balanced diet high in fiber content stimulates peristalsis. b. Sufficient fluid intake is necessary to maintain bowel patterns and promote proper stool consistency. c. Taking advantage of circadian rhythms may aid in establishing a regular defecation schedule.

(continued)

Interventions	**Rationales**

following a meal and remain in the bathroom a suitable length of time.

d. Simulation of the home environment:
- Have client use the bathroom instead of a bedpan if possible; offer a bedpan or a bedside commode if the client cannot use the bathroom.
- Assist into position on the toilet, commode, or bedpan if necessary.
- Provide privacy (e.g., close door, draw curtains around the bed, play a TV or radio to mask sounds, make room deodorizer available).
- Provide for comfort (e.g., provide reading materials as a diversion) and safety (e.g., make a call bell readily available).

d. Privacy and a sense of normalcy can promote relaxation, which can enhance defecation.

e. Proper positioning:
- Assist client to a normal semisquatting position on the toilet or commode if possible.
- Assist onto a bedpan if necessary, elevating the head of the bed to high Fowler's position or to the elevation permitted.
- Stress the need to avoid straining during defecation efforts.

e. Proper positioning uses the abdominal muscles and the force of gravity to aid defecation. Straining can activate Valsalva's response, which may lead to reduced cardiac output.

4. Notify physician if bowel sounds do not return within 6 to 10 hours or if elimination does not return within 2 to 3 days postoperatively.

4. Absence of bowel sounds may indicate paralytic ileus; absence of bowel movements may indicate obstruction.

Documentation

Flow record
  Bowel movements
  Bowel sounds

Activity Intolerance Related to Pain and Weakness Secondary to Anesthesia, Tissue Hypoxia, and Insufficient Fluid and Nutrient Intake

Goal

The client will increase tolerance to activities of daily living (ADLs).

Indicators

➤ Progressive ambulation
➤ Ability to perform ADLs

Interventions	**Rationales**
1. Encourage progress in client's activity level during each shift as indicated.	1. A gradual increase in activity allows the client's cardiopulmonary system to return to its preoperative state without excessive strain.
a. Allow client's legs to dangle first; support client from the side.	a. Dangling the legs helps to minimize orthostatic hypotension.
b. Place the bed in high position and raise the head of the bed.	b. Raising the head of the bed helps to reduce stress on suture lines.
c. Increase client's time out of bed by 15 minutes each time. Allow client to set a comfortable rate of ambulation and agree on a distance goal for each shift.	c. Gradual increases toward mutually established realistic goals can promote compliance and prevent overexertion.
d. Encourage client to increase activity when pain is at a minimum or after pain relief measures take effect.	
2. Increase client's self-care activities from partial to complete self-care as indicated.	2. Client's participation in self-care improves physiologic functioning, reduces fatigue from inactivity, and improves sense of self-esteem and well-being.

(continued)

Interventions	Rationales

3. If client is not progressing at the expected or desired rate, do the following:
  a. Take vital signs prior to activity.
  b. Repeat vital sign assessment after activity.
  c. Repeat again after client has rested for 3 minutes.
  d. Assess for abnormal responses to increased activity:
    • Decreased pulse rate
    • Decreased or unchanged systolic blood pressure
    • Excessively increased or decreased respiratory rate
    • Failure of pulse to return to near the resting rate within 3 minutes after discontinuing activity
    • Complaints of confusion or vertigo
    • Uncoordinated movements
	3. Activity tolerance depends on client's ability to adapt to the physiologic requirements of increased activity. The expected immediate physiologic responses to activity are increased blood pressure and increased respiratory rate and depth. After 3 minutes, pulse rate should decrease to within 10 beats/min of client's usual resting rate. Abnormal findings represent the body's inability to meet the increased oxygen demands imposed by activity.

4. Plan regular rest periods according to client's daily schedule.	4. Regular rest periods allow the body to conserve and restore energy.
5. Identify and encourage client's progress. Keep a record of progress, particularly for a client who is progressing slowly.	5. Encouragement and realization of progress can give client an incentive for continued progression.

Documentation

Flow record
  Vital signs
  Ambulation (time, amount)
Progress notes
  Abnormal or unexpected response to increased activity

Risk for Ineffective Therapeutic Regimen Management Related to Insufficient Knowledge of Care of Operative Site, Restrictions (Diet, Activity), Medications, Signs and Symptoms of Complications, and Follow-up Care

Goals

The goals for this diagnosis represent those associated with discharge planning. Refer to the discharge criteria.

Interventions	Rationales
1. As appropriate, explain and demonstrate care of an uncomplicated surgical wound: a. Washing with soap and water b. Dressing changes using clean technique	1. Uncomplicated wounds have sealed edges after 24 hours and therefore do not require aseptic technique or a dressing; however, a dressing may be applied if wound is at risk for injury.
2. As appropriate, explain and demonstrate care of a complicated surgical wound. a. Aseptic technique b. Handwashing before and after dressing changes c. Avoiding touching the inner surface of the soiled dressing and discarding it in a sealed plastic bag d. The use of sterile hemostats if indicated e. Wound assessment—condition and drainage f. Wound cleaning g. Drainage tubes if indicated h. Dressing reapplication	2. Aseptic technique is necessary to prevent wound contamination during dressing changes. Handwashing helps to prevent contamination of the wound and the spread of infection. Proper handling and disposal of contaminated dressings helps to prevent infection transmission. Daily assessment is necessary to evaluate healing and detect complications.
3. Reinforce activity restrictions as indicated (e.g., bending, lifting).	3. Avoiding certain activities decreases the risk of wound dehiscence before scar formation occurs (usually after 3 weeks).
4. Explain the importance of the following: a. Avoiding ill persons and crowds b. Drinking 8 to 10 glasses of fluid daily c. Maintaining a balanced diet	4. Wound healing requires optimal nutrition, hydration, and rest as well as avoiding potential sources of infection.

(continued)

Interventions	Rationales
5. Review with client and family the purpose, dosage, administration, and side effects of all prescribed medications.	5. Complete understanding can help to prevent drug administration errors.

6. Teach client and family to watch for and report signs and symptoms of possible complications.
  a. Persistent temperature elevation
  b. Difficulty breathing, chest pain
  c. Change in sputum characteristics
  d. Increasing weakness, fatigue, pain, or abdominal distention
  e. Wound changes (e.g., separation, unusual or increased drainage, increased redness or swelling)
  f. Voiding difficulties, burning on urination, urinary frequency, or cloudy foul-smelling urine
  g. Pain, swelling, and warmth in calf
  h. Other signs and symptoms of complications specific to surgical procedure performed
	6. Early detection and reporting danger signs and symptoms enable prompt intervention to minimize severity of complications.

7. Whenever possible, provide written instructions.	7. Written instructions provide an information resource for use at home.
8. Evaluate client's and family's understanding of information provided.	8. Knowledge gaps may indicate need for a referral for assistance at home.

Documentation

Flow records
  Discharge instructions
  Follow-up instructions
Discharge summary record
  Status at discharge (pain, activity, wound healing)
  Achievement of goals (individual or family)

Bibliography

General References

Abrams, A. C. (2004). *Clinical drug therapy* (8th ed.). Philadelphia: Lippincott Williams & Wilkins.

Alfaro-LeFevre, R. (2001). *Applying nursing process: A step-by-step guide* (5th ed.). Philadelphia: Lippincott Williams & Wilkins.

Allender, J., & Spradley, B. (2001). *Community health nursing* (4th ed.). Philadelphia: Lippincott Williams & Wilkins.

American Psychiatric Association. (2000). *DSM IV-TR: Diagnostic and statistical manual of mental disorders* (4th ed., text revision). Washington, DC: Author.

Andrews, M., & Boyle, J. (2003). *Transcultural concepts in nursing* (4th ed.). Philadelphia: Lippincott Williams & Wilkins.

Bennett, J. V., & Brachman, P. S. (Eds.). (1995). *Hospital infections* (3rd ed.). Boston: Little, Brown.

Bickley, B. (2003). *A guide to physical examination and history taking* (8th ed.). Philadelphia: Lippincott Williams & Wilkins.

Boyd, M. A. (2005). *Psychiatric nursing: Contemporary practice* (3rd ed.). Philadelphia: Lippincott Williams & Wilkins.

Carpenito, L. J. (2004). *Nursing care plans and documentation: Nursing diagnoses and collaborative problems* (4th ed.). Philadelphia: Lippincott Williams & Wilkins.

Carpenito, L. J. (1995). *Nurse practitioner and physician discipline specific expertise in primary care.* Unpublished manuscript.

Carpenito-Moyet, L. J. (2006). *Nursing diagnosis: Application to clinical practice* (11th ed.) Philadelphia: Lippincott Williams & Wilkins

Clemen-Stone, E., Eigasti, D. G., & McGuire S. L. (2002). *Comprehensive family and community health nursing* (6th ed.). St. Louis: Mosby Year Book.

Dudek, S. (2006). *Nutrition handbook for nursing practice* (5th ed.). Philadelphia: Lippincott Williams & Wilkins.

Edelman, C. L. & Mandle, C. L. (2001). *Health promotion throughout the lifespan* (5th ed.). St. Louis: Mosby-Year Book.

Giger, J., & Davidhizar, R. (2004). *Transcultural nursing: Assessment and intervention* (5th ed.). St. Louis: Mosby Year Book.

Hickey, J. (2002). *The clinical practice of neurological and neurosurgical nursing* (5th ed). Philadelphia: Lippincott Williams & Wilkins.

Lubkin, J. M. (1995). *Chronic illness: Impact and interventions* (3rd ed.). Boston: Jones & Bartlett.

McMillan, J., De Angelis, C., Feigin, R., & Waishaw, J. (1999). *Oski's pediatrics.* Philadelphia: Lippincott Williams & Wilkins.

Miller, C. (2004). *Nursing for wellness in older adults* (4th ed.). Philadelphia: Lippincott Williams & Wilkins.

Mohr, W. K. (2003). *Psychiatric–mental health nursing: Adaptation and growth* (5th ed). Philadelphia: Lippincott Williams & Wilkins.

Morton, P., Fontaine, D., Hudak, C., & Gallo, B. (2005). *Critical care nursing* (8th ed.). Philadelphia: Lippincott Williams & Wilkins.

North American Nursing Diagnosis Association (2005). *Definitions and Classification 2005-2006.* Philadelphia: NANDA International.

North American Nursing Diagnosis Association (2002). *Nursing diagnosis: Definitions and classification 2001–2002.* Philadelphia: Author.

Oski, F. (2001). *Principles and practice of pediatrics* (3rd ed.) Philadelphia: Lippincott Williams & Wilkins.

Pillitteri, A. (2003). *Maternal and child health nursing* (4th ed.). Philadelphia: Lippincott Williams & Wilkins.

Porth, C. (2002). *Pathophysiology* (6th ed.). Philadelphia: Lippincott Williams & Wilkins.

Smeltzer, S., & Bare, B. (2004). *Brunner and Suddarth's Textbook of medical–surgical nursing* (10th ed.). Philadelphia: Lippincott Williams & Wilkins.

Stuart, G. W., & Sundeen, S. (2002). *Principles and practice of psychiatric nursing* (6th ed.). St. Louis: Mosby–Year Book.

Taylor, C., Lillis, C., & LeMone, P. (2001). *Fundamentals of nursing: The art and science of nursing care* (4th ed.). Philadelphia: Lippincott Williams & Wilkins.

Varcarolis, E. (2002). *Foundations of psychiatric mental health nursing* (4th ed.). Philadelphia: W. B. Saunders.

Weber, J., & Kelley, J. (2003). *Health assessment in nursing* (2nd ed.). Philadelphia: Lippincott Williams & Wilkins.

Wong, D. (2003). *Nursing care of infants and children* (7th ed.). St. Louis: Mosby-Year Book.

Activity Intolerance

Cohen, J., Gorenberg, B., & Schroeder, B. (2000). A study of functional status among elders at two academic nursing centers. *Home Care Provider, 5*(3), 108–112.

Magnan, M. A. (1987, September). *Activity intolerance: Toward a nursing theory of activity.* Paper presented at the Fifth Annual Symposium of the Michigan Nursing Diagnosis Association, Detroit, Michigan.

Sarna, L. & Bialous, S. A. (2004). Why tobacco is a women's health issue. *Nursing Clinics of North America, 39*(1), 165–180.

Anxiety

Blanchard, C. M., Courneya, K. S. & Larng, D. (2001). Effects of acute exercise on state anxiety in breast cancer survivors. *Oncology Nursing Forum, 28*(10), 1617–21.

DeMarco-Sinatra, J. (2000). Relaxation Training as a holistic nursing intervention. *Holistic Nursing Practice, 14*(3), 30–39.

Grainger, R. (1990). Anxiety interrupters. *American Journal of Nursing, 90*(2), 14–15.

Grealish, L., Lomasney, A., & Whiteman, B. (2000). Foot massage. A nursing intervention to modify the distressing symptoms of pain and nausea in patients hospitalized with cancer. *Cancer Nursing, 23*, 237–243.

Lyon, B.A. (2002). Cognitive self-care skills: A model for managing stressful lifestyles. *Nursing Clinics of North America, 37*(2), 285–294.

Stephenson, N. L., Weinrich, S. P., & Tavakoli, A. S. (2000). The effects of foot reflexology on anxiety and pain in patients with breast and lung cancer. *Oncology Nursing Forum, 27,* 67–72.

Tusaie, K. & Dyer, J. (2004). Resilience: A historical review of construct. *Holistic Nursing Practice, 18*(1), 3–8.

Wong, H. L. C., Lopez-Nahas, V. & Molassiotis, A. (2001). Effects of Music Therapy on anxiety in ventilator dependent patients. Heart Lung Journal of Acute Cultural Care. 30(5) 376–87.

Risk for Imbalanced Body Temperature

Andrews, A. (1990). Inadvertent hypothermia: A complication of postoperative cholecystectomy patients. *AORN Journal, 52,* 987–991.

Bernthal, E. (1999). Inadvertent hypothermia prevention: The anaesthetic nurse's role. *British Journal of Nursing, 8*(1), 17–18, 20–25.

DeFabio, D. C. (2000). Fluid and nutrient maintenance before, during and after exercise. *Journal of Sports Chiropractic and Rehabilitation, 14*(2), 21–24, 42–43.

Giuliano, K. K., Giuliano, A. J., Scott, S. S., et al. (2000). Temperature measurement in critically ill adults: A comparison of tympanic and oral methods. *American Journal of Critical Care, 9*(4), 254–261.

Robbins, A. S. (1989). Hypothermia and heat stroke: Protecting the elderly patient. *Geriatrics, 44*(1), 73–79.

Bowel Incontinence

Chassagne, P., Jego, A., & Gloc, P. (2000). Does treatment of constipation improve fecal incontinence in institutionalized elderly patients? *Aging, 29*(2), 159–164.

Demata, E. (2000). Faecal incontinence. *Journal of Wound Care and Enterostomal Therapy, 19*(4), 6–11.

McLane, A., & McShane, R. (1991). Constipation. In M. Maas, K. Buckwalter, & M. Hardy (Eds.). *Nursing diagnoses and interventions for the elderly.* Redwood City, CA: Addison-Wesley Nursing.

Weeks, S. K., Hubbartt, E., & Michaels, T. K. (2000). Keys to bowel success. *Rehabilitation Nursing, 25*(2), 66–69.

Impaired Comfort

Agency for Health Care Policy and Research. (1992). *Acute pain management: Operative or medical procedures and trauma.* Rockville, MD: Author.

DeWitt, S. (1990). Nursing assessment of skin and dermatological lesions. *Nursing Clinics of North America, 25*(1), 235–245.

Eckert, R. M. (2001). Understanding anticipatory nausea. *Continuing Education, 28*(10) 1553–1560.

Ezzone, S., Baker, C., Rosselet, R., & Terepka, E. (1998). Music as an adjunct to antiemetic therapy. *Oncology Nursing Forum, 25*(9), 1551–1556.

Field, T., Peck, M., Hernandez Reif, M., et al. (2000). Postburn itching, pain and psychological symptoms are reduced with massage therapy. *Journal of Burn Care Rehabilitation, 21*(3), 189–193.

Gaston-Johansson, F. (2000). The effectiveness of the comprehensive coping strategy program on clinical outcomes in breast cancer autologous bone marrow transplantation. *Cancer Nursing, 23*(4), 277–285.

Grealish, L., Lomasney, A., & Whiteman, B. (2000). Foot massage. A nursing intervention to modify the distressing symptoms of pain and nausea in patients hospitalized with cancer. *Cancer Nursing, 23*(3), 237–243.

Ladd, L. A. (1999). Symptom management: Nausea in palliative care. *Journal of Hospice and Palliative Nursing, 1*(2), 67–70.

Ludwig-Beymer, P. (1989). Transcultural aspects of pain. In J. Boyle & M. Andrews (Eds.). *Transcultural concepts in nursing.* Glenview, IL: Scott, Foresman.

McGuire, D., Sheidler, V., & Polomano, R. C. (2000). Pain. In S. Groenwald, M. Frogge, M. Goodman, & C. Yarbo (Eds.). *Cancer nursing: Principles and practice* (5th ed.). Boston: Jones and Bartlett.

Perry, S., & Heidrich, G. (1981). Placebos. *American Journal of Nursing, 81,* 721–725.

Porter, J., & Jick, H. (1980). Addiction rate in patients treated with narcotics. *New England Journal of Medicine, 302,* 123.

Zborowski, M. (1952). Cultural components in response to pain. *Journal of Social Issues, 8,* 16–30.

Children

Schechter, N. (1989b). Undertreatment of pain in children: An overview. *Pediatric Clinics of North America, 36,* 795–1045.

Impaired Communication

Iezzoni, L. F., O'Day, B., Keleen, M. A., & Harker, H. (2004). Improving patient care: Communicating about health care: Observations from persons who are deaf or hard of hearing. *Annals of Internal Medicine, 140*(5), 356–362.

Underwood, C. (2004). How can we best deliver an inclusive health service? *Primary Health Care, 14*(9), 20–21.

Confusion

Anderson, C. (1999). Delirium and confusion are not interchangeable terms [letter to editor]. *Oncology Nursing Forum, 26*(3), 497–498.

Blazer, D. G. (1986). Depression: Paradoxically a cause for hope. *Generations, 10*(3), 21–23.

Burnside, I., & Haight, B. (1994). Reminiscence and life review: Therapeutic interventions for older people. *Nurse Practitioner, 19*(4), 55–60.

Dellasega, C. (1998). Assessment of cognition in the elderly. *Nursing Clinics of North America, 33*(3), 395–406.

Dennis, H. (1984). Remotivation therapy groups. In I. M. Burnside (Ed.). *Working with the elderly group: Process and techniques* (2nd ed.). Monterey, CA: Jones & Bartlett.

Feil, N. (1992). Validation therapy. *Geriatric Nursing, 13*(3), 129–133.

Foreman, M. D., Mion, L. C., Tyrostad, L., & Flitcher, K. (1999). Standard of practice protocol: Acute confusion/delirium. *Geriatric Nursing, 20*(3), 147–152.

Gerdner, L. (1999). Individualized music intervention protocol. *Journal of Gerontological Nursing, 25*(10), 10–16.

Hall, G. R. (1988). Care of the patient with Alzheimer's disease living at home. *Nursing Clinics of North America, 23,* 31–46.

Hall, G. R. (1991). Altered thought processes: Dementia. In M. Maas, K. Buckwalter, & M. Hardy (Eds.). *Nursing diagnoses and interventions for the elderly.* Menlo Park, CA: Addison-Wesley.

Hall, G. R. (1994). Caring for people with Alzheimer's disease using the conceptual model of progressively lowered stress threshold in the clinical setting. *Nursing Clinics of North America, 29,* 129–141.

Hall, G. R., & Buckwalter, K. C. (1987). Progressively lowered stress threshold: A conceptual model for care of adults with Alzheimer's disease. *Archives of Psychiatric Nursing, 1,* 399–406.

Janssen, J., & Giberson, D. (1988). Remotivation therapy. *Journal of Gerontological Nursing, 14*(6), 31–34.

Katzman, R. (1988). *Alzheimer's disease as an age dependent disorder, research and the aging population* (CIBA Foundation Symposium 1334). New York: John Wiley & Sons.

Quinn, C. (1994). The four A's of restraint reduction: Attention, assessment, anticipation, avoidance. *Orthopaedic Nursing, 13*(2), 11–19.

Constipation

Schaefer, D. & Cheskin, L. (1998). Constipation in the elderly. *American Family Physician, 58*(4), 907–914.

Shua-Haim, J. Sabo, M., & Ross, J. (1999). Constipation in the elderly: A practical approach. *Clinical Geriatrics, 7*(12), 91–99.

Weeks, S. K., Hubbartt, E., & Michaels, T. K. (2000). Keys to bowel success. *Rehabilitation Nursing, 25*(2), 66–80.

Diarrhea

Bennett, R. (2000). Acute gastroenteritis and associated conditions. In L. R. Barker, J. Burton, & P. Zieve (Eds.). *Principles of ambulatory medicine.* Baltimore: Williams & Wilkins.

Fuhrman, M. P. (1999). Diarrhea and tube feeding. *Nutritional Clinical Practice, 14*(2), 83–84.

Larson, C. E. (2000). Evidence-based practice. Safety and efficacy of oral rehydration therapy for treatment of diarrhea and gastroenteritis in pediatrics. *Pediatric Nursing, 26*(2), 177–179.

Disuse Syndrome

Maher, A. Salmond, S., & Pellino, T. (1998). *Orthopedic nursing* (2nd ed.). Philadelphia: W. B. Saunders.

Maklebust, J., & Sieggreen, M. (2001). *Pressure ulcers: Guidelines for prevention and nursing management* (3rd ed.). Springhouse, PA: Springhouse.

McKinley, W. O., Jackson, A. B., Cardenas, D. D., & Devivo, M. J. (1999). Long-term medical complications after traumatic spinal cord injury. *Archives of Physical Medical Rehabilitation, 80*(11) 1402–1410.

Interrupted Family Processes

Clark, J., & Gwin, R. (2001). Psychological responses of the family. In S. Groenwald, M. Frogge, M. Goodman, & C. Yarbo (Eds.). *Cancer nursing: Principles and practice* (3rd ed.). Boston: Jones and Bartlett.

Smith-DiJulio, K. (1998). Families in crisis: Family violence. In E. M. Varcarolis (Ed.). *Foundations of psychiatric mental health nursing* (3rd ed.). Philadelphia: W. B. Saunders.

Fatigue

Adinolfi, A. (2001). Assessment and treatment of HIV-related fatigue. *Journal of the Association of Nurses in AIDS Care, 12*(Suppl.), 33–39.

Crosby, L. (1991). Factors which contribute to fatigue associated with rheumatoid arthritis. *Journal of Advanced Nursing, 16,* 974–981.

Dzurec, L. C. (2000). Fatigue and relativeness experiences of inordinately tired women: Fourth quarter. *Journal of Nursing Scholarship, 32*(4), 339–345.

Hart, L., Freel, M., & Milde, F. (1990). Fatigue. *Nursing Clinics of North America, 25,* 967–976.

Jiricka, M. K. (2002). Alterations in activity tolerance. In C. M. Porth (Ed.), *Pathophysiology: Concepts of altered health states* (6th ed.). Philadelphia: Lippincott Williams & Wilkins.

Nail, L., & Winningham, M. (1997). Fatigue. In S. Groenwald, M. Frogge, M. Goodman, & C. Yarbo (Eds.). *Cancer nursing: Principles and practice* (4th ed.). Boston: Jones and Bartlett.

Rhoten, D. (1982). Fatigue and the postsurgical patient. In C. Norris (Ed.). *Concept clarification in nursing.* Rockville, MD: Aspen Systems.

Deficient and Excess Fluid Volume

Maughan, R., Leiper, J., & Shirreffs, S. (1997). Factors influencing the restoration of fluid and electrolyte balance after exercise in the heat. *British Journal of Sports Medicine, 31*(3), 175–182.

Sansevero, A. (1997). Dehydration in the elderly: Strategies for prevention and management. *Nurse Practitioner: American Journal of Primary Health Care, 22*(4), 41–42, 51–52, 54–57.

Terry, M., O'Brien, S., & Derstein, M. (1998). Lower-extremity edema: Evaluation and diagnosis. *Wounds: A Compendium of Clinical Research and Practice, 10*(4), 118–124.

Delayed Growth and Development

Bergland, Adel (2001). Thriving-a useful theoretical perspective to capture the experience of well-being among frail elderly in nursing homes? *Journal of Advanced Nursing* 36(3), 426–432.

Haight, Barbara K. (2002). Thriving: A life span theory. *Journal Of Gerontological Nursing* 14–22.

Kimball, M. J., & Williams-Burgess, C. (1995). Failure to thrive: The silent epidemic of the elderly. *Archives of Psychiatric Nursing, 9*(2), 99–105.

Newbern, V. B., & Krowchuk, H. V. (1994). Failure to thrive in elderly people: A conceptual analysis. *Journal of Advanced Nursing,* 840–849.

Wagnild, G. & Young H. M. (1990) Resilience among older women. *Image: Journal of Nursing Scholarship* 22,252–255.

Ineffective Health Maintenance

Allen, K. M., & Phillips, J. M. (1997). *Women's health across the life span.* Philadelphia: J. B. Lippincott.

Edelman, C. L., & Mandle, C. L. (2001). *Health promotion throughout the lifespan* (5th ed.). St. Louis: Mosby-Year Book.

Hanson, S. M., & Boyd, S. T. (1996). *Family health care nursing: Theory, practice and research.* Philadelphia: W. B. Saunders.

Moore, S. M., & Charvat, J. M. (2002). Using the CHANGE intervention to enhance long-term exercise. *The Nursing Clinics of North America, 37*(2), 273–281.

Rankins, S., & Stallings, K. D. (2001). *Patient education: Issues, principles, practices* (4th ed.). Philadelphia: Lippincott Williams & Wilkins.

Gerontologic

Allison, M., & Keller, C. (1997). Physical activity in the elderly: Benefits and intervention strategies. *Nurse Practitioner, 22*(8), 53–54, 56, 58, 63, 64.

Tobacco Use

DuRant, R., & Smith, J. (1999). Adolescent tobacco use and cessation. *Primary Care, 26*(3), 553–576.

Pletsch, P. K. (2002). Reduction of primary and secondary smoke exposure for low-income black pregnant women. *The Nursing Clinics of North America, 37*(2), 315–326.

Obesity

Buiten, C., & Metzger, B. (2000). Childhood obesity and risk of cardiovascular disease: A review of the science. *Pediatric Nursing 26*(1), 13–18.

Dennis, K. (2004). Weight management in women. *Nursing Clinics in North America, 39*(14), 231–241.

Wiereng, M. E., & Oldham, K. K. (2002). Weight control: a lifestyle-modification model for improving health. *The Nursing Clinics of North America, 37*(2), 303–311.

Health-Seeking Behaviors

See also References/Bibliography for *Ineffective Health Maintenance.*

Leon, L. (2002). Smoking cessation—Developing a workable program. *Nursing Spectrum, FL9*(18), 12–13.

Tusaie, K. & Dyer, J. (2004). Resilience: A historical review of construct. *Holistic Nursing Practice, 18*(1), 3–8.

Risk for Infection/Infection Transmission

Bertin, M. L. (1999). Communicable diseases: Infection prevention for nurses at work and at home. *Nursing Clinics of North America, 34*(2), 509–526.

Centers for Disease Control and Prevention. (2000). Guidelines for prevention of transmission of human immunodeficiency virus and hepatitis B virus to health-care and public safety workers. *MMWR, 49*, 5–15.

Risk for Injury

Baumann, S. L. (1999). Defying gravity and fears: The prevention of falls in community-dwelling older adults. *Clinical Excellence for Nurse Practitioners, 3*(5), 254–261.

Schoenfelder, D. P. (2000). A fall prevention program for elderly individuals. *Journal of Gerontological Nursing, 26*(3), 43–45.

Ineffective Therapeutic Regimen Management

Bandura, A. (1982). Self-efficacy mechanism in human agency. *American Psychology, 37*(3), 122–147.

Edelman, C. L., & Mandle, C. L. (2001). *Health promotion throughout the lifespan.* (5th ed.). St. Louis: Mosby-Year Book.

Rakel, B. A. (1999). Interventions related to teaching. In G. Bulechek & J. McCloskey (Eds.). *Nursing interventions* (4th ed.). Philadelphia: W. B. Saunders.

Zimmerman, G., Olsen, C. & Bosworth, M. (2000). A "Stages of Change" approach to helping patients change behavior. *American Family Physicians, 61*(5), 1409–1416.

Impaired Physical Mobility

Addams, S. & Clough, J. A. (1998) Modalities for mobilization. In A. B. Mahler, S. Salmond, & T. Pellino (Eds.). *Orthopedic nursing.* Philadelphia: W. B. Saunders.

Levin, R. F., Krainovitch, B. C., Bahrenburg, E., & Mitchell, C. A. (1989). Diagnostic content validity of nursing diagnoses. *Image, 21*(1), 40–44.

Pellino, T., Polacek, L. P., Preston, A., Bell, N., & Evans, R. (1998). Complications of orthopedic disorders and orthopedic surgery. In A. Maher, S. Salomond, & T. Pellino (Eds.). *Orthopaedic nursing* (2nd ed.). Philadelphia: W. B. Saunders.

Imbalanced Nutrition: Less than Body Requirements

Evans-Stoner, N. (1997). Nutrition assessment. *Nursing Clinics of North America, 32*(4), 637–650.

Risk for Peripheral Neurovascular Dysfunction

Bourne, R. B., & Rorabeck, C. H. (1989). Compartment syndrome of the lower leg. *Clinical Orthopaedics and Related Research, 240,* 97–104.

Fahey, V., & Milzarek, A. (1999). Extra-anatomic bypass surgery. *Journal of Vascular Nursing, 17*(3), 71–75.

Kracun, M. D., & Wooten, C. L. (1998). Crush injuries: A case of entrapment. *Critical Care Nursing Quarterly, 21*(2), 81–86.

Pellino, T., Polacek, L. P., Preston, A., Bell, N., & Evans, R. (1998). Complications of orthopedic disorders and orthopedic surgery. In A. Maher, S. Salomond, & T. Pellino (Eds.). *Orthopaedic nursing* (2nd ed.). Philadelphia: W. B. Saunders.

Ross, D. (1991). Acute compartmental syndrome. *Orthopaedic Nursing, 10*(2), 33–38.

Ineffective Protection

Agency for Health Care Policy and Research [AHCPR] Panel for the Prediction and Prevention of Pressure Ulcers in Adults. (1992, May). *Pressure ulcers in adults: Prediction and prevention.* Clinical Practice Guidelines Number 3, AHCPR, Bulletin No. 92-0047. Rockville, MD: Agency for Health Care Policy & Research, Public Health Services, U.S. Department of Health and Human Services.

Boynton, P. R., Jaworski, D., & Paustian, C. (1999). Meeting the challenges of healing chronic wounds in older adults. *Nursing Clinics of North America, 34*(4), 921–932.

Maklebust, J., & Sieggreen, M. (2000). *Pressure ulcers: Guidelines for prevention and nursing management* (3rd ed). Springhouse, PA: Springhouse.

Wysocki, A. (1999). Skin anatomy, physiology and pathophysiology. *Nursing Clinics of North America, 34*(4), 777–798.

Impaired Oral Mucous Membrane

Beck, S. L. (2001). Mucositis. In S. L. Groenwald, M. Goodman, M. H. Frogge, C. H. Yarbro, (Eds.). *Cancer symptom management* (4th ed.). Boston: Jones & Bartlett Publishers.

Kemp, J., & Brackett, H. (2001). Mucositis. In R. A. Gates, R. M. Fink (Eds.). *Oncology nursing secrets* (pp. 245–249). Philadelphia: Hanley & Belfus.

Relocation Stress

Rodgers, B. L. (1997). Family members' experiences with the nursing home placement of an older adult. *Applied Nursing Research, 10*(2), 57–63.

Rosenkoetter, M. M. (1996). Changing life patterns of the resident in long-term care and the community-residing spouse. *Geriatric Nursing, 17*(6), 267–272.

Smider, N. A., Essex, M. J., & Ryff, C. D. (1996). Adaptation to community relocation: The interactive influence of psychological resources and contextual factors. *Psychology of Aging, 11*(2), 362–372.

Vernberg, E. M. (1990). Experiences with peers following relocation during early adolescence. *American Journal of Orthopsychiatry, 60*, 466–472.

Wilson, S. A. (1997). The transition to nursing home life: A comparison of planned and unplanned admissions. *Journal of Advanced Nursing, 26*(5), 864–871.

Self-Care Deficit Syndrome

Chang, B., Uman, G., & Hirsh, M. (1998). Predictive power of clinical indicators for self-care deficit. *Nursing Diagnosis, 9*(2), 71–81.

Maher, A. B., Salmond, S. W., & Pellino, T. (1998). *Orthopedic nursing* (2nd ed.). Philadelphia: W. B. Saunders.

Impaired Urinary Elimination

Dougherty, M. (1998). Current status of research on pelvic muscles strengthening techniques. *Journal of Wound, Ostomy and Continence, 25*(3), 75–83.

Fanti, J. A., Newman, D. K., & Colling, J. (1996). *Urinary incontinence in adults: Acute and chronic management, Clinical practice guidelines No. 2*. Rockville, MD: U.S. Department of Health and Human Services.

Sampselle, C., & DeLancey, J. (1998). Anatomy of female continence. *Journal of Wound, Ostomy and Continence Nursing, 25*(3), 63–74.

Scardillo, J., & Aronovitch, S. A. (1999). Successfully managing incontinence-related irritant dermatitis across the lifespan. *Ostomy Wound Management, 45*(4), 36–44.

Steeman, E., & Defever, M. (1998). Urinary incontinence among elderly persons who live at home. *Nursing Clinics of North America, 33*(3), 441–455.

Collaborative Problems

Refer to General References.

Index

Page numbers followed by "f" denote figures; those followed by "t" denote tables